D1344595

Practical
Radiotherapy
Planning

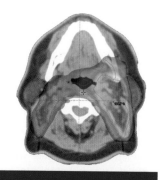

Practical Radiotherapy Planning

Fourth Edition

Ann Barrett MD, FRCP, FRCR ■
Professor Emeritus of Oncology,
University of East Anglia, Norwich

Jane Dobbs MA, FRCP, FRCR ■
Consultant Emeritus in Clinical Oncology,
Guy's and St Thomas' NHS Foundation Trust

Stephen Morris MRCP, FRCR ■
Consultant Clinical Oncologist,
Guy's and St Thomas' NHS Foundation Trust

Tom Roques MRCP, FRCR ■
Consultant Clinical Oncologist,
Norfolk and Norwich University Hospital NHS Foundation Trust

Illustrations editor:
Jonathan Harrowven BSc (Hons),
Radiographer, Norfolk and Norwich University Hospital
NHS Foundation Trust

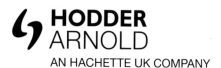

HODDER
ARNOLD

AN HACHETTE UK COMPANY

Hodder Arnold, an imprint of Hodder Education, an Hachette UK Company
338 Euston Road, London NW1 3BH

http://www.hoddereducation.com

British Library Cataloguing in Publication Data
A catalogue record for this book is available from the British Library

Library of Congress Cataloging-in-Publication Data
A catalog record for this book is available from the Library of Congress

ISBN   978 034 0927731

3 4 5 6 7 8 9 10

Commissioning Editor: Gavin Jamieson
Project Editors: Eva Senior and Joanna Silman
Production Controller: Joanna Walker
Cover Designer: Helen Townson
Indexer: Jan Ross

Typeset in 10/12 Galliard by Macmillan Publishing Solutions
Printed and bound in Italy

What do you think about this book? Or any other Hodder Arnold title?
Please visit our website: www.hoddereducation.com

Contents

Preface

Since the last edition of *Practical Radiotherapy Planning* in 1999, the practice of radiotherapy has changed radically. Advances in imaging have been integrated with technological developments in radiotherapy delivery so that 3D planning of volumes has replaced 2D field arrangements. Major developments in tumour localisation have included the publication of ICRU reports on target definition (Report 62 in 1999 and Report 71 in 2004) and the possibility of registration of different imaging modalities including CT, MRI and PET. In treatment delivery, multi-leaf collimation has enabled treatments to be shaped to tumours and intensity-modulated dose plans have provided solutions to previous planning dilemmas. Accuracy of treatment delivery has been ensured by development of portal imaging and daily image-guided and adaptive radiotherapy techniques.

This is therefore a completely new book, with new introductory chapters and a changed structure within each tumour site chapter. We have been able to make much more use of clinical images to illustrate important planning concepts. The aim of the book, however, remains unchanged: to provide a guide to radiotherapy treatment planning that is based on sound pathological and anatomical principles. Complexity of treatment planning has increased greatly but this new edition continues to emphasise the underlying principles of treatment, which can be applied to conventional, conformal, and novel treatments, taking into account advances in imaging and treatment delivery.

Much treatment is now given according to local, national or international protocols and these should always be consulted and used when appropriate. Details of drug and of some radiotherapy regimens are not given as they change frequently. Again we have largely excluded recommendations for treatment of benign disease.

The ICRU report proposed a colour convention for outlining target volumes, but with regret we have chosen different colours to ensure optimal reproduction of plans. We have used the following scheme in all illustrations:

GTV	dark blue
CTV	cyan (light blue)
CTV2	magenta (purple)
PTV	red
PTV2	lime green
OAR	yellow, light yellow, light green, dark green

Two authors from the first three editions have been joined by two younger colleagues from our departments to ensure that we continue to reflect the most up-to-date approach to treatment planning. It would have been impossible to produce a book like this one, in the age of site-specialised practice and multidisciplinary team working, without relying very heavily on expert colleagues within our respective departments. We are most grateful to them for the time and effort they have put in to ensuring the accuracy and appropriateness of what we have written. Special thanks are due to Anna Winship, George Mikhaeel, David Convery and Kim Ball at Guy's and St Thomas' Hospital, Mark Gaze at University College Hospital, Richard Benson at Addenbrooke's Hospital, and at the Norfolk and Norwich University Hospital: Dinos Geropantas, Suat Loo, Adrian Harnett, Max Dahele, Rob Wade, Jenny Tomes, and our radiological colleagues. We would like to acknowledge our radiographer colleagues in both departments who have helped us to find illustrations and plans. The work was supported in part by a sabbatical leave award to Jane Dobbs from the Clinical Oncology Dean's Fund of the Royal College of Radiologists, London, whom we thank.

This small textbook cannot describe all the research which has been undertaken to develop treatment schedules. We aim always to use evidence-based solutions where they exist and have suggested, in a short list of information sources at the end of each chapter, where more detailed data may be found. Some fields of research, such as the use of gating and adaptive therapy, 3D rotational arc therapy, and stereotactic radiotherapy are still undergoing evaluation and are therefore beyond the scope of this book. We give a brief introduction to the principles and practice of brachytherapy but details must be found elsewhere. Commonly used abbreviations have been spelled out only at first mention in the book but are included in the appendix for further reference.

Trainees in radiation oncology and radiographers, working within a multidisciplinary team, will, we hope, continue to use our book to produce safe and appropriate plans for common tumours.

Ann Barrett; Jane Dobbs; Stephen Morris; Tom Roques

2008

What you need to know before planning radiotherapy treatment

Introduction

Radiotherapy treatment can only produce good effects if it is delivered in an appropriate clinical context. Attempting radical treatment for a patient with metastatic disease, or one who is likely to die soon from cardiac or lung disease is inappropriate. These decisions require a fine balance of judgement between therapeutic optimism and nihilism and must be firmly based in good clinical history taking and examination. The clinician must then be able to synthesise all the information about the patient, tumour, investigations and previous treatment to make a decision about whether radiotherapy should be given and if so, with radical or palliative intent. Comorbidities, such as diabetes or vascular disease, which would affect the toxicity of treatment, must also be considered.

Sometimes the decision to offer radiotherapy may be relatively simple if the disease is common, the treatment effective and standardised, the histological features well categorised, and imaging easy to interpret. Some breast cancers fit well into this category. In contrast, decisions may be very difficult if there is no treatment of proven benefit, the prognosis is uncertain, the patient's general performance status is poor, imaging is of limited usefulness or there is histological uncertainty. Clinical experience and judgement is then critically important. This expertise is built on the foundation of good history taking which enables us to set the patient's disease in the context of their own ideas, concerns and expectations. Have other family members had radiotherapy with good or bad outcomes? Are they so claustrophobic that they will not go into a scanner or treatment room? Do they have other problems which would affect the feasibility of radiotherapy – arthritis which limits joint movement, shortness of breath which prevents them lying flat, heart valves or prostheses which may affect dose delivery?

Clinicians may consider that the new era of cross-sectional and functional imaging has made examination of the patient irrelevant but it remains the essential foundation of appropriate clinical judgements; for example, detection of a lymph node in the axilla, otherwise overlooked in imaging, or the progression of tumour since the last scan, may change a decision taken earlier in a multidisciplinary team meeting.

Classification systems

Many classification systems have been developed to ensure that clinicians throughout the world share a common language as they describe patients, tumours, and their treatment. This is essential to allow effective cancer registration and comparisons of incidence, prognosis and outcome of treatments. Many protocols for treatment are also based on such classification systems.

Pathological classification

The International Classification of Disease (ICD) version 10 of the World Health Organization (WHO) has been in use since 1994. It is the international standard diagnostic classification for epidemiology and health management. It is used in hospital records and on death certificates, which in turn are the basis for compiling mortality and morbidity statistics nationally and internationally. There is a subclassification, the International Classification of Disease for Oncology version 3 (ICD-O-3) which is used in cancer/tumour registries to code site (topography) and type (morphology) of neoplasms from the histopathology report.

Information about malignancy (malignant, benign, *in situ* or uncertain) and differentiation is also coded. In the UK, this information is abstracted from clinical notes by trained coders. The introduction of computerised systems suggests that clinicians will be required to develop greater awareness of this classification, at least in their own areas of expertise, especially if the information becomes essential data before income is assured. ICD 10 and ICD-O-3 are available online.

The morphological information for ICD-O-3 coding comes from the pathologist whose expertise is essential to establish a precise diagnosis and choose appropriate treatment volumes. A pathology report will contain a description of the macroscopic appearance of the gross tumour specimen, its size, margins and anatomical relationships. It will describe the microscopic appearance after appropriate staining of cut sections of the tumour, including features such as areas of necrosis. Recognition of the tissue of origin and grading of the tumour will then often be possible.

There has been an explosion of new techniques in pathology, such as immunocytochemical staining, immunophenotyping and fluorescence *in situ* hybridisation, which may help to remove uncertainties about diagnoses following conventional histopathological examination. Oncologists must be in constant dialogue with their colleagues in pathology to ensure that they understand the significance of results of these special investigations and know how to assess the degree of certainty of the report.

Staging

Tumour stage, histological classification and grading determine prognosis and treatment decisions. An internationally agreed system of staging is essential to interpret outcomes of treatment and compare results in different treatment centres. The behaviour of tumours in different sites is determined by the anatomical situation, blood supply and lymphatic drainage, as well as the histological classification and grading. Any staging system must take into account this variability. The most commonly used systems are the UICC (Union Internationale Contre le Cancer) TNM, AJCC (American Joint Committee on Cancer) and FIGO (Federation Internationale de Gynecologie et d'Obstetrique) for gynaecological malignancy. The TNM system describes the tumour extent (T) nodal involvement (N) and distant metastases (M). This defines a clinical classification (cTNM) or a pathological one (pTNM) which incorporates information derived from an excised tumour and any draining lymph nodes that are also removed or sampled. Details of this system are given in the TNM atlas which should be available and used wherever patients are seen or results of investigation are correlated.

T staging includes measurement of the tumour either clinically, by imaging techniques or by macroscopic examination of an excised specimen. Correct pathological T staging can only be assured if the pathologist receives a completely excised tumour with a rim of surrounding tissue. The tumour should not be cut into or fixed except by the pathologist. Examination of the whole specimen is needed to determine the highest grade of tumour (as there is frequently inhomogeneity across the tumour), any vascular or lymphatic invasion or invasion of adjacent tissues. Spread into a body space such as the pleural or peritoneal cavity affects T stage as it changes prognosis.

Numbers are added to indicate extent of disease. T0 implies no primary tumour (as after spontaneous regression of a melanoma). Categories T1–4 indicate tumours of increasing size and/or involvement of lymphatic vessels or surrounding tissue. If it is impossible to ascertain size or extent of primary tumour, it is designated Tx.

N classification describes whether there is lymph node involvement and if so, how many nodes are involved. Pathological staging requires adequate excision of the relevant lymph node compartment and a minimum number of nodes which indicates that this has been achieved may be defined for each site. If there are positive nodes, the ratio of negative to positive is of prognostic significance. For example, one node positive out of four removed indicates a worse prognosis than one out of 12. The size of tumour in the nodes must be recorded as well as any extension through the capsule. Micrometastases are classified differently from tumour emboli in vessels and this affects the N staging.

Identification and sampling of a sentinel node may give useful prognostic information about other potential node involvement and help to choose appropriate treatment strategies. In breast cancer, for example, it appears highly predictive (>90 per cent) for axillary node involvement.

M category indicates presence (M1) or absence (M0) of metastases to distant sites.

For some sites, other staging systems have proved clinically more useful. These include the FIGO system for gynaecological malignancy and Dukes' classification of colonic tumours. Useful atlases of patterns of lymph node involvement have been devised for several tumour sites. These are included in subsequent chapters where relevant. Recommendations for the most appropriate imaging techniques for staging in different sites have been published.

Residual tumour after surgical excision is an important poor prognostic factor. Examination of resection margins assigns tumours to categories: R0, no residual tumour; R1, histologically detectable tumour at margins; and R2, macroscopic evidence of residual tumour. Where serum markers (S) convey important prognostic information, as in tumours of the testis, an S category has been introduced to the TNM system.

TNM categorisation is often used to group tumours subsequently into stages indicating local and metastatic extent and correlating with likely outcome.

Grading is defined by degree of differentiation as: G1, resemblance to tissue of origin; G2, moderately well differentiated; G3, poorly differentiated; and G4, undifferentiated tumours; with Gx used when it is not possible to determine grading, as for example from a damaged specimen. GB signifies a borderline malignant tumour (for example in the ovary). Grading systems have been agreed to reduce the subjective element of these assessments.

Performance status

Performance status measures attempt to quantify cancer patients' general wellbeing. They are used to help to decide whether a patient is likely to tolerate a particular treatment such as chemotherapy, whether doses of treatment need to be adjusted or whether palliative treatment has been effective. The status of all patients should be recorded using one of these scores at presentation and with any change in treatment or the disease. They are also used as a measure of quality of life in clinical trials.

There are various scoring systems, of which the most commonly used are the Karnovsky and WHO scales for adults, and the Lansky score for children. The SF-36 is a short form (SF) survey of overall health (originally with 36 questions, now 12) which gives a profile of mental and physical health. It has produced statistically reliable and valid results in many reported studies. There are modifications of this questionnaire for specific tumour sites. Another commonly used scale in quality of life assessment is the HADS (Hospital Anxiety and Depression Scale) which is used to measure changes in mental and emotional wellbeing during treatment or with progression of disease.

Prognostic factors

All possible information which may help in predicting prognosis should be collected in order to advise the patient and help make the most appropriate treatment decision.

Screen detected cancers may have a better prognosis than tumours presenting symptomatically because diagnosis is made earlier (breast and oesophagus). However, in other situations, screening is as yet of unproven benefit (for example chest X-ray for detecting early lung cancer).

Histological tumour type, grading and staging are most influential in determining outcome for an individual patient, and new techniques of tumour examination are yielding more information on gene function and expression which may affect prognosis. Other factors which must also be considered include epidemiological ones such as age, sex, lifestyle factors such as smoking, alcohol and other drug use, obesity, and family history of disease. Other biological factors such as performance status, which may reflect comorbidities, must be considered.

Biochemical tumour markers may be specific enough to give prognostic information by their absolute value, as for example β subunit of human chorionic gonadotrophin (β-hCG) levels in testicular cancer. However, they may be only relatively poorly correlated with tumour volume, such as carcinoembryonic antigen (CEA) in bowel cancer, but still be useful to indicate treatment response or disease progression by their rise or fall.

One of the most important prognostic factors is whether there is effective treatment for the condition. Because new treatments are being introduced all the time, prognostic predictions must also be constantly reviewed and validated in prospective controlled clinical trials.

Predictive tools based on population datasets are available for some tumours such as 'Adjuvant! On line' for breast cancer, and Partin tables and the Memorial Sloane Kettering nomogram for prostate cancer.

Predictive indicators are variables determined before treatment which give information on the probability of a response to a specific treatment. Predictive indices based on multiple indicators give an individual score which may help to make decisions. These tools can only be developed by painstaking retrospective analysis and careful prospective studies, but it is likely that their use will increase steadily. They are important in determining strategies for treating different tumour subsets in guidelines and protocols.

Increasingly, specific genetic profiles are correlated with natural history of disease or outcome of treatment. Examples are the predictive value of MYCN amplification in neuroblastoma, oestrogen/HER2 receptor status and response to hormone therapy or trastuzumab, and predilection of patients with Li–Fraumeni syndrome to development of second tumours. Microarray technology will provide more genetically determined prognostic factors which will have to be taken into account in planning treatment.

Influence of other treatments on radiotherapy

Surgery is most commonly used as a primary treatment for cancer. If performed before radiotherapy, it removes the gross tumour volume (GTV) so that a clinical target volume (CTV) must be used for planning (see Chapter 2).

If it is known from the time of diagnosis that both treatments will be needed, the best sequencing has to be decided. If the tumour is initially inoperable, radiotherapy first may produce tumour shrinkage which makes complete excision possible, thereby improving outcome. Radiotherapy may increase surgical complications if the interval between the two treatments is not optimal. Surgery before radiotherapy will alter normal anatomy, causing problems for planning unless pre- and postsurgical image co-registration is used.

Effective chemotherapy may produce complete resolution of the primary tumour (no residual GTV), and potentially increased acute normal tissue effects. The treatment the patient receives will be the best possible only if all these potential interactions are taken into consideration by all members of the team working together.

A true therapeutic gain from chemotherapy and radiotherapy together requires either more cell kill for the same level of normal tissue damage (which is useful in radio-resistant tumours) or the same cell kill with reduced normal tissue effects (useful for tumours cured with low dose radiotherapy). Concurrent chemoradiotherapy is now used for many tumours. It may improve outcomes by promoting spatial cooperation in cell killing, where the chemotherapy kills metastatic cells, and the radiotherapy those cells in the local tumour, or in-field cooperation where exploitation of differing molecular, cellular or tissue effects produces more cell kill than when the two agents are given sequentially.

Patients themselves may be using alternative therapies with possible effects on efficacy and complications of surgery, chemotherapy and radiotherapy. Antioxidants may interfere with free radical production which effects cell kill. St John's wort, used for depression, may affect the metabolism of some drugs. Aspirin and gingko biloba may increase risk of bleeding, and phyto-oestrogens may affect hormonally sensitive cancers. Lifestyle factors such as smoking or eating many vegetables during radiotherapy may influence the severity of acute treatment side effects such as mucositis or diarrhoea.

Systems for recording outcomes of treatment

In the past, various systems have been used for recording outcomes of treatment, including the WHO and European Organisation for Research and Treatment of Cancer (EORTC) criteria. Following advances in imaging techniques and improvements in treatment, a new set of tumour response criteria have been agreed – the Response Evaluation Criteria in Solid Tumours (RECIST). Other outcomes are recorded as the time to a specific event: time to progression for tumours with partial response (progression-free survival), time to local recurrence where there has been a complete remission (relapse-free survival), time to distant metastases, time to death from any cause (overall survival), time to second malignancy. The start and end dates for these time periods must be clearly defined and stated as, for example, date of first treatment, date of randomisation, date of imaging of relapse, or date of histological proof of relapse. There is still no clear convention for defining these dates.

Quality of life measures are also essential for assessing treatment effects. Standardised scales such as the EORTC, QLQ-C36 and C30 have been validated and can be used for many cancer sites and in many countries.

Acute side effects can be recorded using the NCI-CTC 3 (Common Toxicity Criteria version 3). This is a complex and comprehensive system that has only partially been adopted. Late effects are recorded either using the Radiation Therapy Oncology Group (RTOG) criteria or the European LENT-SOMA classification or other simpler schemes for individual body sites such as gynaecological tumours. Use of the NCI-CTC 3 is recommended until a more concise system gains international recognition.

Clinical anatomy

Modern radiotherapy planning requires a comprehensive knowledge of cross-sectional anatomy and the ability to visualise structures in three dimensions. Formal teaching in anatomy should be part of training, using standard atlases, various online resources, e.g. the Visible Man, and three-dimensional (3D) images, which have become more accessible with picture archiving and conservation systems (PACS). We attempt to give some relevant anatomical details in the following chapters, but collaboration with a diagnostic radiologist will be essential for accurate GTV delineation. Oncologists will tend to develop expertise in their own specialist area, but are unlikely to be familiar with all the possible normal variants and anomalies which may occur.

Protocols and guidelines

In the UK, there has been a proliferation of guidance, guidelines and protocols for the management of cancer. Some, such as Improving Outcomes Guidance (IOG) and decisions of the National Institute for Health and Clinical Excellence (NICE) have a mandatory element which ensures their adoption. The firmest base for clinical decision-making is evidence of effectiveness of treatment from well-designed prospective randomised clinical trials (RCTs). Where this is lacking, careful analysis of outcomes data can be very informative and has the advantage of wider generalisability. National and international trial protocols offer useful information for treatment planning, as they represent current consensus on best practice, as for example, how to scan lung cancer for treatment planning, or what quality assurance programme to use. Departments will have their own written protocols for treatment at different sites to ensure consistency and quality and to avoid errors.

Not all patients' circumstances will fit within standardised guidelines and protocols, although these should be followed whenever possible for best outcomes. However, with the rate of change in treatment in oncology, there should be a constant cycle of writing guidelines and using, auditing, challenging and rewriting them.

Information sources

Adjuvant! Online. www.adjuvantonline.com (accessed 26 November 2008).

Clark A, Fallowfield LJ (1986) Quality of life measurement in patients with malignant disease. *Royal Soc Med* **79**:165–9.

Cochran AJ, Roberts AA, Saida T (2003) The place of lymphatic mapping and sentinel node biopsy in oncology. *Int J Clin Oncol* **8**: 139–50.

Common Toxicity Criteria for Adverse Events v3.0 (CTCAE) (2006) http://ctep.cancer.gov/forms/CTCAEv3.pdf (accessed 26 November 2008).

Dukes CE (1949) The surgical pathology of rectal cancer. *J Clin Path* **2**: 95–8 and at www.emedicine.com.

ECOG/WHO Oken MM, Creech RH, Tormey DC *et al.* (1982) Toxicity and response criteria of the Eastern Oncology Cooperative Group. *Am J Clin Oncol* **5**: 649–55.

Ernst E, Cassileth BR (1998) The prevalence of complementary/alternative medicine in cancer. *Cancer* **83**: 777–82.

Gipponi M, Solari N, Di Somma FC *et al.* (2004) New fields of application of the sentinel node biopsy in the pathological staging of solid neoplasms: Review of the literature and surgical perspectives. *J Surg Oncol* **85**: 171–9.

Imaging for Oncology: *Collaboration Between Clinical Radiologists and Clinical Oncologists in Diagnosis, Staging, and Radiotherapy Planning*. (2004) Royal College of Radiologists, London.

Karnovsky DA, Burchenal JH (1949) The clinical evaluation of chemotherapeutic agents in cancer. In: MacLeod CM (ed) *Evaluation of Chemotherapeutic Agents*. Columbia University Press, New York, p. 196 and at http://en.wikipedia.org/wiki/Performance_status.

Kattan MW, Eastham JA, Stapleton AM *et al.* (1998) A prospective nomogram for disease recurrence following radical prostatectomy for prostate cancer. *J Natl Cancer Inst* **90**: 766–71.

Lansky SB, List MA, Lansky LL *et al.* (1987) The measurement of performance in childhood cancer patients. *Cancer* **60**: 1651–6.

NICE guidance. www.nice.org.uk.

Partin AW, Mangold LA, Lamm DM *et al.* (2001) Contemporary update of prostate cancer staging nomograms (Partin tables) for the new millennium. *Urology* **58**: 843–8.

Pecorelli S, Ngan HYS, Hacker NF (2006) *Staging Classifications and Clinical Practice Guidelines for Gynaecological Cancers*. Reprinted from *Int J Gynae Obstet* 2002; **70**: 207–312 at www.figo.org/docs/staging_booklet.pdf (accessed 2 December 2008).

QLC-30. http://groups.eortc.be/qol/questionnaires_qlqc30.htm (accessed 26 November 2008).

Recommendations for Cross-sectional Imaging in Cancer Management (2006). Royal College of Radiologists, London.

Seiwert TY, Joseph K, Salama JK *et al.* (2007) The concurrent chemoradiation paradigm – general principles. *Nat Clin Pract Oncol* **4**: 86–100.

SF36. www.pdmed.bham.ac.uk/trial/Clinicians/SF36%20Questionnaire.pdf (accessed 2 December 2008).

Sobin LH, Wittekind CH (2002) *TNM Classification of Malignant Tumours*, 6th edn. John Wiley, Chichester.

Therasse P, Arbuck SG, Eisenhauer EA *et al.* (2000) New guidelines to evaluate the response to treatment in solid tumours. *J Natl Cancer Inst* **92**: 205–16 and at http://ctep.cancer.gov/forms/TherasseRECISTJNCI.pdf (accessed 26 November 2008).

The Visible Human Project, National Library of Medicine 1989–1995. www.nlm.nih.gov/research/visible/visible_human.html (accessed 2 December 2008).

Radiation Therapy Oncology Group. www.rtog.org/hnatlas/main.html.

Wittekind CH, Hutter R, Greene FL *et al.* (2005) *TNM Atlas: Illustrated Guide to the TNM Classification of Malignant Tumours*, 5th edn. John Wiley, Chichester.

World Health Organization (2007) International Classification of Disease – Version 10, Chapter 2 Neoplasms. www.who.int/classifications/apps/icd/icd10online (accessed 26 November 2008).

Zigmond AS, Snaith RP (1983) Hospital Anxiety and Depression Scale. *Acta Pyschiatr Scand* **67**: 361–70 and at www.sign.ac.uk/guidelines (Guideline 57).

Principles of radiotherapy planning

The practice of radiotherapy requires not only excellent clinical skills but also appropriate technical expertise. Chapter 1 considered some factors contributing to making good clinical judgements; Chapter 2 outlines the specialist knowledge required to plan radiotherapy treatment.

Target volume definition

A common international language for describing target volumes is found in International Commission on Radiation Units (ICRU) published recommendations Report 50 (1993), 62 (1999) and 71 (2004). These contain clear definitions (Fig. 2.1) to enable centres to use the same criteria for delineating tumours for radiation so that their treatment results can be compared.

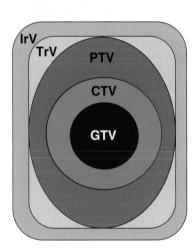

Figure 2.1 ICRU target volume definitions showing GTV, CTV, PTV, treated and irradiated volume. Reproduced with permission from ICRU (1993) *Prescribing, Recording and Reporting Photon Beam Therapy*. ICRU report 50.

■ Gross tumour volume

Gross tumour volume (GTV) is the primary tumour or other tumour mass shown by clinical examination, at examination under anaesthetic (EUA) or by imaging. GTV is classified by staging systems such as TNM (UICC), AJCC or FIGO. Tumour size, site and shape may appear to vary depending on the imaging technique used and an optimal imaging method for each particular tumour site must therefore also be specified. A GTV may consist of primary tumour (GTV-T) and/or metastatic lymphadenopathy (GTV-N) or distant metastases (GTV-M). GTV always contains the highest tumour cell density and is absent after complete surgical resection.

■ Clinical target volume

Clinical target volume (CTV) contains the GTV when present and/or subclinical microscopic disease that has to be eradicated to cure the tumour. CTV definition is based on histological examination of post mortem or surgical specimens assessing extent of tumour cell spread around the gross GTV, as described by Holland *et al.* (1985) for breast cancer. The GTV-CTV margin is also derived from biological characteristics of the tumour, local recurrence patterns and experience of the radiation oncologist. A CTV containing a primary tumour may lie in continuity with a nodal GTV/CTV to create a CTV-TN (e.g. tonsillar tumour and ipsilateral cervical nodes). When a potentially involved adjacent lymph node which may require elective irradiation lies at a distance from the primary tumour, separate CTV-T and CTV-N are used (Fig. 2.2), e.g. an anal tumour and the inguinal nodes.

CTV can be denoted by the dose level prescribed, as for example, CTV-T50 for a particular CTV given 50 Gy. For treatment of breast cancer, three CTVs may be used for an individual patient: CTV-T50 (50 Gy is prescribed to the whole breast); CTV-T66 (66 Gy to the tumour bed); and CTV-N50 (50 Gy to regional lymph nodes).

Variation in CTV delineation by the clinician ('doctor's delineation error') is the greatest geometrical uncertainty in the whole treatment process. Studies comparing outlining by radiologists and oncologists have shown a significant inter-observer variability for both the GTV and/or CTV at a variety of tumour sites. This is greater than any intra-observer variation. Published results for nasopharynx, brain, lung, prostate, medulloblastoma and breast all show significant discrepancies in the volumes outlined by different clinicians. Improvements can be made with training in radiological anatomy which enables clinicians to distinguish blood vessels from lymph nodes and to identify structures accurately on computed tomography (CT) and magnetic resonance imaging (MRI). Joint outlining by radiologists and oncologists can improve consistency and ensure accurate interpretation of imaging of the GTV. Consensus guidelines such as those for defining CTV for head and neck nodes (Gregoire *et al.* 2000) and pelvic nodes (Taylor *et al.* 2005) have improved CTV delineation greatly. Protocols for outlining GTV and CTV at all tumour sites are needed and suggestions are made in each individual chapter.

■ Planning target volume

When the patient moves or internal organs change in size and shape during a fraction of treatment or between fractions (intra- or inter-fractionally), the position of the CTV may also move. Therefore, to ensure a homogeneous dose to the CTV throughout a fractionated course of irradiation, margins must be added around the CTV. These allow for physiological organ motion (internal margin) and variations in patient positioning and alignment of treatment beams (set-up margin), creating a geometric planning target volume. The planning target volume (PTV) is used in treatment planning to select appropriate beams to ensure that the prescribed dose is actually delivered to the CTV.

■ Organ motion/internal margin

Variations in organ motion may be small (e.g. brain), larger and predictable (e.g. respiration or cardiac pulsation), or unpredictable (e.g. rectal and bladder filling).

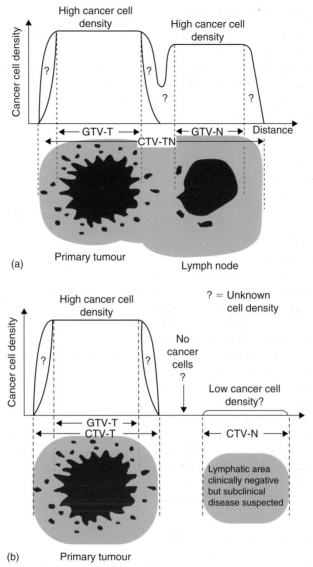

Figure 2.2 ICRU illustrations to show (a) GTV-T plus GTV-N in continuity (CTV-TN) and (b) CTV-T and CTV-N at a distance. Reproduced with permission from ICRU (2004) *Prescribing, Recording and Reporting Electron Beam Therapy*. ICRU report 71.

When treating lung tumours, the displacement of the CTV caused by respiration can be dealt with in several ways: by increasing the CTV-PTV margin eccentrically to include all CTV positions during a respiratory cycle; by using suspended respiration with a technique such as the active breathing control (ABC) device; or by delivery of radiation using gating or respiratory correlated CT scanning and treatment.

Protocols for minimising effects on the CTV of variations in bladder and rectal filling are described in relevant chapters. Uncertainties from organ motion can also be reduced by using fiducial markers, and published results are available for lung, prostate and breast tumours. Radio-opaque markers are inserted and imaged at localisation using CT or MRI, and at treatment verification, using portal films, electronic portal imaging devices (EPIDs) or online cone beam CT image-guided radiotherapy (IGRT).

The internal margin therefore allows for inter- and intra-fractional variations in organ position and shape which cannot be eliminated.

■ Set-up variations/set-up margin

During a fractionated course of radiotherapy, variations in patient position and in alignment of beams will occur both intra- and inter-fractionally, and a margin for set-up error must be incorporated into the CTV-PTV margin. Errors may be systematic or random.

Systematic errors may result from incorrect data transfer from planning to dose delivery, or inaccurate placing of devices such as compensators, shields, etc. Such systematic errors can be corrected.

Random errors in set-up may be operator dependent, or result from changes in patient anatomy from day to day which are impossible to correct. Accuracy of set-up may be improved with better immobilisation, attention to staff training and/or implanted opaque fiducial markers, such as gold seeds, whose position can be determined in three dimensions at planning, and checked during treatment using portal imaging or IGRT. Translational errors can thereby be reduced to 1 mm and rotational errors to 1°.

Each department should measure its own systematic and random errors for each treatment technique by comparing portal imaging and digitally reconstructed radiographs (DRRs). These measurements are then incorporated into the CTV-PTV margin using the formula devised by Van Herk, where the CTV is covered for 90 per cent of the patients with the 95 per cent isodoses:

$$\text{PTV margin} = 2.5\Sigma + 0.74\sigma$$

where Σ = total standard deviation (SD) computed as the square root of the sum of the squared individual SD values of all systematic errors for organ motion and set-up; and σ = total SD of all random errors combined quadratically in a similar way.

This provides a population-derived standard CTV-PTV margin for a particular technique in a given centre and can be non-isotropic in cranio-caudal, transverse and anteroposterior (AP) directions. Accurate treatment delivery depends on reducing or eliminating systematic errors and requires a high level of awareness of all staff throughout the many different work areas from localisation through to treatment.

Other theories about how to incorporate organ motion and the uncertainty of the 'mean' position of the CTV on a snapshot CT scan used for localisation have been proposed. Van Herk suggests a volume large enough to contain the mean position of the CTV in 90 per cent of cases, called the systematic target volume (STV) (British Institute of Radiology 2003). Collection of data on the precise CT location of tumour recurrences in relation to the original target volume is important to improve margin definition.

Treated volume

This is the volume of tissue that is planned to receive a specified dose and is enclosed by the isodose surface corresponding to that dose level, e.g. 95 per cent. The shape, size and position of the treated volume in relation to the PTV should be recorded to evaluate and interpret local recurrences (in field versus marginal) and complications in normal tissues, which may be outside the PTV but within the treated volume.

Conformity index

This is the ratio of PTV to the treated volume, and indicates how well the PTV is covered by the treatment while minimising dose to normal tissues.

Irradiated volume

This is the volume of tissue that is irradiated to a dose considered significant in terms of normal tissue tolerance, and is dependent on the treatment technique used. The size of the irradiated volume relative to the treated volume (and integral dose) may increase with increasing numbers of beams, but both volumes can be reduced by beam shaping and conformal therapy.

Organs at risk

These are critical normal tissues whose radiation sensitivity may significantly influence treatment planning and/or prescribed dose. Any movements of the organs at risk (OAR) or uncertainties of set-up may be accounted for with a margin similar to the principles for PTV, to create a planning organ at risk volume (PRV). The size of the margin may vary in different directions. Where a PTV and PRV are close or overlap, a clinical decision about relative risks of tumour relapse or normal tissue damage must be made. Shielding of parts of normal organs is possible with the use of multi-leaf collimation (MLC). Dose–volume histograms (DVHs) are used to calculate normal tissue dose distributions.

Immobilisation

The patient must be in a position that is comfortable and reproducible (whether supine or prone), and suitable for acquisition of images for CT scanning and treatment delivery. Immobilisation systems are widely available for every anatomical tumour site and are important in reducing systematic set-up errors. Complex stereotactic or relocatable frames (e.g. Gill–Thomas) are secured to the head by insertion into the mouth of a dental impression of the upper teeth and an occipital impression on the head frame, and are used for stereotactic radiotherapy with a reproducibility of within 1 mm or less. Perspex shells reduce movement in head and neck treatments to about 2 mm. The technician preparing the shell must have details of the tumour site to be treated, e.g. position of the patient (prone, supine, flexion or extension of neck, arm position, etc.). An impression of the relevant area (made using quick setting dental alginate or plaster of Paris) is filled with plaster and this form is used to make a Perspex shell by vacuum moulding. The shell fits over the patient and fastens to a device on the couch with Perspex straps and pegs in at least five places. Alternatively, thermoplastic shells can be made by direct moulding of heat-softened material on the patient and these have a similar degree of accuracy.

Relocatable whole body fixation systems using vacuum moulded bags of polystyrene beads on a stereotactic table top restrict movement to 3–4 mm and are used to immobilise the trunk and limbs with markings on the bag instead of on the patient's skin. Where the patient has kyphosis, scoliosis or limitation of joint movement, extra limb pads or immobilisation devices may be required. Metallic prostheses, abdominal stomata and the batteries of pacemakers must be located and excluded from the radiation volume where possible. Details of immobilisation devices are discussed in each tumour site chapter.

Parameters of limb rests, thoracic or belly boards, foot rests and leg restraints, Perspex shells and skin tattoos should be clearly recorded to avoid transfer errors between the planning process and subsequent treatment. Gantry and couch top flexibility should be measured and couch sag avoided by using rigid radiolucent carbon fibre tables. Table tops must have fixtures for immobilisation devices and laser light systems are essential in CT, simulator and treatment units (Fig. 2.3). Protocols for bladder and rectal filling, respiration and other patient parameters must be documented at localisation, and reproduced daily during treatment to minimise uncertainties.

CT scans taken for localisation are only a single snapshot, and the CT scan should be repeated daily on several days to measure variation in organ motion and systematic set-up errors for an individual patient. These values can then be used to inform the CTV-PTV margin on an individual basis rather than using population derived margin values. This is known as adaptive radiotherapy (ART). Kilovoltage (kV), cone beam CT, and megavoltage (MV) imaging on treatment machines make it possible to obtain CT images immediately before treatment. While

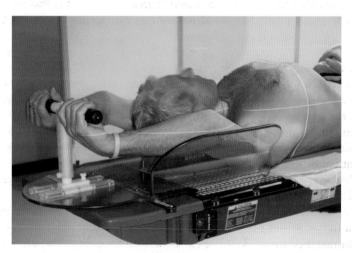

Figure 2.3 Patient positioned to show immobilisation on the CT scanner with arms up and laser lights used to prevent rotational set-up errors.

resolution is not as good as with diagnostic CT, the use of fiducial markers and image registration protocols enables daily online IGRT. With this technique only intra-fractional variations and the doctor's CTV delineation error remain.

Data acquisition

Accurate 3D data about tumour, target volumes and organs at risk are acquired in relation to external reference points under exactly the same conditions as those used for subsequent treatment. Optimal diagnostic imaging modalities are chosen for each tumour site according to protocols developed with diagnostic radiologists. Multi-slice CT, MR with dynamic scanning, 3D ultrasound, positron emission tomography (PET) and single photon emission computed tomography (SPECT) have provided a wealth of anatomical, functional and metabolic information about the GTV. These MRI and PET images are fused with CT planning scans to optimise tumour localisation using a CT scanner with virtual simulation. Alternatively, when these are unavailable, a simulator or simulator CT is used for 2D planning.

■ CT scanning

CT scanning provides detailed cross-sectional anatomy of the normal organs, as well as 3D tumour information. These images provide density data for radiation dose calculations by conversion of CT Hounsfield units into relative electron densities using calibration curves. Compton scattering is the main process of tissue interaction for megavoltage beams and is directly proportional to electron density. Hence CT provides ideal density information for dose corrections for tissue inhomogeneity, such as occurs in lung tissue. Clinical studies have shown that 30–80 per cent of patients undergoing radiotherapy benefit from the increased accuracy of target volume delineation with CT scanning compared with conventional simulation. It has been estimated that the use of CT improves overall 5-year survival rates by around 3.5 per cent, with the greatest impact on small volume treatments.

CT scans taken for radiotherapy treatment planning usually differ from those taken for diagnostic use. Ideally, planning CT scans are taken on a dedicated radiotherapy CT scanner by a therapy trained radiographer. The scanner should have the largest possible aperture to aid positioning of the patient for treatment. The standard diagnostic CT aperture is 70 cm but 85 cm wide-bore scanners are available, which are helpful for large patients and those being treated for breast cancer, who lie with both arms elevated on an inclined plane that can be extended up to around 15°. The CT couch must be flat topped with accurate couch registration to better than 1 mm. The patient is positioned using supporting aids and immobilisation devices and aligned using tattoos and midline and lateral laser lights identical to those used for subsequent radiotherapy treatment. A tattoo is made on the skin over an immobile bony landmark nearest to the centre of the target volume (e.g. pubic symphysis). It is marked with radio-opaque material such as a catheter or barium paste for visualisation on the CT image. Additional lateral tattoos are used to prevent lateral rotation of the patient and are aligned using horizontal lasers (see Fig. 2.3).

Oral contrast medium is used in small concentrated dose to outline small bowel as an organ at risk (e.g. for pelvic intensity-modulated radiotherapy [IMRT] treatment), but care must be taken to avoid large quantities which may cause diuresis and overfill the bladder. Intravenous contrast is given for patients with lung and mediastinal tumours to differentiate between mediastinal vascular structures, tumour and lymph nodes, and in the pelvis to enhance blood vessels for CTV delineation of lymph nodes. Structures such as the vulva, vaginal introitus, anal margin, stomata and surgical scars may be marked with radio-opaque material. Patients with locally advanced tumours should be examined in the treatment position and tumour margins clearly marked. Protocols to reduce organ motion, for example by emptying the bladder before bladder radiotherapy and the rectum before prostate treatment, need to be in place. Patients are given information leaflets to explain the importance of, and rationale for, these procedures.

Multi-slice CT scanners perform a scan of the entire chest or abdomen in a few seconds with the patient breathing normally. Scanning for lung tumours can involve 'slow' CT scans, respiratory correlated CT scans, gating, or use of the ABC device to cope with the effect of respiratory movement.

Protocols for CT scanning are developed with the radiologist to optimise tumour information, to ensure full body contour in the reconstruction circle and scanning of relevant whole organs for DVHs. DRRs are produced from CT density information and are compared with electronic portal images (EPIs). Contiguous thin CT slices are obtained at 2–5 mm intervals for the head and 3–10 mm for the body.

■ Contouring

CT scans are transferred digitally to the target volume localisation console using an electronic network system which must be compliant with DICOM 3 and DICOM RT protocols (Fig. 2.4). The GTV, CTV, PTV, body contour and normal organs are outlined by a team of radiation oncologist, specialist radiologist and planning technician, with appropriate training. Where MRI is the optimal imaging modality for tumours such as the prostate, uterus, brain, head and neck and sarcomas, it is incorporated into target volume definition by image fusion. Treatment planning based on MR images alone is reported, but more commonly CT and MR images are co-registered, ideally scanning using a flat MRI couch top to aid matching. PET or PET-CT images may give additional information for head and neck tumours, lymphomas, lung and gynaecological tumours, and SPECT for brain tumours. Multimodality image fusion of all these images in the treatment planning process is ideal for accurate delineation of the target.

Departmental protocols for target volume delineation are essential for each tumour site; these should define optimal window settings, how to construct the CTV, 3D values for CTV-PTV margins, type of 3D expansion software and method of outlining for each OAR to be used. 'Doctor's delineation errors' resulting from contouring are said to be the most uncertain part of the whole planning process and training in, and validation of these procedures is essential.

Contouring starts with definition of the GTV on a central slice of the primary tumour and then on each axial CT image moving superiorly and then inferiorly. Involved nodes can then be defined in the same way. Viewing the GTV on coronal and sagittal DRRs ensures consistency of definition between slices so that no artificial steps in the volume are created. A volume should not be copied or cut and pasted onto sequential slices for risk of pasting an error: it is more accurate to redraw the GTV on each slice. If there are slices where the GTV cannot be defined – for example

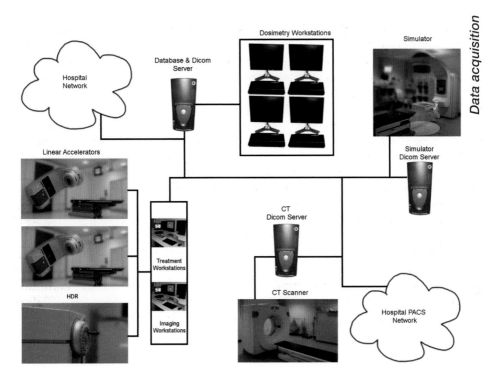

Figure 2.4 Network for transferring data between steps in the radiotherapy planning process.

due to dental artefact – the planning software will usually allow the missing contours to be interpolated from those either side.

■ CT virtual simulation

Using CT data, software generates images from a beam's eye perspective, which are equivalent to conventional simulator images. External landmarks are used to define an internal isocentre for treatment set-up. The CT simulator provides maximal tumour information as well as full 3D capabilities (unlike the simulator CT facility). It is particularly useful for designing palliative treatments such as for lung and vertebral metastases, as well as for some breast treatments using tangential beams, which can be virtually simulated and then 3D planned. The ability to derive CT scans, and provide target volume definition, margin generation, and simulation all on one workstation, provides a rapid solution.

■ Conventional simulator

For palliative treatments, a simulator may still be used to define field borders following the 50 per cent isodose line of the beam, rather than a target volume. A simulator is an isocentrically mounted diagnostic X-ray machine which can reproduce all the movements of the treatment unit and has an image intensifier for screening. The patient is prepared in the treatment position exactly as described above for CT scanning. The machine rotates around the patient on an axis centred on a fixed point, the isocentre, which is 100 cm from the focal spot and is placed at the centre of the target volume. Digital images or radiographs are used to record the field borders chosen by reference to bony landmarks. The simulator is commonly used either for palliative single field treatments of bone metastases or to define opposing anterior and posterior fields for palliative treatment to locally advanced tumour masses.

■ Simulator-CT

A CT mode attached to the simulator gantry can be used to produce images with a relatively limited resolution during the simulation process. This provides both external contouring and some normal anatomical data, such as lung and chest wall thickness, for simple inhomogeneity corrections. Images do not give detailed tumour information or accurate CT numbers. These scans are time consuming to obtain, and are therefore usually limited to the central, superior and inferior levels of the target volume.

Dose solutions

When the PTV and normal organs have been defined in 3D, the optimal dose distribution for treating the tumour is sought. Consultation with a dosimetrist is vital to select the best parameters. For example, a treatment machine must be chosen according to percentage depth dose characteristics and build up depth which will vary with energy and beam size as shown in Table 2.1. These can be used to calculate doses for treatment using single fields and to learn the construction of isodose distributions using computer modelling. Other factors to be considered in the choice of machine are the effect of penumbra on beam definition, the availability of independent or multi-leaf collimators, facilities for beam modification and portal imaging.

Table 2.1 Data from treatment machines in common use, showing variation of D_{max} and percentage depth dose (DD) with energy

Machine	Energy (MV)	FSD (cm)	10 × 10 cm field*	
			D_{max} depth (cm)	% DD at 10 cm
Cobalt-60	1.25	100	0.5	58.7
Linear accelerator	6	100	1.5	67.5
	10	100	2.3	73
	16	100	2.8	76.8

*Maximum field size at 100 cm is 40 × 40 cm.

Three levels of dose planning and treatment are described here:

■ **Conventional** treatment uses single or opposing beams, with or without 2D dose distributions, with compensators and simple shielding.
■ **Conformal** treatment involves target volume delineation of tumour and normal organs according to ICRU principles with 3D dose calculations using MLC to shape beams.

- **Complex** treatment includes the use of IMRT to shape the fluence of the beam, dynamic treatments, IGRT and 3D or 4D delivery.

Most dose computation is done using 3D computerised treatment planning systems which are programmed with beam data from therapy machines. These systems require careful quality control programmes. Following production of a satisfactory isodose distribution to a given target volume using 2D or 3D algorithms, the calculations are checked by a physicist and detailed instructions for delivery are prepared by radiographers on the therapy unit.

■ Conventional treatment

Single fields may be used with borders defined by the 50 per cent isodose for bone metastases. Parallel opposing beams are used for speed and ease of set-up for palliative treatments (e.g. lung), for target volumes of small separation (e.g. larynx) or tangential volumes (e.g. breast). Isodose distributions show that the 95 per cent isodose does not conform closely to the target volume, the distribution of dose is not homogeneous and much normal tissue is irradiated to the same dose as the tumour. Beam modification with the use of wedges alters the dose distribution to compensate for missing tissue, obliquity of body contour or a sloping target volume, and may produce a more homogeneous result.

For many tumours seated at depth, a radical tumour dose can only be achieved with a combination of several beams if overdose to the skin and other superficial tissues is to be avoided. When multiple beams are chosen for a plan, variable wedges can be used to attenuate the beam and thereby avoid a high dose area at beam intersections. To achieve the same dose at the patient, the number of monitor units set will have to be increased compared with those for an open field. Computerised dose planning systems are used to construct an isodose distribution with beams of appropriate energy, size, weighting, gantry angle and wedge to give a homogeneous result over the target volume.

■ Inhomogeneity corrections

Attenuation of an X-ray beam is affected by tissue density, being less in lung than bone. This variation affects both the shape of the dose distribution and the values of the isodoses. Lung tissue should therefore be localised when planning treatment for tumours of the thorax (e.g. lung, breast, oesophagus, mediastinum). The relative electron density of lung compared with water is in the range 0.2–0.3 and these values are used to correct for inhomogeneity.

When 2D conventional planning is used, correction is only valid at the planned central slice of the target volume, e.g. breast treatment planned with a simulator using central lung distance (CLD). Using CT scanning, the whole lung is localised in 3D and a pixel by pixel correction made for all tissue densities by conversion of CT numbers into relative electron densities using calibration curves. CT numbers are affected by contrast agents but dose distributions in the chest and abdomen are not significantly changed by the quantities used in most CT scanning protocols. However, large amounts of gas in the rectum can cause organ motion of the prostate and uterus as well as affecting CT densities.

■ Beam junctions

When treatment is given to target volumes that lie adjacent to one another, consideration must be given to the non-uniformity of dose in the potential overlap regions caused by divergence of the adjacent beams. If the beams abut on the skin surface, they will overlap with excess dose at depth. If there is a gap between beams at the skin, there will be a cold area in the superficial tissues. Clinical examples of this problem include treatment of (a) adjacent vertebrae with single posterior fields which may be separated in time, where there is a risk of overlap of dose at the underlying spinal cord, (b) primary breast cancer and adjacent lymph nodes, where a single isocentric technique centred at the junction can be used (see Chapter 22), (c) primary head and neck tumours and their regional nodes which can be treated with IMRT or matched photon and electron fields to avoid overlap over the spinal cord (see Chapter 8) and (d) primary central nervous system (CNS) tumours such as medulloblastoma, where beams are matched at the anterior spinal cord and junctions between beams shifted during the course of treatment (see Chapter 18).

Various techniques have been developed to minimise dose heterogeneity at beam junctions in these different clinical situations. Half beam blocking using shielding or independent collimator jaws can be used to eliminate divergence up to the match line, but accuracy is then dependent on precise immobilisation and reliability of skin marks to reproduce the match perfectly. Couch rotation can be used to remove beam divergence when matching breast and lymph node irradiation. However, for some sites, it is still common to match beams by using a gap between beams so that the beam edges converge at a planned depth (Fig. 2.5). The dose in the triangular gap (x) below the skin surface will be lower than at the point P where the beams converge because it lies outside the geometric margins of both beams. Doses at (y) are higher because they include contributions from both beams. The positioning of point P anatomically will vary according to the aim of treatment. If treatment is for medulloblastoma, a homogeneous dose is required to potential tumour cells within the spinal cord which is therefore placed at point P, and point P is moved in a cranio-caudal direction at regular intervals to prevent any risk of overdose at

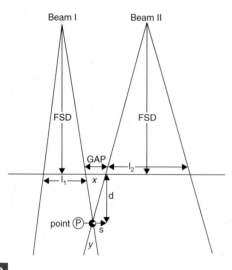

Figure 2.5 Technique for matching two beams I and II (length l_1 and l_2) at a point P at depth d by allowing a gap on the skin surface (x, y, s – see text).

junctions. Where treatment is aimed at metastases in adjacent vertebral bodies, it is important to avoid overdosage at the spinal cord which is therefore placed in the superficial cold triangle (x) with point P anterior to it. The gap on the skin is the sum of the beam divergence of each beam. It is calculated as the distance from the edge of the beam as defined by the 50 per cent isodose to the point of convergence P measured perpendicular to the central axis and marked (s) spread (beam divergence) for each beam. Graphs have been drawn up expressing beam divergence as a function of the depth below the skin for different field sizes and focus skin distance (FSD). Once the gap has been calculated, it may be necessary to increase it slightly to allow for possible movement of patient or skin tattoos, to ensure that there is no overdosage. Whenever possible, a patient should be treated in the same position (supine or prone) for matching adjacent fields.

When planning a new treatment for metastatic disease in the spine, previous treatment fields should be reconstructed from films and records and the patient placed in the same position to ensure there is no overlap.

■ Electron therapy

Electron therapy may be used to treat superficial tumours overlying cartilage and bone (for example nose, ear, scalp and dorsum of hand), in preference to superficial or orthovoltage therapy where there is increased bone absorption due to the photoelectric effect. There is a sharp fall in dose beyond the 90 per cent isodose (4–12 MeV) and electron energy is chosen so that the target volume is encompassed by the 90–95 per cent isodose at the deep margin. Electrons at higher energies (15–25 MeV) may be used for treating cervical lymph nodes overlying spinal cord, parotid tumours and in mixed beams with photons.

The effective treatment depth in centimetres is about one-third of the beam energy in MeV and the total range about half (Fig. 2.6) but this is dependent on field size (especially at <40 mm). Different tissue densities such as bone and air (as found in ribs overlying lung and facial bones containing air filled sinuses) cause inhomogeneous dose distributions. Doses beyond air cavities may be higher than expected even after density corrections and this limits the usefulness of electrons for treating in these clinical situations. Electron beam edges do not diverge geometrically due to lateral scatter, which is greater at low energies with the characteristic shape shown in Figure 2.7. Wider margins must be added when choosing the beam width for adequate treatment of tumours at depth. Where there is tumour infiltration of skin, the skin sparing characteristics of electron beams below 16 MeV should be removed by adding bolus material, which can also be used to provide tissue equivalent material for an irregular contour such as the nose or ear. Beam sizes <40 mm should be avoided because of inadequate depth of penetration and loss of beam flatness.

■ Conformal treatment

3D conformal radiotherapy (CFRT) links 3D CT visualisation of the tumour with the capability of the linear accelerator to shape the beam both geometrically and by altering the fluence of the beam (IMRT). This encloses the target volume as closely as possible while reducing dose to adjacent normal tissues. The radiation oncologist and dosimetrist agree the final PTV, which has been created using 3D

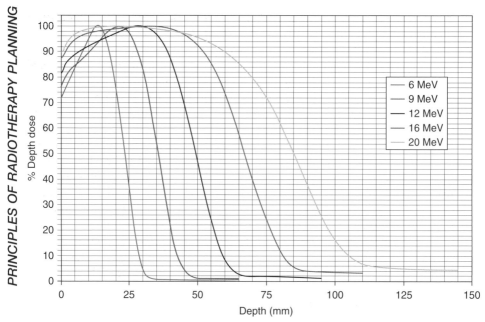

Figure 2.6 Percentage depth dose of varying electron energies for 10 × 10 cm applicator.

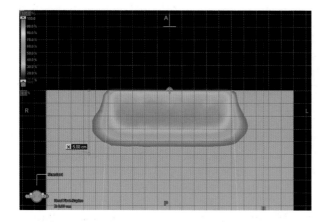

Figure 2.7 9 MeV electron dose distribution.

growth algorithm software and departmental protocols, taking into consideration OAR. Discussions between oncologist and dosimetrist include an understanding of the tumour cell density pattern within the PTV, requirements for homogeneity of dose distribution, dose constraints to adjacent OAR, avoidance of maximum or minimum dose spots in 3D and review of a preliminary plan of likely beam arrangements. Basic CFRT may consist of coplanar and static beams with MLC or conformal blocks shaping the volume. For coplanar non-standard configuration of beams, DVHs may aid selection of the best plan, but they do not indicate which part of the organ is receiving a high or low dose; DVHs of the PTV, CTV and all PRVs are needed to allow subsequent correlation with clinical outcome. Selection of the final dose plan is made at the treatment-planning terminal by inspecting

3D physical dose distributions and DVHs. Good communication is important between radiographers, dosimetrist, physicist and clinician to avoid transfer errors occurring between CT, treatment planning and treatment machine.

Conformal therapy may involve the use of mixed beams combining photons and electrons for part of the treatment. Beams can be modified using bolus, wedges, compensators, MLCs and shielding blocks. Optimisation of skin dose is achieved by skin sparing using higher megavoltage energies, or by maximising skin dose with tissue equivalent bolus. Higher beam energies (10–18 MV) are preferred for pelvic treatments, to increase dose to the centre and reduce dose to skin and subcutaneous tissues. Lower energies (6–8 MV) are used for breast and head and neck treatments to avoid excess skin sparing and treat the relatively superficial target volume.

Treatment is delivered using beam shaping with MLCs which have multiple leaves or shields which can block part of the radiation beam. Typical MLCs have 20–80 leaves arranged in opposing pairs which can be positioned under computer control to create an irregular beam conforming to the target shape. As well as eliminating the hazards of production and use of alloy blocks, this system allows rapid adjustment of shaping to match the beam's eye view of the PTV.

■ Complex treatment

IMRT

IMRT is created using MLC to define the beam intensity independently in different regions of each incident beam, to produce the desired uniform distribution of dose, or a deliberate non-uniform dose distribution, in the target volume. The position of the leaves of the MLC can be varied in time with a fixed or moving gantry. IMRT can be delivered using dose compensation, multiple static fields, step-and-shoot, dynamic MLC or tomotherapy.

A sequence of static MLC fields can be used with the beam being switched off between changes in position – the step-and-shoot technique. Alternatively, there may be automatic sequencing of beam segments without stopping treatment – dynamic MLC. Other methods include tomotherapy and other devices where there is intensity modulated rotational delivery with a fan beam.

Forward planned or segmental IMRT provides simple tissue compensation with a beam's eye view of the PTV and sub-segments which are shaped with different MLC to create a uniform dose in the PTV. Inverse planning requires specification of dose prescription to GTV, PTV and PRV in terms of dose–volume constraints, fluence optimisation and 3D dose planning. Very careful quality assurance must be developed to assure accuracy of the beam. Verification of an IMRT plan requires either measurement of the dose distribution in a phantom, or an independent monitor unit calculation with portal dosimetry. Dose delivery is verified throughout the course of treatment using radiographic film or adapted EPIDs or transit dosimetry. Accurate patient positioning, target volume delineation and reduction of organ and patient motion uncertainties, especially respiration, are critical for safe IMRT.

IMRT techniques modulate the intensity of the beam as well as its geometric shape, delivering complex dose distributions, using forward or inverse treatment planning. Plans can be produced with concave shapes, and critical structures at sites such as head and neck (eye or spinal cord), prostate (rectum) and thyroid (spinal cord) avoided. Late toxicity can be reduced significantly for tumour sites such as prostate, pelvis, breast and head and neck. Dose escalation studies in prostate cancer show an improvement in biochemical relapse-free survival using IMRT with reduced late rectal toxicity. There is proof of sparing of salivary gland function with IMRT for head and neck cancer with no loss of tumour control. Late fibrotic changes in the breast can be reduced, and IMRT pelvic treatments, more conformal to the tumour lymph node drainage, have reduced bone marrow and acute bowel and bladder toxicity. However, integral dose may be greater with some IMRT solutions, with increased risk of late malignancies. IMRT dose plans with steep dose gradients may risk underdosage of tumour if margins are close and organ motion still present.

It is difficult to produce evidence of benefit from new technology until it is widely enough available to conduct RCTs, preferably on a multicentre basis. Often, pioneering groups develop and test the technology from the physical viewpoint and clinical implementation goes from pilot (phase 1 type) studies to routine use without a rigorous evidence base of efficacy. A further problem of particular relevance for radiotherapy is that unwanted late effects of treatment cannot be quantified for many years, so that determination of therapeutic ratio – the true test of efficacy – is delayed.

IGRT

Organ motion during treatment makes it necessary to consider the fourth dimension of time. IGRT refers to all techniques in which cross-sectional, X-ray or ultrasound images obtained during treatment are used to check that the actual treatment delivered matches that which has been planned. Ideally the moving tumour outline is imaged during treatment using daily EPIs or real time cone beam CT. Alternatively, EPIs can be taken on the first few days of treatment and used to adjust treatment volumes where necessary.

Variations in overall positioning of the body during treatment can be monitored using optical imaging devices, sometimes in association with markers attached to the skin. To avoid respiratory motion, treatment may be delivered while the patient holds his or her breath using the ABC device. This demands cooperation from the patient and may be difficult in those with lung diseases. Treatment may be gated to a specific phase of the respiratory cycle, usually expiration, using optical devices or X-ray fluoroscopic measurements. CT scans obtained by imaging devices on the linear accelerator can be compared with respiration-correlated spiral CT planning images. Treatment delivery is triggered when the two images match.

These techniques may reduce the PTV and restrict the dose to normal lung but are time consuming. Some evidence is accumulating that respiratory gating may be of limited benefit overall since, although it reduces organ movement effects, it prolongs treatment time. Composite multi-field conformal plans delivered in multiple fractions may have a similar overall effect in a more cost effective way. Further randomised trials are needed to assess 4D treatment delivery.

Adaptive radiotherapy (ART) involves regular changes (weekly or daily) to treatment delivery for an individual patient based on analysis of images taken before treatment or ideally during treatment. Linear accelerator mounted imaging devices are essential for this technique. One integrated approach is to use rotational IMRT or tomotherapy. The MLC is linked to a machine-mounted CT scanner with images taken during therapy used to gate treatment to the correct body slice.

Special techniques

■ Protons

Some radiation oncologists consider that many of the advantages of IMRT could be better obtained by using the superior dose distributions of protons. There are some indications where the benefits seem to be established firmly enough for this to be the treatment of choice (some paediatric and skull-based tumours, and radio-resistant tumours in difficult sites, such as vertebral chondrosarcoma). At present the cost of installing proton facilities precludes widespread use, but guidelines for referral to specialist centres have been drawn up.

■ Stereotactic radiotherapy

This technique is only available in a limited number of centres but has been used for many years, mainly for the treatment of small brain tumours and arteriovenous malformations. Accuracy of patient positioning to approximately 1 mm is maintained using a stereotactic frame attached to the patient's skull. Radiotherapy may be delivered as a single or multiple fractions and may be considered as an alternative to surgery. The gamma knife device uses multiple cobalt sources arranged around a half circle, which irradiate a very conformal volume by blocking selected collimator openings with different collimation helmets for different time intervals. Alternatively, a linear accelerator with specialised collimators can be used to deliver multiple arc therapy.

This technique requires very careful quality assurance because of steep dose gradients and problems of electron equilibration with very small beams. It also requires close collaboration within a team of people with relevant expertise in imaging, neuroanatomy, tumour management and physics. This approach may also be beneficial for some small volume lung and liver tumours.

Dose-fractionation

Prescription of radiotherapy treatment is the responsibility of the radiation oncologist and usually follows agreed guidelines, taking into consideration individual patient factors, such as the expected risk–benefit ratio of treatment, comorbidities and consideration of scheduling of other treatment modalities. Radiotherapy regimens vary internationally. Fractions of 2 Gy or less delivered 5 days a week are the standard of care in much of North America and Europe. Regimens given in this book are safe evidence-based schedules but national and international protocols or trials should be used as appropriate.

Alternative fractionation schedules using fewer larger fractions in a shorter overall time (hypofractionation) have been developed, especially in the UK and Canada, driven initially by resource constraints, but now supported by extensive published clinical data, e.g. for breast and prostate cancer as well as for palliative treatments. Accelerated fractionation gives the same overall dose in a shorter time, often using smaller fraction sizes to reduce toxicity, and has been used successfully in head and neck cancer trials. Hyperfractionation regimens deliver treatment twice or three times a day using smaller fraction sizes, thereby increasing the total dose and remaining within tolerance for late toxicity (see Table 3.2, p. 42).

The linear quadratic (LQ) model of radiation-induced cell killing is currently the most useful for comparing different fractionation schedules (see Chapter 3), taking into account the effect of dose per fraction and repopulation on tumour and normal tissue late effects. Clinical outcome depends on the total dose, dose per fraction, overall treatment time, volume of tumour and normal tissues irradiated, dose specification points and quality control procedures. If treatment has to be stopped unexpectedly for operational or clinical reasons causing an unscheduled gap in treatment, the dose-fractionation schedule may need to be altered (see Chapter 3).

Dose specification

All dose distributions are inhomogeneous and so the dose throughout the PTV varies. The biological effect of a given dose is difficult to predict because of variations in cell density at the centre and periphery of the CTV, heterogeneity of tumour cell populations and inadequate knowledge of cellular radio-sensitivity. Nevertheless, one must attempt to specify a dose which is representative of the absorbed dose in the target volume as a whole, to assess effectiveness of treatment.

To facilitate understanding and exchange of precise and accurate radiotherapy treatment data, it is important that all centres report their results using the same volume concepts and prescribing definitions.

The ICRU reports 50 and 62 recommend that the radiation dose should be reported, and hence is also best prescribed, at or near the centre of the PTV, and when possible at the intersection of the beam axes (ICRU reference dose). This ICRU reference point for prescription is selected because it is clinically relevant, usually situated where there is maximum tumour cell density, easy to define, often lies on the central axis of the beam where dose can be accurately determined, and is not in a region of steep dose gradient. It is essential that this dose specification point is accompanied by a statement of the homogeneity of the irradiation as defined by at least the maximum and minimum doses to the PTV. The maximum target dose is the highest dose in the target volume which is clinically significant (to a volume greater than $15 \, mm^3$ unless in a critical tissue where special considerations apply). The minimum target dose is an important parameter because it correlates with the probability of tumour control. Additional information, such as average dose and its standard deviation, DVHs and an accurate description of dose to OAR, is also very important (Fig. 2.8).

Superficial treatment machines, with energies ranging from 50 kV to 150 kV and appropriate filtration which defines percentage depth dose characteristics, are used to treat superficial skin tumours. The dose prescription point is at D_{max}, the maximum dose, which is at the skin surface. An appropriate energy is selected from tables for different beam sizes for a given FSD to encompass the target volume both on the skin and at depth with a 90 per cent isodose.

When a single megavoltage beam is used, dose is prescribed to the ICRU point at the centre of the target volume rather than to D_{max}. For example, for bone metastases, the prescription point may be at the centre of the vertebra e.g. 40–50 mm depth for a thoracic vertebra. Alternatively, for palliative treatments, the ICRU point may be chosen at the dose-limiting structure, such as the spinal cord, and a dose prescribed to maximum tolerance.

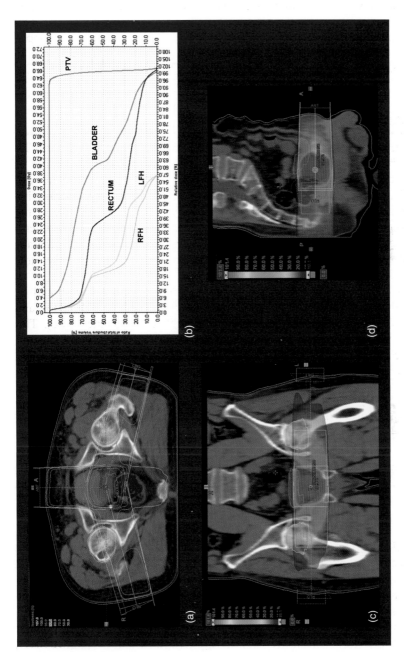

Figure 2.8 Dose distribution to treat carcinoma of the prostate showing (a) axial view with isodoses, ICRU point (100 per cent): maximum = 101 per cent; minimum = 95 per cent. (b) DVH showing PTV, and doses to bladder, rectum, left (LFH) and right (RFH) femoral head. (c) Coronal view with dose colourwash. (d) Sagittal view with dose colourwash.

For co-axial opposing lateral or AP beams, the dose is specified at the midplane dose (MPD) on the central axis of the beam, as recommended by ICRU. In subsequent chapters of this book, these ICRU dose specification conventions have been followed for all dose distributions and prescriptions.

Verification

Verification is needed of the geometrical set-up of the treatment and the dose being delivered. Electronic portal imaging is available on most linear accelerators and images can be compared with DRRs obtained from the treatment planning system. Image evaluation software tools can be used to match predefined bony landmarks on both images noting displacements of beam borders, to match the edges of beams measuring the change in position of bony structures or to match fiducial markers. Errors may be systematic or random. Repeating the portal image daily for the first few days will identify any systematic errors, which can then be corrected. Random errors in set-up may be reduced by better patient immobilisation or staff education, or the CTV-PTV margin may have to be increased if correction is impossible.

Image matching of EPIs with DRRs is usually carried out by the treating radiographers after appropriate training. Verification protocols, both online and off-line, will define the level of action for any deviation. EPIs or portal films should be signed by the clinician, verifying and recording any actions taken.

Verification of the dose delivered to the patient is essential using semiconductor silicon diodes with instant readout, or thermo-luminescent dosimetry (TLD) with delayed readout, and is performed on the first day of each patient's treatment. Transit dosimetry uses a transmission portal image to measure the dose delivered to the patient, which can be compared with the planned dose distribution. Equally important are the mechanical checks of MLC that are required to ensure safe delivery of treatments. These must include examination of the stability of leaf speed, accuracy of leaf position and transmission through and between leaves.

Patient care during treatment

Response to treatment, both in terms of tumour and acute side effects, should be monitored regularly. Weekly clinics are held, often led by a therapy radiographer or radiotherapy clinical nurse specialist, to check for early acute side effects, and to answer patients' questions and give them and their carers psychological and emotional support. Information sheets listing common and uncommon side effects for each tumour site are discussed with individual patients when they give informed consent. Protocols for scoring acute side effects, such as NCI-CTC-3 or RTOG, should be used to document acute reactions and guide appropriate investigations.

The radiation oncologist states on the radiotherapy prescription sheet any specific imaging or blood tests that are required during treatment and is responsible for supervising the review clinics and seeing the patient at appropriate intervals. Patients receiving concurrent radiochemotherapy may experience increased side effects and require special interventions. Specific instructions for dealing with different acute reactions are dealt with in each individual tumour site chapter.

Quality assurance

A comprehensive quality assurance programme is needed to ensure that the best possible care is delivered to the patient by defining and documenting all procedures involved in radiotherapy treatments. A quality assurance policy must be formulated by a radiotherapy manager with overall responsibility for implementation, although large parts of this responsibility may be delegated to other appropriately trained and qualified members of the radiotherapy team. Internal quality assurance systems are supplemented by external accreditation visits. Individual treatment techniques may be checked before trials begin, by requiring participants to submit sample treatment plans and descriptions of methods of beam matching, techniques used for tissue compensation and beam data for verification of output and flatness. Phantom measurements are routinely used to give a composite check of all factors, including dose homogeneity and beam matching. Any internal or external system must be periodically reviewed with documentation of all activity according to a defined protocol. Reference values must be specified with tolerances and action to be taken if these are exceeded. A departmental procedure for investigation of deviations or errors must be in place for every part of the system.

■ Practical considerations

Routine checks of the following must be included in the quality assurance protocol:

- machine checks
- dosimetry protocols
- planning checks
- patient documentation.

Machine checks

During installation and acceptance of new equipment, calibration data are obtained to provide reference against which subsequent checks are made. Inter-comparisons between different institutions or with national or international standards are useful for detecting systematic errors. Quality control should then ensure that a unit performs according to its specification and is safe for both patients and staff. It should guarantee accuracy of dose delivered, prevent major errors, minimise downtime for machines and encourage preventative machine maintenance. There should be a specific quality control protocol for each unit, which outlines the test to be performed, the methods to be used to ensure consistency in the performance of each unit, parameters to be tested, frequency of measurement, staff responsibilities, reference values, tolerances, action to be taken in case of deviation and rules for documentation. Daily, weekly and extended testing of dosimetry beam alignment and safety checks are necessary. Regular checks include tests of optical, mechanical and computer hardware and software systems. Action levels are defined where correction is needed before treatment can proceed. Similar checks must be carried out for all imaging equipment and treatment planning systems. The results of daily checks must be recorded in the control room of the treatment units and radiographers must also record any problems in machine functioning. All other checks, actions and maintenance work are recorded in a separate log book. Good cooperation is needed between all staff groups. A physicist who coordinates all quality control activity checks that tests are up to standard and reports any major deviations to the clinician.

Dosimetry protocols

These include dose monitor calibration checks, checks of beam quality and symmetry and evaluation of beam flatness. *In vivo* dosimetry systems such as TLDs and silicon diodes must also be regularly checked and calibrated.

Planning checks

Treatment prescriptions are now mostly electronic, and recording of treatment delivery parameters is automatic by computer systems attached to treatment machines. Reports of activity obtained from these systems can be used for audit, and central collection of these output data may give very useful information about patterns of radiotherapy delivery. Individual weekly review of patients' treatment records should verify that treatment is being delivered as planned.

Patient documentation

Electronic systems are being used increasingly. Radiation treatment records are usually kept separately from other hospital documents to ensure reliable rapid access. Records should identify the patient, give clinical history and examination findings, histological diagnosis, staging of the tumour and proposed treatment plan. There should be written treatment policies for specific tumour sites and data should be recorded to enable subsequent evaluation of the outcome of treatment. Written consent for treatment is required. At the end of treatment, a summary detailing actual treatment parameters must be prepared and appropriate continuing care of the patient assured.

Staffing

A quality programme as described above is essential for the safe delivery of treatment. It can only be achieved if each member of the team understands clearly the boundaries of responsibility and if there is excellent coordination of all quality control activity by a highly qualified physicist acting with the person responsible for overall management of the radiotherapy department. Careful training of all staff members must therefore be an integral part of any effective quality assurance system.

Information sources

Bel A, Bartelink H, Vijbrief RE *et al.* (1994) Transfer errors of planning CT to simulator: a possible source of set up inaccuracies? *Radiother Oncol* **31**: 176–80.

Bel A, van Herk M, Bartelink H *et al.* (1993) A verification procedure to improve patient set-up accuracy using portal images. *Radiother Oncol* **29**: 253–60.

BIR Working Party (2003) *Geometric Uncertainties in Radiotherapy: Defining the Planning Target Volume.* British Institute of Radiology, London.

Chao KSC, Majhail N, Huang C-J *et al.* (2001) Intensity-modulated radiation therapy reduces late salivary toxicity without compromising tumor control in patients with oropharyngeal carcinoma: a comparison with conventional techniques. *Radiother Oncol* **61**: 275–80.

Development and Implementation of Conformal Radiotherapy in the United Kingdom (2002) Royal
College of Radiologists, London.

Dobbs HJ, Parker RP, Hodson NJ *et al.* (1983) The use of CT in radiotherapy treatment planning.
Radiother Oncol **1**: 133–41.

Gregoire V, Coche E, Cosnard G *et al.* (2000) Selection and delineation of lymph node target
volumes in head and neck conformal therapy. Proposal for standardising terminology and
procedure based on the surgical experience. *Radiother Oncol* **56**: 135–50.

*Guidelines for the Management of Unscheduled Interruption or Prolongation of a Radical Course of
Radiotherapy*, 2nd edn. (2002) Royal College of Radiologists, London.

Holland R, Veling S, Mravunac M *et al.* (1985) Histologic multifocality of Tis, T1–2 breast
carcinomas. Implications for clinical trials of breast-conserving surgery. *Cancer* **56**: 979–90.

Hurkmans CW, Remeijer P, Lebesque JV *et al.* (2001) Set-up verification using portal imaging:
review of current clinical practice. *Radiother Oncol* **58**: 105–20.

International Commission on Radiation Units and Measurements (1993) *Prescribing, Recording and
Reporting Photon Beam Therapy ICRU: Report 50*. ICRU, Bethesda, Maryland, USA.

International Commission on Radiation Units and Measurements (1999) *Prescribing, Recording and
Reporting Photon Beam Therapy (supplement to ICRU Report 50): ICRU Report 62*. ICRU,
Bethesda, Maryland, USA.

International Commission on Radiation Units and Measurements (2004) *Prescribing, Recording and
Reporting Electron Beam Therapy: ICRU Report 71*. ICRU, Bethesda, Maryland, USA.

LENT-SOMA Tables (1995). *Radiother Oncol* **35**: 17–60.

McKenzie AL, van Herk M, Mijnheer B (2000) The width of margins in radiotherapy treatment plans.
Phys Med Biol **45**: 3331–42.

McKenzie AL, van Herk M, Mijnheer B (2002) Margins for geometric uncertainty around organs at
risk in radiotherapy. *Radiother Oncol* **63**: 299–307.

National Cancer Guidance (2008) *Proton Referral-Treatment Abroad*. Royal College of Radiologists,
London.

Radiotherapy Dose-Fractionation. (2006) Royal College of Radiologists, London.

Seddon B, Bidmead M, Wilson J *et al.* (2000) Target volume definition in conformal radiotherapy for
prostate cancer: quality assurance in the MRC RT-01 trial. *Radiother Oncol* **56**: 73–83.

Suter B, Shoulders S, Maclean M *et al.* (2000) Machine verification radiographs: an opportunity for
role extension. *Radiography* **6**: 245–51.

Taylor A, Rockall AG, Reznek RH *et al.* (2005) Mapping pelvic lymph nodes: guidelines for
delineation in intensity-modulated radiotherapy. *Int J Rad Oncol Biol Phys* **63**: 1604–12.

van Herk M, Remeijer P, Rasch C *et al.* (2000) The probability of correct target dosage:
dose-population histograms for deriving treatment margins in radiotherapy. *Int J Rad Oncol
Biol Phys* **47**: 1121–35.

Webb S (2005) *Contemporary IMRT: Developing Physics and Clinical Implementation*. Institute of
Physics Publishing, London.

Wong JW, Sharpe MB, Jaffray DA *et al.* (1999) The use of active breathing control (ABC) to reduce
margin for breathing motion. *Int J Radiat Oncol Biol Phys* **44**: 911–19.

World Health Organization (1988) *Quality Assurance in Radiotherapy*. WHO, Geneva.

Yan D, Ziaja E, Jaffray D *et al.* (1998) The use of adaptive radiation therapy to reduce setup error: a
prospective clinical study. *Int J Radiat Oncol Biol Phy* **41**: 715–20.

Zelefsky MJ, Fuks Z, Hunt M *et al.* (2002) High-dose intensity modulated radiation therapy for
prostate cancer: early toxicity and biochemical outcome in 772 patients. *Int J Radiat Oncol
Biol Phys* **53**: B1111–16.

3 Radiobiology and treatment planning

Radiation and cell kill

Ionising radiation causes wide-ranging molecular damage throughout cells by the production of ionised atoms, which cause breakage of chemical bonds, production of free radicals and damage to DNA. Most clinically significant effects of radiotherapy are due to irreparable DNA lesions which result in sterilisation – a loss of proliferative cells' ability for sustained cell division. In tumours, loss of proliferative ability by all the cells of the tumour is a necessary condition for tumour cure. Partial sterilisation of the tumour cell population results in tumour stasis or regression, giving a clinical remission, followed by regrowth of the tumour from those cells which have retained their proliferative ability. In self-renewing normal tissues, sterilisation of proliferative cells leaves the tissues unable to provide replacements for cells that are ordinarily being lost at a constant rate from the tissue, and initiates a rundown of the mature cells of the tissue. Proliferative sterilisation is often referred to as cell kill, with those cells that retain long-term proliferative ability being described as survivors.

Cell survival curves

Cell culture techniques have been very important in allowing the proliferative sterilisation of cells to be investigated quantitatively. For an irradiated cell population, the proportion of cells that still retain the ability to proliferate (relative to an unirradiated control population) is called the surviving fraction, and a plot of log surviving fraction against single radiation dose gives a *survival curve* for the cells concerned. Typically, survival curves are continuously bending, with a slope that steepens as the dose increases. Mathematically a continuously bending curve is most simply described by a *linear quadratic* (LQ) equation of the form:

$$SF = Exp\,(-\alpha d - \beta d^2) \tag{3.1}$$

where SF is the surviving fraction, d is the given single dose and α and β are parameters characteristic of the cells concerned. The ratio α/β gives the relative importance of the linear dose term and the quadratic dose term for those cells, and controls the shape of the survival curve (Fig. 3.1). When α/β is large, the linear term predominates, so a plot of log (SF) against d is relatively straight, while if α/β is small, the quadratic term is more important, giving a plot with greater curvature. For cells whose survival curves have a lower α/β ratio, doubling the dose leads to more than doubling of the effect on log (SF). Such cells will be particularly sensitive to changes in fraction size when radiation is given as a fractionated schedule.

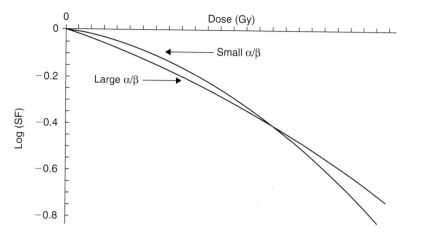

Figure 3.1 Two contrasting survival curves for irradiated cells, with log of the surviving fraction (SF) plotted against single radiation dose. The more steeply curving survival curve has the lower α/β ratio when fitted to the linear-quadratic equation.

Acute and late effects on tissues

The dose–response relationship for normal tissue injury depends on the survival curves of the tissue stem cells. The timing of expression of injury depends on the rate of turnover of mature cells in the tissue. Epithelial and haemopoietic tissues have rapid turnover, and so manifest acute effects (with a timescale of days or weeks). Late effects (with a timescale of months or years) occur in tissues and organs with slow turnover (e.g. endothelial and neuroglial tissues, and parenchymal tissues of lung, liver and kidney). The risk of major late effects is usually dose-limiting in radiotherapy. Stem cells of late-responding tissues have been found to have much more curved survival curves (low α/β ratio) than cells of acute-responding tissues (higher α/β ratio, less curved survival curve). Radiobiologically, this difference may be related to slow cell turnover in late-responding tissues, allowing many stem cells to remain in resting states where they are highly proficient in the repair of damage caused by small doses. Consequently, late-responding tissues are particularly sensitive to changes in fraction size, larger fractions being more damaging to these tissues, but small fractions being well tolerated. Acute and late-responding tissues are also affected differentially by changes in the overall treatment time. Because surviving stem cells of acute-responding tissues initiate repopulation during the course of radiotherapy, the time over which the radiation is distributed makes a difference to the final level of damage. Late-responding tissues do not experience repopulation during the course of radiotherapy and are relatively unaffected by the overall treatment time. Expression of late effects will also be influenced by the organisation of functional subunits within the organ. Serially arranged subunits, such as are found in the bowel, mean that damage to some units will lead to change in the whole organ, whereas in those organs where subunits are arranged in parallel, such as the kidney, each subunit acts independently and continuing function is possible if only some of the subunits are damaged.

The linear quadratic model for tissues

Differences between acute- and late-responding tissues and typical tumours are important when we consider the biological consequences of replacing one treatment schedule with a different one. From experience, radiation oncologists developed 'rules of thumb' for altering a treatment schedule, e.g. a substantial dose reduction might be necessary if fraction size was increased, increased treatment time improved skin tolerance, etc. It is now recognised that tissues react differently to changes in schedule structure and there is better understanding of how changes in scheduling will affect different tissues. The application of the LQ model is based on the idea that the severity of tissue damage is inversely proportional to stem cell survival, and that stem cell survival can be calculated by mathematical development of the LQ survival curve equation to allow it to be applied to fractionated treatments. In particular, two different schedules will have equal biological effects on a tissue (i.e. they will be 'isoeffective' for the tissue) if each schedule produces the same level of stem cell survival.

We shall not attempt to derive the mathematics of the LQ model in detail, but will state some results which are useful in practice. Consider two treatment schedules, namely total dose D_1 or D_2 given as fractions sized d_1 or d_2. We shall assume for now that both schedules are given in the same overall time period. For a tissue whose cells have a survival curve described by the LQ parameters α and β, it can be shown that the two schedules are isoeffective, for that tissue, when:

$$D_1 (\alpha/\beta + d_1) = D_2 (\alpha/\beta + d_2) \tag{3.2}$$

Notice that the survival curve parameters appear as a ratio in this expression, which means that only this single number for a tissue need be known in order to apply the equation. In fact, α/β estimates have been made and tabulated for many tissues. Late-responding tissues are usually found to have low values of α/β (about 3 Gy), while acute-responding tissues have higher values (about 10 Gy). (This means that the cells of late-responding tissues have more steeply curving survival curves.) Tumours are more variable; many are like acute-responding tissues, with α/β values of 10 Gy or more, but recent estimates for breast tumours suggest lower values. In practice, Equation 3.2 is often used to compare an unfamiliar schedule with a standard schedule which would have the same effect. Most usefully, the unfamiliar schedule can be assessed by asking what total dose, given as 2 Gy fractions, would have the same effect (on that tissue) as the unfamiliar schedule. This is helpful for determining whether the unfamiliar schedule is 'hot' or 'cold'. For example, consider a schedule which consists of 10 twice-weekly fractions of 4 Gy to a total dose of 40 Gy in 5 weeks. In Equation 3.2, let d_1 be 4 Gy and D_1 be 40 Gy. If we now set $d_2 = 2$ Gy, and calculate D_2 (for a particular choice of tissue α/β), we shall get the total dose given as 2 Gy fractions which would have the same effect on that tissue as the schedule D_1, d_1. Notice, however, that the calculation depends on the assumed value of α/β. For this example, we shall repeat the calculation for acute-responding and late-responding tissues. For acute-responding tissues ($\alpha/\beta = 10$ Gy) we find that $D_2 = 47$ Gy, while for late-responding tissues ($\alpha/\beta = 3$ Gy), we find that $D_2 = 56$ Gy. Therefore, the new schedule is expected to be 'hotter' in terms of its effects on late-responding than on acute-responding tissues, but it is no 'hotter' than a conventional radical regimen (e.g. 60 Gy in 2 Gy fractions).

It should be noted that the simple LQ model does not allow for differences in total time between the schedules, which are therefore presumed to be given in the same overall time (5 weeks in this case), despite their different fractionation patterns. This restriction is not so important for late-responding tissues (for which the total time is a minor variable), but the results for acute-responding tissues (for which the time factor can be significant) need to be interpreted cautiously with this limitation of the model borne in mind.

In recent years, the LQ model has been developed extensively and applied to more complex schedules, including brachytherapy. The standard schedule with which an unfamiliar schedule is to be compared is not necessarily one using 2 Gy fractions. A rather abstract standard schedule, more appealing to mathematicians than to clinicians, is a hypothetical regimen in which a very large number of small fractions are given (mathematically, an infinite number of zero-sized fractions are given, but to a finite total dose). The equivalent total dose calculated for such a schedule is called the biological effective dose (BED). It is usually quite a large dose (e.g. 100 Gy for a typical radical regimen) because it represents the limit of tissue sparing by fractionation, i.e. the total dose that could be given if the individual fraction size were vanishingly small. Linear quadratic calculations performed using BED are mathematically equivalent to those performed with the standard regimen taken to be one using 2 Gy fractions, although the latter has the advantage of clinical familiarity. An important feature of the LQ model in its various forms is the recognition that the cells of different tissues differ in their survival curve shape and therefore respond differently to changes in fraction size. Since a target volume may contain several tissue types as well as the tumour, a change of fractionation regimen will affect these components differently. There is therefore no such thing as a regimen which is 'generally equivalent' to some other regimen – the regimens can only be matched (by choice of total dose) for equivalent effects on each specific tissue.

Volume effects

Together with the total dose and fractionation schedule, target volume is a major variable in radiotherapy. For a given fractionation regimen, higher doses can usually be given when volumes at the same site are small rather than large. Normal tissues are required to perform orchestrated functions, which can be impaired in various ways by irradiation. Most normal tissues also cannot regenerate from a single surviving cell. However, tissue recovery may be assisted by immigration of unirradiated neighbouring cells, particularly if the treatment volume is small. Volume is also an important determinant of normal tissue response to a given dose, first because larger volumes provide less opportunity for tissues to draw on their 'functional reserve' and second because larger irradiated volumes make it more likely that a critical volume element will exceed some upper dose limit. These factors differ according to tissue structure, and vary from one treatment to another.

In general, the normal tissue complication probability (NTCP) increases with dose (for a given fractionation regimen) and with the irradiated volume. It is important to know, at least approximately, how changes in irradiated volume at a particular site will affect the tolerance dose which can safely be given. The 'tolerance dose' may arbitrarily be defined as that dose which gives no more than 5 per cent incidence of significant side effects, based on clinical experience. A body of data has been amassed which provides some simple 'rules of thumb' concerning the trade-off between treatment volume and tolerance dose, but these need to be used very cautiously. Tolerance is affected not only by volume, but also by radiation sensitivity and fraction size, and tolerance to the various new schedules in use must be carefully confirmed by clinical studies. In some cases, radiation injury may result from an excessively high dose to a small tissue element within the treatment volume. The possibility of ensuring better homogeneity of dose distribution with IMRT may help to ameliorate this problem.

Radiation dose and tumour cure probability

In radical radiotherapy, the objective is complete sterilisation of any tumour cells present, which must be achieved without incurring an unacceptably high risk of serious injury to normal tissues.

Radiation kills cells randomly, which means that each tumour cell has the same probability of surviving irradiation, that probability depending on the given dose. Suppose that SF_2 is the probability of any cell surviving a single dose of 2 Gy, the most commonly used fraction size. For example, SF_2 might be 0.5 for a typical carcinoma. After the first 2 Gy fraction, 50 per cent of the cells survive; after the second dose, 50 per cent of those survivors still survive (i.e. 25 per cent of the original population); after the third dose, 50 per cent of *those* survivors still survive (i.e. 12.5 per cent of the original population), and so on. Generally, after F fractions, the final survival probability will be $(SF_2)^F$. Therefore, for a conventional treatment regimen consisting of 30 treatments of 2 Gy, the final survival probability (in this example) would be 0.5^{30} or 9×10^{-10}.

These relationships have some interesting clinical implications. First, there is no dose which gives zero probability of cell survival – even after a large dose there will be some probability, possibly very small, of survival of each cell. However, a visible tumour will contain a large number of cells, so even if each cell individually only has a small chance of surviving, there may be a good chance that at least one cell will survive and could regenerate the tumour. We therefore need to know the relationship between the given dose and the probability that a whole cell population will be sterilised with not a single cell surviving – the basic requirement for tumour cure. This can be computed using the theory of Poisson statistics. We can then calculate the number of treatments necessary to achieve some value of cure probability, such as 90 per cent (remember that 100 per cent cure probability cannot be achieved by any finite dose).

We can repeat the calculation for tumours of different sizes (different cell population numbers) for our example of $SF_2 = 0.5$, and also for other values of SF_2 representing more sensitive or less sensitive tumour types. Figure 3.2 shows these relationships. Although we have used a rather simple model for these calculations, we can observe some features which also turn up in more complex and realistic models.

First, note that the relationship between tumour cell number and number of treatments is logarithmic, i.e. a large change in cell number corresponds to a rather

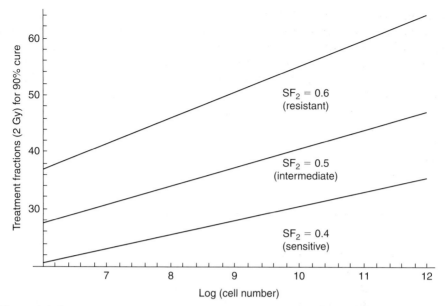

Figure 3.2 Shows the calculated number of 2 Gy fractions to achieve 90 per cent cure probability, as a function of tumour cell population number, for differing values of cellular intrinsic radiosensitivity (expressed as the surviving fraction following a single 2 Gy treatment, SF_2). Moderate variation of SF_2, as seen between cells of different tumour types, leads to large differences in the number of 2 Gy treatment fractions required for 90 per cent cure probability. In some cases, the predicted number of fractions required is much larger than could be safely given.

modest change in the number of treatments and hence the total dose required. For example, the number of treatments required for a tumour of 10^4 cells is just half the number required for 10^8 cells. It is because of this logarithmic relationship that quite high total doses have to be given to regions containing only microscopic spread (in fact often about half the dose given to the bulk tumour). Within regions of microscopic spread it is likely that the tumour cell density will gradually decrease, on average, with increasing distance from the visible edge. This suggests that the radiotherapy dose should similarly decrease with distance, roughly in proportion to log cell density. Although the cell density distribution will not be known in detail, it is possible that a tapering dose distribution, such as occurs in a conventional plan with a peripheral dose gradient, or achieved with IMRT and deliberate dose modulation within the volume, could be advantageous. A second feature of the model is that a small change in SF_2 has quite a large effect on the required total dose (compare the three curves shown in Fig. 3.2). Small variations in the intrinsic radiosensitivity of tumour cells could result in a tumour being easily curable, or completely incurable, by a radiotherapy regimen.

Another feature of the dose–cure relationship is the steepness of the increase in tumour cure probability with total dose, illustrated in Figure 3.3. In this figure, the solid curves show the dose–cure relationships for a series of tumours with slightly different parameters, and they can be seen to be increasing steeply with total dose in all cases. This implies that relatively small differences in total dose

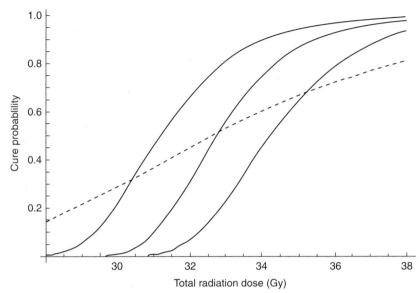

Figure 3.3 The solid lines in this figure show the expected relationship between total radiation dose and cure probability for individual tumours with differing radiosensitivity and cell number. The curves are sigmoid in shape, located at different positions on the dose axis, and each is quite steep. The broken line shows the much shallower dose-response usually seen when proportion cured is plotted against dose for groups of tumours, as in clinical trial studies. The shallower response is thought to result from the heterogeneity of the tumours in each dose group.

could make a significant difference to cure probability for each tumour. However, these steep relationships are not seen in the dose–cure relationships for treatment of groups of tumours with differing parameters, such as occur in clinical studies with patient groups. The broken line in Fig. 3.3 shows the much shallower gradient which is typically observed in such studies. The shallow gradient of the curve for tumour groups is the resultant of a series of steep curves for individual tumours with differing radiosensitivities. This has some significance when we consider the importance of moderate changes in total dose when treating individual patients. The importance of a dose increment in treating an individual tumour depends on how close the treatment regimen has come to achieving cure. For a large or resistant tumour (such as glioblastoma) with cure probability close to zero, a modest dose increment will make little difference. Conversely, for a small or highly sensitive tumour (such as seminoma) with cure probability close to unity, a small dose increment again makes little difference. However, if the treatment regimen achieves a cure probability close to 50 per cent (such as head and neck tumours), it is in this situation that the dose–response curve is as steep as that calculated from the Poisson model. This means that for any individual patient there is some probability, usually unknown, that a large change in tumour control probability will result from a small change in delivered dose. Even where the average dose–response curve for patient groups is known to be shallow, a minority of patients may benefit substantially from small changes in the given dose. It is these patients for whom the choice of treatment plan may be especially critical.

Tumour radiobiology

It is believed that the main factors controlling tumour response to fractionated radiotherapy are the so-called 'five Rs' of radiobiology (Table 3.1). Currently, the most important of these factors are thought to be the intrinsic radiosensitivity of cells and the kinetics of repopulation of surviving cells.

Intrinsic radiosensitivity varies between different tumour cell lines in culture, with cell lines derived from clinically resistant tumour types having a statistical tendency towards higher SF_2 values. SF_2 measurements on tumours are technically

Table 3.1 Radiobiological factors controlling response to fractionated radiotherapy (the 'five Rs') and their clinical relevance

Radiobiological factor	Mechanism of effect on response	Clinical relevance
Radiosensitivity	Intrinsic radiosensitivity differs between cells of tumours and normal tissue types, and strongly determines final surviving fraction	Can account for variable response of tumours Curative dose is proportional to the log of cell number (so subclinical disease needs smaller dose)
Repair	Cells differ in their capacity to repair DNA damage, particularly after small doses of radiation	Repair is maximal in late-responding tissues given small fractions. Hyperfractionation may be advantageous
	Repair is usually more effective in non-proliferating cells. The repair process takes at least 6 h to complete	Treatments need to be well separated in order to avoid compromising repair
Repopulation	Surviving cells in many tumours and in acute-responding (but not in late-responding) normal tissues proliferate more rapidly once treatment is in progress	Shortened treatment times (accelerated therapy) may be advantageous for some tumours. Acute (but not late) effects will be increased. Gaps should be avoided
Reoxygenation	Hypoxic cells, which occur especially in tumours, are relatively resistant to radiation. Hypoxic surviving cells reoxygenate, becoming radiosensitive, as treatment proceeds	Very short treatment times could lead to resistance due to persistence of hypoxic cells. Treatment of anaemia is essential to optimise tumour response
Redistribution	Cells in certain phases of the proliferative cycle (e.g. late S) are relatively resistant and survive preferentially. With time between fractions, cells redistribute themselves over all phases of the cycle	Closely spaced treatment fractions could lead to resistance due to persistence of cells in less sensitive phases

difficult and time-consuming, and techniques are not yet clinically available to help predict radiosensitivity of tumour and normal tissues in individual patients.

Although tumours are very diverse, the radiobiological properties of most tumours are similar to those of acute-responding tissues, i.e. a high α/β ratio, moderate sensitivity to changes in fraction size, and some dependence on total treatment time. The role of treatment time has been controversial, but it is now widely believed that many tumours repopulate rapidly during the latter part of a course of radiotherapy, and that any factor which prolongs time in treatment could lead to significantly reduced tumour cure probability. Attempts are currently being made to identify which tumours are most capable of rapid repopulation by measuring kinetic parameters. Measurements of tumour kinetics to detect those most capable of rapid repopulation are possible using thymidine analogues, but these tests are not yet available to use as predictive tools for individual patients.

Avoidance of gaps during treatment

The occurrence of rapid repopulation in irradiated tumours, sometimes with doubling times as short as 3–4 days, has important implications for interruptions of treatment. Unscheduled gaps occur not infrequently in radiotherapy schedules because of machine breakdown or patient intercurrent illness or non-attendance. (We shall exclude from consideration patients whose treatment is deliberately stopped because of unusually severe acute reactions.) Gaps are important because they may lead to prolongation of the total treatment time, allowing opportunities for rapid repopulation for surviving tumour cells towards the end of the schedule. Although prolongation will often spare acute normal tissue reactions, the risk of late effects is not reduced. It has been shown for squamous carcinomas of the head and neck that reductions in cure probability of 1–2 per cent may result from each day of prolongation. If gaps occur, the best management strategy is 'post-gap acceleration', i.e. the use of twice daily treatments (separated by more than 6 h) or weekend treatments to enable 'catching up' so that treatment is nevertheless completed within the originally intended period. This does not require any changes to fraction size or total dose. However, this approach is not always feasible in practice. Now that the deleterious effect of prolongation is recognised, avoidance of gaps is an important consideration for all radiotherapy departments.

Treatment scheduling

Conventionally, radiotherapy schedules have consisted of multiple fractions of 2 Gy delivered for 5 days a week over several weeks. The total dose is usually limited by anticipated risk of injury to late-responding tissues, although there are situations where acute responses (e.g. mucosal reactions) are the main concern. Treatment schedules with this structure probably take advantage of differences between the survival curves of cells in late-responding tissues (low α/β ratio and fraction size sensitivity) and the survival curves of those in typical tumours (with higher α/β ratios). This means that late-responding tissues are spared to a greater extent than most tumours by the use of small fractions, giving a favourable therapeutic ratio. Late responses are not strongly influenced by overall treatment time, and it would be desirable to make the latter as short as possible in order to minimise the opportunities for tumour repopulation. However, this must be balanced by the need to allow time for reoxygenation of hypoxic cells during therapy, and there also may be an adverse effect of reduced treatment time on acute-responding tissues (which also have reduced opportunities for repopulation).

There is now considerable experience with different schedules of treatment (for details, see Table 3.2). All these changes in scheduling may bring important gains in tumour control. However, tumours are known to be extremely heterogeneous with regard to cell survival parameters and growth kinetics, as well as other properties. It is unlikely that any one schedule is ideal for treatment of all tumours, even those of a single pathological type, and it would be highly desirable to select treatment schedules for individual patients on the basis of the radiobiological and kinetic parameters for each tumour. Predictive tests are not yet sufficiently reliable to be used in this way, but individualised scheduling based on biological assay is a likely development for the future.

Treatment plan, schedules and 'double trouble'

The design of physical treatment plans usually proceeds without regard to treatment schedule. However, there may be interplay between dose distributions and treatment schedules, which gives an altered biological effect sometimes described as 'double trouble'. Consider a treatment plan in which the spread of dose within the target volume is 10 per cent, so if the intended treatment is 30 fractions of 2 Gy to give 60 Gy in total, the spread of dose will be from 57 Gy to 63 Gy. However, the low-point and high-point doses will not have been delivered as 2 Gy fractions (the dose variation of 10 per cent affects each dose fraction, so the fraction size will range from 1.9 Gy to 2.1 Gy). A treatment schedule of 30×2.1 Gy = 63 Gy is what is 'seen' by cells located close to the high-dose point in this example, and this 63 Gy dose is more damaging, especially to late-responding tissues with a low α/β ratio, than 63 Gy given as 2 Gy fractions (which is what is implied when only the physical total dose is cited). Therefore, the spread of radiobiological damage within a target volume has two components, namely that due to variation in the total dose, and that due to variation in the fraction size by which that total dose is given. The 'double trouble' effect is most marked for late-responding tissues, for large treatment volumes with considerable dose variation, and for intended treatment schedules where the prescribed fraction size is sometimes large (radiotherapy of breast cancer may be such a situation). Although not yet routine, radiobiological considerations need to be included in the analysis of the dose–response relationship in patients who are experiencing side effects.

Two ways of accounting for 'double trouble' can be envisaged. First, IMRT makes it possible to ensure homogeneity of dose distribution across a treatment volume and this approach is being used clinically after it has been shown, for example, to reduce late normal tissue effects of fibrosis after treatment for breast cancer. Second, radiobiological dose plans may be constructed with the physical dose mathematically replaced by some radiobiological equivalent which includes the effect of variation in fraction size. For example, the physical dose at each point in the dose matrix could be replaced by a dose calculated by the LQ model to have

Table 3.2 Effects of alterations in scheduling of radiotherapy on tumour and normal tissues

Fractionation scheme	Rationale	Mode of delivery	Effect on tumour	Effect on acute-responding tissues	Effect on late-responding tissues
Hyperfractionation	Tumours resemble acute-reacting tissues with high α/β ratio	Multiple daily fractions of less than 2 Gy using an increased number of fractions to give an increased total dose	Increased tumour cell kill	Increased	Increased
Accelerated	High rate of repopulation in tumours may eliminate proliferation. Time factor for late effects relatively unimportant	Reduced overall treatment time. Same fraction size, 6 h interval between treatments if used with hyperfractionation. Six or seven times a week for daily fractions	Increased tumour cell kill	Increased	Minimal Increase
Accelerated hyperfractionation (CHART, concomitant boost)	Combines the advantages of hyperfractionation and acceleration	Benefit of this approach either with reduced total dose or shorter overall treatment time	Increased tumour cell kill	Increased	Decreased or same
Hypofractionation	May help to overcome radio-resistance. Is possible for some sites where normal tissue reactions are not dose limiting. Reduces overall time eliminating proliferation	Decreased number of fractions of increased fraction size. Suitable for small volume, high-precision treatments	Same or increased cell kill	Same or increased	Increased if total dose is unchanged. Same if dose is decreased

the same effect on late-responding tissues when given as 2 Gy fractions. Isodose curves can be constructed using the 'radiobiological dose' and compared with more conventional isodose plots using the physical dose. Algorithms have been developed which can be incorporated in commercial treatment planning systems and used to compute radiobiological treatment plans. Alternatively, LQ transformed DVHs (which incorporate the biological effects of changing fraction size within the volume) can be computed and the biologically equivalent dose to the hottest and coldest parts of the volume calculated.

Future directions

Careful analysis of data from clinical trials of novel fractionation schemes after long-term follow up of late effects will permit refinement of understanding of the LQ model. This will stimulate further investigation, particularly of shortened courses of radiotherapy, which, if isoeffective with conventional fractionation, would bring benefits to both patients and healthcare providers. Widespread use of IMRT with functional imaging makes it possible to improve homogeneity within a treatment volume or to plan for inhomogeneity according to defined biological characteristics of the tumour.

Information sources

Ling CC, Humm J, Larson S (2000) Towards multi-dimensional radiotherapy (MD-CRT): biological imaging and biological conformality. *Int J Radiat Oncol Biol Phys* **47**: 551–60.

Royal College of Radiologists (2008) The Timely Delivery of Radical Radiotherapy: standards and guidelines for the management of unscheduled treatment interruptions. Royal College of Radiologists, London.

Steel GG (ed) (2002) *Basic Clinical Radiobiology*, 3rd edn. Hodder Arnold, London.

4 Organs at risk and tolerance of normal tissues

Therapeutic ratio

When considering how to achieve the best outcome from radiotherapy in the treatment of tumours, it is critical to understand the concept of therapeutic ratio. Cure is always achieved at some cost in terms of normal tissue damage. There must be a balance between trying to ensure that all tumour cells receive a lethal dose of radiation and that acute and late effects are tolerable. The total dose, dose per fraction, treated volume and addition of drugs (radiochemotherapy) will all affect this balance, as will individual factors for each patient (e.g. age, comorbidity and intrinsic tissue radiosensitivity).

In some clinical situations, the frequency or severity of late effects drives a reduction in radiotherapy dose. For example, concern about the high incidence of second malignancies after radiotherapy for Hodgkin lymphoma has led to chemotherapy being used in preference. In some paediatric tumours with high cure rates (Wilms', germ cell tumours), research has focused on lowering radiotherapy dose to see if late effects can be reduced without compromising cure.

More commonly, a desire to increase radiotherapy dose to improve cure rates may be limited by the response of normal tissues to radiation. However, although the optimal balance of cure and side effects may have been reached for one radiotherapy technique, further dose escalation may be possible with more precise treatment delivery or better patient support. If a more conformal technique is used, the dose to critical structures may be reduced and dose hot-spots or cold-spots in individual sites or in parts of tumours can be minimised. Improvements in patient support, such as using gastrostomy tubes for feeding patients undergoing head and neck radiotherapy, may make acute effects more tolerable. A better understanding of the mechanisms of late effects is helping to produce a less nihilistic approach to their management. There are specialist teams now providing a multidisciplinary therapeutic approach to the management of late effects of pelvic and breast radiation.

Any change to a treatment regimen, such as the use of IMRT, a dose increase or addition of chemotherapy or biological agents, will change the therapeutic ratio. The challenge for the radiation oncologist is to ensure that this change improves the ratio and that an increase in dose is not counteracted by an increase in unmanageable acute or serious late effects. TCP (tumour control probability) and NTCP (normal tissue complication probability) are mathematical models used to predict effects of such changes. However, to know whether a new treatment has really produced better outcomes overall, and to inform and improve the reliability of these modelling estimates, good clinical data must be collected, not only for outcome measures relating to tumour control, but also for acute and late normal tissue damage.

Normal tissue effects can be specified in relation to the probability of them occurring, their severity and their timing. Radiation injury may be expressed soon after treatment (early effects) or after 6 months up to many years later (late effects). Subsequent treatment, as for example with anthracyclines, may reveal latent, previously asymptomatic, damage. Expression of damage may depend on genetic susceptibility. It has been estimated that 20 per cent of the observed variation in normal tissue sensitivity to radiation is random and 80 per cent deterministic, including that due to genetic variations. No single gene has been isolated but several conditions are known to predispose to abnormal radiation sensitivity. These include ataxia telangiectasia, Fanconi's anaemia and Bloom's syndrome.

Underlying all normal tissue damage, there is a mechanism of dysregulated repair of the radiation injury. Fibroblastic proliferation and extracellular matrix deposition are influenced by cytokine and growth factor release and may lead to endothelial proliferation and subsequent fibrosis. This is common in soft tissues such as skin, breast, bowel, lung, kidney and liver. Alternatively, cell death may lead to atrophy or necrosis of tissues as may occur with bone, nerves or brain.

Late damage will also depend on the hierarchical organisation of the irradiated tissue at risk – whether the cells are serial in arrangement (e.g. spinal cord) or parallel (e.g. liver).

Organs at risk

The ICRU defines OAR as those normal tissues which lie adjacent to tumours and may therefore be included within treated volumes, with a risk that the radiation may impair their normal functioning. Preparation of a treatment plan involves outlining in three dimensions not only tumour and its potential extensions, but also any OAR.

OAR should be outlined according to protocols so that dose can be correlated with end effect and comparisons made between institutions. For example in lung cancer, the OAR volume for the normal lung is variously defined as the whole of both lungs, lungs with GTV subtracted or lungs with PTV subtracted. The volume of OAR can be expanded in three dimensions to take account of organ movement and of systematic and random errors in treatment delivery. This will create a PRV in the same way that a CTV is expanded to form a PTV.

There is a risk that the increasing awareness of organ motion and treatment delivery errors will lead to larger PTVs and larger PRVs, which may overlap when a dose solution is chosen. While it may be theoretically correct to generate a PRV for each organ so that with each fraction the true location of that organ will be within the PRV, in practice, dose limits for organs at risk are usually applied to the OAR as defined on the planning images. One exception is the spinal cord where a more conservative approach is often taken because of the potential severity of late effects (paralysis). The cord itself can be contoured and a 3–5 mm margin added isotropically to produce a PRV. Alternatively, the spinal canal is contoured as the organ at risk which effectively adds a margin to the OAR. This approach also makes it possible to make comparisons with data derived from 2D planning where the spinal canal was considered to represent the cord.

For some tumours, the PTV can be treated with a plan where accepted tolerance doses to normal tissues are not exceeded. But sometimes the clinician may need to make a value judgement about the relative risks of possible normal tissue damage and loss of tumour control. It is important to consider the type and severity of the effect, the possible consequences of a local tumour recurrence and how an individual patient may tolerate radiotherapy. For example, late damage to the spinal cord resulting in paralysis may be catastrophic, whereas an oesophageal stricture or a cataract may be treatable. It may be acceptable to irradiate one kidney to high dose if the contralateral one is functioning normally, but not in the presence of hypertensive nephropathy. In postoperative radiotherapy for a tumour close to the optic nerve, using a lower dose of radiation to try to keep within accepted tolerance may increase the risk of blindness from a local recurrence. In trying to prevent blindness, the risk of not giving adequate dose to the PTV may be greater than the risk of normal tissue damage. In the same patient, the acceptable dose to the ipsilateral and contralateral optic nerves may therefore be different.

Tolerance doses

There are very few prospective dose escalation studies of radiation, analogous to phase 1 studies of new drugs, to help determine the maximum tolerated dose of radiotherapy. The tables of tolerance doses which are used in clinical practice are often extrapolated from laboratory or animal studies or at best relate to radiotherapy given many years ago with techniques and technology which have been superseded by 3D planning and treatment delivery. In addition, the fraction size, dose rate, volume treated, concomitant therapy and comorbidity will all affect the probability of late effects occurring in an individual. A tolerance dose needs to be interpreted in this context. Moreover tolerance doses will change over time as 3D dose distributions are correlated with late effects in the modern era. Nevertheless it is possible to give guidance as to the chance that a given dose will produce a given side effect and to define safe limits to use when devising a plan.

Correlating the risk of side effects with 2D dose distributions led to the production of TD5/5 tables which are still used clinically today. These provide an estimate of the dose which gives a 5 per cent probability of a given late effect 5 years after treatment. Similarly a TD50/5 is the dose giving a 50 per cent risk of a particular effect at 5 years. From these point estimates, models to predict probability of normal tissue complications were developed such as the Lyman-probit and the Kallman-relative seriality models.

While point doses such as TD5/5 may be useful for some serial organs such as the spinal cord where exceeding a dose threshold at any point can compromise whole organ function, they are less useful in organs composed of parallel subunits. The advent of 3D planning has made it possible to describe the dose given to a volume of tissue and to correlate it with acute and late effects. This description is usually in the form of a DVH.

A DVH is a plot of dose of radiation on the x-axis and per cent volume of the structure of interest on the y-axis. The shape and area under the DVH curve are used to ensure that the target volume is adequately covered with a homogeneous dose and that dose to critical structures is within acceptable limits. A 3D planning system can calculate the dose in each pixel of the organ outlined and sum these to produce a DVH. From this, the percentage of the volume of an organ receiving a given dose (d) can be read – Vd. From the x-axis, the mean, median doses, etc. can be calculated. Figure 4.1 shows a DVH for a lung plan where the V20 (volume of lung receiving more than 20 Gy) is 7.89 per cent and the mean lung dose (total lung volume – PTV) is 6 Gy. DVHs can also be used to evaluate dose given to a PTV. A plan should ideally produce a steep curve showing that the dose within the PTV varies from no more than 95 per cent to 107 per cent of that prescribed in accordance with ICRU50 (Fig. 4.2); DVHs for multiple volumes can be plotted on the same axes.

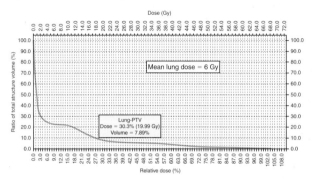

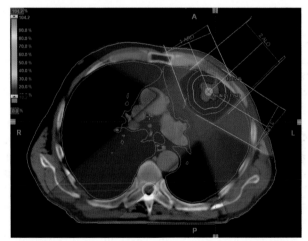

Figure 4.1 DVH for a lung plan for a small peripheral tumour receiving 66 Gy in 33 fractions where the V20 (volume of lung receiving more than 20 Gy) is 7.89 per cent and the mean lung dose (total lung volume – PTV) is 6 Gy.

Figure 4.2 Plan with dose colourwash showing dose within the PTV varying from 95 per cent to 103.2 per cent of that prescribed, in accordance with ICRU50.

If DVHs are obtained from a series of patients in whom acute or late effects are recorded, points on the DVH can be correlated with the probability of these effects occurring. Thus, for parotid sparing IMRT, the chance of producing long-term xerostomia correlates best with a mean dose to the contralateral parotid gland of more than 24 Gy. For lung radiotherapy, the chance of symptomatic lung fibrosis correlates best with a V20 of >32 per cent. These are the usual limits for an acceptable plan. It must be remembered that these limits essentially still simplify a 3D dose distribution into a single dose, albeit the dose that is best correlated with effect measured in a series of patients.

It is therefore essential to view and record the whole DVH for a volume rather than just one dose point. This can be particularly useful when comparing two plans for the same patient. Consider DVHs for the PTV and the lung in two possible plans for a stage 3 lung cancer. Plan A conforms better to the PTV but with a V20 of 35 per cent. Plan B underdoses more of the PTV but has a V20 of 30 per cent. The clinician must decide whether it is preferable to risk lung fibrosis to optimise PTV coverage or whether, for this patient, a higher risk of fibrosis is unacceptable and PTV coverage must be compromised.

DVH calculations do not take into account all the biological variables which may determine a treatment outcome and the concept of BED has been developed by Withers and colleagues (see Wilson 2007), based on the LQ model (see Chapter 3) to allow comparison of equivalent doses delivered to a particular structure for other dose/fractionation schedules. The formula for BED is:

$$BED = \{n*d\,[1 + d/(\alpha/\beta)]\} - [(0.693*T)/(\alpha*Tp)] \qquad (4.1)$$

where n = number of treatments, d = dose per fraction, T = treatment time and α/β = 3 Gy (for late effects). Tp (potential doubling time), and α (linear component of cell killing) are taken from published data for each tumour.

Equivalent uniform dose (EUD) is another method of summarising and reporting inhomogeneous dose distributions which assumes that any two dose distributions are equivalent if they cause the same radiobiological effect. A project, known as Quantec, has recently been established to try to summarise 3D dose/ volume/outcome data in a clinically useful manner.

Individual organ tolerances

Suggested dose thresholds and dose–volume constraints for commonly irradiated organs are given in Table 4.1. They assume radiation is prescribed at 2 Gy per fraction.

■ Spinal cord

Because a possible consequence of late radiation damage is irreversible paralysis, treatments have been cautious and there is a shortage of clinical data on which to base estimates of spinal cord tolerance. The constraints employed are therefore necessarily conservative.

The spinal cord should either be defined with a 5 mm margin to produce a PRV or the spinal canal contoured as a PRV. Dose to any part of the cord should be less than 46 Gy. A small part ($<$1 cm^3) may receive up to 50 Gy. If more than 15 cm length of cord is treated, the dose to any part of the cord should be less than 44 Gy. If dose per fraction is increased due to inhomogeneity of the plan (e.g. 103 per cent to spinal cord) and/or hypofractionation schedules are used, total dose to the spinal cord must be lowered.

When palliative radiotherapy is repeated – for example, for spinal cord compression or when the prognosis is short – a higher dose may be used if withholding treatment is more likely to give a poor outcome than exceeding a theoretical dose limit.

■ Brain and peripheral nerves

For primary brain tumours, high doses of radiation are usually employed only where there is a high risk of local recurrence with consequent brain injury, or when prognosis is poor. The TD5/5 for brain necrosis varies with the volume irradiated. For the whole brain TD5/5 = 45 Gy, for $<$1/3 of the brain TD5/5 = 60 Gy.

Table 4.1 Estimated tolerance doses for various organs expressed as different parameters with dose delivered with 2 Gy/fraction. These have wide confidence limits and vary with age, individual sensitivity, vascular status and with other treatments given

OAR	TD5/5 (Gy)	TD50/5 (Gy)	DVH Vx % or mean dose in Gy	Tolerance dose (Gy)
Spinal cord	5 cm 50 10 cm 50 20 cm 47	70 70		45–50 40–44 (>15 cm) EUD = 52.5
Brain	Whole 45 <1/3 60			50–60
Brainstem	1/3 60 2/3 53 3/3 50	65	V60 < 0.9 mL	54 1% up to 60
Peripheral nerves				60
Pituitary gland (hormone production)				20–24
Permanent hair loss				45–55
Optic nerve				50–55
Optic chiasm				50
Lacrimal gland				32–35
Lens				10
Retina	Whole 45			45–50 Small volume <60
Cornea				<48
Cochlea				50
Parotid	2/3 32 3/3 32	46 46	V30 <45%	24
Epiphyses before fusion in children				10
Femoral heads			V50 <50	
Heart	1/3 60 2/3 45 3/3 40	70 55 50	V40 <30 V30 <40–45 V20 <50	D_{max} <60
Lung	1/3 45 2/3 30 3/3 17.5	65 40 24.5	V30 <10–15 V20 <25 Mean 10	
Kidney	1/3 50 2/3 20–30 3/3 23	40 28	Mean 17.5 Gy	

(Continued)

Table 4.1 Continued

OAR	TD5/5 (Gy)	TD50/5 (Gy)	DVH Vx % or mean dose in Gy	Tolerance dose (Gy)
Oesophagus			V50 <32	
			58 (max)	Surface dose <32 Gy
			34 (mean)	50 Gy <8–12 cm
Small bowel	1/3 50			<45 (250 cm³)
Rectum			V74 <3	65 Gy
			V70 <15–25	
			V60 <50	
			V50 <60	
Liver	1/3 50	55	V30 <60	1/3 40–80
	2/3 35	45	Mean 30–35 Gy	2/3 30
	3/3 30	40		3/3 25
Testis:				
hormone production				25–35
spermatogenesis			Transient 0.2 Gy; count down for 2–3 years 2–3 Gy; permanent sterility >6 Gy	
Ovary			Menses >1.5 Gy Ovarian failure 6–15 Gy	
Bladder	Whole 65		V74 <5	Whole 50–55
	2/3 80		V60 <25	Partial 65–75
			V50 <50	

Data taken from multiple sources including personal records, Emani *et al.* (1991), Milano *et al.* (2007).

EUD, equivalent uniform dose; TD, total dose.

The use of tolerance doses is more applicable to head and neck cancers where the PTV is close to neural tissue. If the brain is not part of the target volume, dose to any part should not exceed 60 Gy.

The brainstem is traditionally regarded as more radiosensitive than the cerebrum. It should not receive more than 54 Gy (1 per cent up to 60 Gy). For peripheral nerves such as the brachial plexus, dose should be limited to <60 Gy.

■ Optic nerves and orbital tissues

Tolerance doses to optic structures are usually approached when the PTV is close to those structures. Underdosing the PTV and increasing the risk of local recurrence may threaten sight more than potentially overdosing the optic pathway.

- Optic nerve – dose to any point <50 Gy. Accept <55 Gy if the PTV is very close to one optic nerve

- Optic chiasm – dose to any point <50 Gy
- Lacrimal gland – dose to any part <35 Gy
- Lens – dose to any part <10 Gy. The late normal tissue effect (cataract) can be treated successfully, so this dose may be exceeded with patient consent in some tumours
- Retina – dose to whole retina <45 Gy (TD5/5 for visual damage). Dose to a small volume <60 Gy

■ Mucosa

Volume irradiated should be minimised to reduce acute mucositis. To prevent oesophageal stricture, the length of oesophagus in the treated volume is kept as short as possible and ideally <10 cm.

■ Lung

Late fibrosis is best correlated with V20 with a target of <32 per cent of the lung-PTV volume receiving more than 20 Gy. Other DVH parameters including mean lung dose are also sometimes used.

■ Kidney

TD5/5 for the whole kidney is 23 Gy. Dose to two-thirds of one kidney (and ideally both) should be below 20 Gy.

■ Liver

If the whole liver is irradiated, dose should be <30 Gy to avoid radiation hepatitis. V30 should be below 60 per cent.

■ Testes and ovaries

For the testis, 0.2 Gy can cause transient brief oligospermia; 2–3 Gy can lower sperm counts for 2–3 years. Doses of more than 6 Gy cause permanent sterility and of more than 20 Gy affect hormone production.

Menses are suppressed at >1.5 Gy, and 6–15 Gy causes permanent ovarian failure. Increasing age lowers the threshold for these effects.

■ Second malignancies

Any radiation dose increases the risk of second malignancy so no safe dose limits can be given. In principle, the irradiated volume should be kept as small as possible. Techniques such as IMRT which use multiple beams may increase the volume of normal tissue irradiated and theoretically increase the risk of second malignancy. It will take decades before data on the incidence of second malignancies is obtained so the possible increase can only be estimated from biological modelling. Clinical experience with radiotherapy for Hodgkin lymphoma, where the absolute incidence of second malignancies after mantle radiotherapy is 30 per cent at 30 years, shows the importance of long-term follow-up and data collection in the assessment of late effects, particularly when a new treatment technique is introduced.

Measurement of late effects

Local control and survival are usually relatively easy to assess with clinical examination, imaging and population databases. In contrast, estimation of the frequency and severity of late effects is often haphazard and incomplete and will depend on the sensitivity of the test used for their detection. Over time treatments change frequently, making it difficult to evaluate the role of each component of treatment to the outcome.

Adverse outcomes of treatment are often poorly documented by physicians and data are often only collected retrospectively. Pressurised doctors prioritise care of the patient before recording outcomes and there is no simple internationally standardised measure of late effects. Most scales involve grading of late effects from the physician's perspective and have been shown to underestimate late effects from the patient's point of view.

Existing scales include the RTOG/EORTC, the French/Italian scheme for gynaecological cancer, LENT-SOMA (late effects of normal tissues – subjective, objective, measured and analytic) and the NCI-CTC (common toxicity criteria) v3 – the National Cancer Institute of USA terminology criteria for adverse events recording with a severity scale for each item. This is used widely for clinical trials but is rather complex for day to day clinic use. Studies of simpler scales for routine use by physicians or for self-reporting by patients are in progress.

Most endpoints in these scales are clinical. Modern imaging modalities will be more sensitive at detecting abnormalities than are ascertained by clinical signs and symptoms or laboratory markers. Currently, imaging is rarely used for the documentation of late effects of radiation, unless subclinical damage progresses to a clinical problem, there is some early preventative intervention possible or the patient is being treated within a trial of a new modality.

Treatment of late effects

Until recently, little attempt has been made to modify any radiation associated damage although prevention may be possible in some cases. Restricting aggravating factors to damage by stopping smoking, maintaining good control of blood pressure and blood sugar levels, and avoiding use of fibrogenic drugs such as bleomycin may help. Control of acute inflammation by corticosteroids or anti-inflammatory drugs may reduce late effects. Vascular-directed therapies such as pentoxifylline, hyperbaric oxygen and angiotensin-converting enzyme inhibitors are being studied with some promising results. Anti-oxidant therapies such as superoxide dismutase and vitamin E have also been tried. Established radionecrosis has been treated with antibiotics, anti-inflammatory agents, bisphosphonates (bone) and hyperbaric oxygen with variable outcomes. Further improvement in preventing or treating late effects will come from collaborative research by specialised multidisciplinary teams.

Information sources

Chan L, Xia P, Gottschalk M *et al.* (2008) Proposed rectal dose constraints for patients undergoing definitive whole pelvic radiotherapy for clinically localised prostate cancer. *Int J Radiat Oncol Biol Phys* **72**: 69–77.

Chon BH, Loeffler JS (2002) The effect of nonmalignant systemic disease on tolerance to radiation therapy. *Oncologist* **7**: 136–43.

Drzymala RE, Mohan R, Brewster L *et al.* (1991) Dose-volume histograms. *Int J Radiat Oncol Biol Phys* **21**: 71–8.

Emani B, Lyman J, Brown A *et al.* (1991) Tolerance of normal tissue to irradiation. *Int J Radiat Oncol Biol Phys* **21**: 109–22.

Franklin JG, Paus MD, Pluetschow A *et al.* (2006) Second malignancy risk associated with treatment of Hodgkin's lymphoma: meta-analysis of the randomised trials. *Ann Oncol* **17**: 1749–60.

Larrier NA, Marks LB (2007) What radiation dose is safe in non-small cell lung cancer? *Nat Clin Pract Oncol* **4**: 80–1.

Lee SP, Leu MY, Smathers JB *et al.* (1995) Biologically effective dose distribution based on the linear quadratic model and its clinical relevance. *Int J Radiat Oncol Biol Phys* **33**: 375–89.

Marks L (2008) MO-D-AUD A-02: A clinician's view of Quantec. *Med Phys* **35**: 2863–4.

Milano MT, Constine LS, Okunieff P (2007) Normal tissue tolerance doses. *Semin Radiat Oncol* **17**: 131–40.

Niemerko A (1997) Reporting and analyzing dose distributions: a concept of equivalent uniform dose. *Med Phys* **24**: 103–10.

Wilson G (2007) Cell kinetics. *Clin Oncol* **19**: 370–84.

5 Principles of brachytherapy

Introduction

Brachy is from the Greek word for 'short' so brachytherapy (also known as sealed source radiotherapy) roughly translated means short-distance therapy. A radioactive material is inserted directly into or next to a tumour and concentrates the dose there. The dose falls off very rapidly according to the inverse square law, and surrounding normal tissues receive substantially lower doses than the tumour. When 65 Gy are delivered at 0.5 cm from the source, the dose at 2 cm is only 4.06 Gy.

As well as its physical advantages, there are also biological advantages. Low dose rate (LDR) brachytherapy is a type of extreme hyperfractionation and is therefore relatively sparing to normal tissues. The dose rate may be low but it is delivered continuously, which shortens overall treatment time and reduces the opportunity for tumour repopulation during treatment. Conversely, high dose rate (HDR) brachytherapy must be fractionated to avoid normal tissue morbidity. Three dose rate bands are defined: LDR ($<$1 Gy/h), medium dose rate (MDR) ($>$1 to $<$12 Gy/h) and HDR ($>$12 Gy/h). It is important to remember that if the dose rate is increased, a dose reduction is needed to give a biologically isoeffective dose. When changing from low to medium dose rate (e.g. changing from LDR intracavitary brachytherapy to MDR), a dose correction of approximately minus 15 per cent is needed. Other advantages of brachytherapy include the accurate localisation and immobilisation of the tumour, which removes the problems of organ movement and set-up errors seen with external beam radiotherapy (EBRT).

The disadvantages of brachytherapy are the operative nature of the procedures often needed to access the tumour, the requirement for skilled personnel, and the radiation protection measures needed to protect patient, staff and general public.

Brachytherapy is considered whenever possible for accessible localised tumours of relatively small volume. It is contraindicated where tumour infiltrates bone, where the margins of the tumour or target volume are not clearly identifiable and where there is active infection in the tissues. Brachytherapy is used as a radical single modality treatment or in combination with EBRT to deliver a boost dose. It can be used after surgical excision to irradiate a tumour bed. Isotopes used for brachytherapy are shown in Table 5.1.

■ Delivery systems

With interstitial brachytherapy, sources are inserted directly into tissue. Iridium-192 wire is ideal and can be cut to any length and curved as required. It is used as hair pins to treat cancer of the anterior tongue, or looped to treat base of tongue

Table 5.1 Isotopes for brachytherapy

Source	Form	Dose rate	Emissions	Half-life
Radium-226	Tubes, needles	LDR	2.45 MV gamma	1620 years
Caesium-137	Tubes, needles; afterloading pellets	LDR	0.662 MV gamma	30 years
Cobalt-60	Tubes; afterloading pellets	HDR	1.17, 1.33 MV gamma	5 years
Iridium-192	Wires; afterloading pellets	LDR HDR	0.38 MV gamma	74 days
Iodine-125	Seeds	LDR	27.4, 31.4, 35.5 kV	60 days
Palladium-103	Seeds	LDR	21 kV	17 days
Ruthenium-106/106 Rhenium	Eye plaques	LDR	3.54 MeV	373 days
Strontium-90	Eye plaques	HDR	0.546 MeV	28.9 years

tumours. Prostate cancer brachytherapy with iodine-125 or palladium-103 seeds is also classed as interstitial therapy.

Intracavitary brachytherapy places applicators inside a body cavity such as the uterine canal or vagina. These applicators can then be afterloaded with radioactive sources. Caesium-137 is the isotope of choice for low dose rate treatments, and small iridium-192 sources for HDR afterloading systems. Surface applicator brachytherapy can be used for very superficial lesions less than 1 mm thick such as strontium-90 eye plaque therapy after resection of pterygium.

Mould brachytherapy uses sealed sources held in a fixed arrangement and distance from the surface by a custom-made mould. It is usually used to treat superficial lesions of skin, mouth or vagina. Intraluminal brachytherapy places applicators loaded with radioactive sources in a lumen such as the bronchus or oesophagus.

For tumour sites where it would be difficult to remove the sources, or where very low dose rate is preferred, a permanent implant can be performed with sources such as iodine-125 seeds for prostate cancer. High dose rate intracavitary afterloading systems place sources temporarily using flexible catheters. Temporary interstitial HDR prostate implants are also possible.

To reduce radiation dose to staff, techniques of afterloading have been developed which involve the initial implantation of non-radioactive applicators, catheters or carriers into the patient. The radioactive sources can then be 'manually afterloaded' by the operator into the applicators, or 'remotely afterloaded' by a machine under computer control. Remote afterloading reduces the doses to staff, patients and visitors to a minimum and, with appropriately shielded rooms, can be used for LDR continuous, and HDR fractionated, treatments.

Clinical use

Table 5.2 shows some of the common sites treated with brachytherapy techniques.

Table 5.2 Clinical uses of brachytherapy

Site	Indications	Technique	Source and dose rate
Anterior tongue	Small T1/T2	Hair pins	Iridium-192 LDR
Buccal mucosa	Small T1/T2	Plastic tube	Iridium-192 LDR
Base of tongue	Boost after EBRT	Loop	Iridium-192 LDR
Lip	Small T1/T2;boost after EBRT	Needle	Iridium-192 LDR
Nasopharynx	Boost after EBRT; re-treatment	Moulds; NPC applicators	Iridium-192; LDR or HDR
Recurrent disease in neck	Re-treatment	Plastic tube	Iridium-192; LDR or HDR
Uterine tumours	Postoperative; palliative	Vaginal applicator; Tube and ovoids	HDR or LDR
Cervical tumours	Boost after EBRT	Tube and ovoids	HDR or LDR
Vagina	Small stage 1; boost after EBRT; palliative	Perineal template	HDR or LDR
Vulva	Boost after EBRT; palliative	Perineal template	HDR or LDR
Anal	Small T1; boost after EBRT; palliative	Perineal implant through template	HDR or LDR
Breast	Boost after EBRT; palliative	Plastic tubes; Needles; Bridge template	HDR or LDR
Prostate	Low risk disease; boost after EBRT	Permanent seeds; Perineal template	LDR I-125 or Pd-103; HDR

Dosimetry

The spatial configuration of brachytherapy sources in a target volume is chosen to achieve as homogeneous a dose as possible. The dose distribution is inherently inhomogeneous with high doses around each source, which can cause necrosis, and low doses between sources, which can result in recurrence. An established set of rules for implantation must be followed to achieve good dose distributions. Several systems have been used to calculate and describe the dose distributions of brachytherapy implants. The Manchester system is widely used for gynaecological implants. However the GEC-ESTRO group has recently published recommendations on target volume concepts and plan evaluation using DVHs (see Chapter 32). The Paris system was specifically designed for use with iridium wire afterloading techniques. Both these systems use traditional dose formalism for manual calculations with reference to precalculated data such as Paterson–Parker tables for needle implants, and the cross-line graphs or escargot curves for iridium wire. These systems have been adapted for computer calculations which follow the TG43 formalism, published in 1995 by the American Association of Physicists in Medicine (AAPM) Task group 43. The sources must be distributed according to the particular dosimetry system used and the method of dose specification and prescription adhered to. Previously it was always important to plan in advance the number and distribution of radioactive sources. With modern implant and dosimetry techniques, it is now possible to perform dynamic intraoperative dosimetry, e.g. for prostate seed implants, which reduces the amount of preplanning needed and avoids repositioning errors. An estimate of the volume to be implanted and the number of sources still needs to be made and the sources must be distributed according to the system used.

The Manchester system for interstitial implants

This was based on the use of radium sources with dose tables that gave the amount of radium and time needed (mg h tables) to give 1000 roentgens (1000 cGy) to the treated surface. The Paterson–Parker rules provide sets of distribution rules for planar or volume implants. For a simple planar rectangular implant, the sources must be parallel and the distance between sources should not exceed 10 mm. The end of rows of parallel needles is crossed by needles at right angles with two-thirds of the sources at the periphery and one-third in the central area. If an end is not crossed, 10 per cent is deducted from the area when reading from the mg h tables.

The Paris system for iridium wire implants and afterloading techniques

The Paris system was developed for iridium-192 wire implants and can also be used to calculate doses for computer-based HDR systems. The distribution rules for iridium-192 implants are as follows:

- Active sources should be parallel and straight.
- The lines should be equidistant.
- The line or plane on which the mid-point of the sources lies (central plane) should be at right angles to the axis of the sources.
- The linear activity should be uniform along the length of each line, and identical for all lines.
- The separation of sources may be varied from one implant to another. A minimum of 8 mm separation is acceptable for the smallest volumes, rising to 20 mm for the largest.
- For volume implants, the distribution of sources in cross-section (central plane) should be either in equilateral triangles or in squares.
- Because it is not usual to cross the ends of the sources, the average length of active wire must be longer than the target volume by 25–30 per cent depending on the number and separation of sources used.

A Paris implant can be a single plane with regularly spaced wires, a circular arrangement of needles/catheters, or a multiple plane arrangement to treat thicker tumours. The multiple plane arrangement can be triangular, rectangular or square. The dose calculation is then based on the distribution of sources in the central plane, that is, the plane which is at right angles to the axis of the mid-point of the sources. An example of a rectangular implant is when hairpins are used to treat anterior tongue tumours. Here the central plane should be half way down the legs of the hairpin ignoring the cross piece. Computer systems can now allow rotation of the implant in 3D to visualise the implant and central plane.

The calculation then uses the basal dose rate, which is the dose in the middle of the implanted volume where the dose rate is lowest. The basal dose rate at a point is the summation of dose rate contributions from each source according to the distance of the source from the point. In the case of a large implant, there may be several basal dose rate points, and a mean basal dose rate is taken for the implant as a whole (Fig. 5.1).

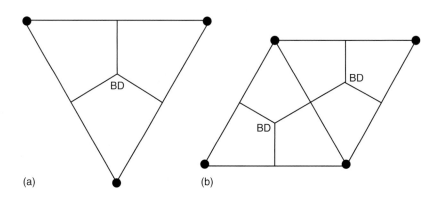

(a)   (b)

Figure 5.1 Basal dose rate point for two different volume implants arranged in (a) one and (b) two equilateral triangles.

Once the basal dose rate at the centre of the implant is known, the reference dose is taken as 85 per cent of the basal dose rate. This is then used to calculate the duration of the implant and the 85 per cent isodose defines the treated volume. The time needed for the implant is derived by dividing the prescribed dose by the reference dose rate and takes into account the activity of the wire used and radioactive decay during the implant. An example is shown in Table 5.3.

It is important to know the relationship between volume treated and length and separation of sources used when performing an implant. The following apply to implants according to the Paris system:

- the length of the treated volume is approximately 70 per cent of the length of the active sources (Fig. 5.2)
- the thickness of the treated volume in a single-plane implant is approximately 50 per cent of the separation between the sources
- the treatment margin around a volume implant performed in triangles is 30–40 per cent of the distance between the sides of the triangle
- the ratio of treated volume to source length or separation increases as more sources are used.

With the increased use of computer programmes for dose calculation, there is a tendency to prescribe to computer-derived isodoses. The isodose for prescription is chosen where the dose gradient is very steep, and there may be wide variation between the dose at the periphery and that at the centre of the target volume. A considerable proportion of the implanted volume may therefore receive a higher

Table 5.3 Calculation for breast implant

Two-plane implant to deliver 25 Gy
Superficial plane = 5-cm wires × 2
Deep plane = 7-cm wires × 3
Separation between sources = 18 mm
Activity of wire (midway through treatment) = air kerma rate 0.5 µGy/h/mm at 1 m (0.1193 mG/mm)

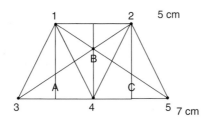

Wire	A		B		C	
	Distance (mm)	Dose rate (Gy/h)	Distance (mm)	Dose rate (Gy/h)	Distance (mm)	Dose rate (Gy/h)
1	10.4	0.1245	10.4	0.1245	20.8	0.0465
2	20.8	0.0465	10.4	0.1245	10.4	0.1245
3	10.4	0.1340	20.8	0.0555	27.5	0.0365
4	10.4	0.1340	10.4	0.1340	10.4	0.1340
5	27.5	0.0365	20.8	0.0555	10.4	0.1340
Total		0.4755		0.4940		0.4755

$$\text{Mean basal dose rate} = \frac{0.4755 + 0.4940 + 0.4755 \text{ Gy/h}}{3}$$

$$= 0.4817 \text{ Gy/h}$$

Reference dose rate $= 0.4817 \times 0.85$

(85%) $= 0.4095$ Gy/h

$$\text{Treatment time} = \frac{25.00}{0.4095}$$

$$= 61.05 \text{ h}$$

$$= 2 \text{ days } 13 \text{ h}$$

dose than that at the periphery. For safe treatment, it is advised that the central dose should be no more than 20 per cent higher than the peripheral dose.

Dose reporting

The ICRU report 38 (1985) gives guidance on reporting absorbed doses and volumes for intracavitary brachytherapy. It recommends that a combination of total reference air kerma, description of the reference volume and absorbed dose at reference points be used to specify intracavitary applications for cervix carcinoma.

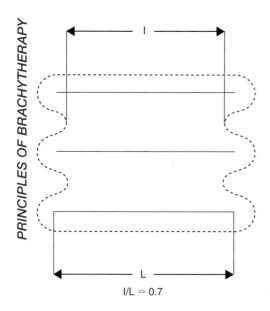

I/L ≃ 0.7

Figure 5.2 Relationship between treated volume (l) and length of active sources (L).

The ICRU report 58 (1997) recommends that the following information should be reported following an interstitial implant:

- Description of volumes:
  - gross tumour volume
  - clinical tumour volume
  - treated volume
- Description of sources and techniques:
  - description of time pattern
  - total reference air kerma (TRAK) (the sum of the products of the reference air kerma rate and irradiation time for each source)
- Description of doses:
  - prescribed dose
  - mean central dose in the central plane (equivalent to basal dose in the Paris system)
  - peripheral dose (equivalent to the reference dose in the Paris system)
- Description of high and low dose volumes.

A highly skilled and trained team is essential to perform brachytherapy implants safely. Everyone in the team should be trained in the principles of radiation safety so that the patient, staff and public are not at risk of unnecessary irradiation. Protective measures should be in place to keep dose levels as low as reasonably practicable (ALARP).

Legislation pertaining to brachytherapy

The following legislation governs the use of sealed brachytherapy sources in hospitals in the UK:

- Health and Safety at Work Act 1974

- Ionising Radiations Regulations 1999
- Ionising Radiation (Medical Exposure) Regulations 2000 (IR(ME)R)
- Medicines (Administration of Radioactive Substances) Regulations 1978 (amendment 1995)
- Radioactive Material (Road Transport) Regulations 2002
- Radioactive Substances Act 1993

The IR(ME)R practitioner for brachytherapy must be authorised under the Medicines (Administration of Radioactive Substances) regulations and hold a valid ARSAC licence before being able to administer radioactive sources for brachytherapy. The regulations allow for the safe implementation of brachytherapy in clinical practice.

Information sources

Gerbaulet A, Pötter R, Mazeron J-J *et al.* (2002) *The GEC ESTRO Handbook of Brachytherapy.* ESTRO, Brussels.

Hoskin P, Coyle C (2005) *Radiotherapy in Practice.* Oxford University Press, Oxford.

International Commission on Radiation Units and Measurements (1985) *Dose and Volume Specification for Reporting Intracavitary Therapy in Gynaecology, ICRU Report 38.* Bethesda, Maryland, USA.

International Commission on Radiation Units and Measurements (1997) *Dose and Volume Specification for Reporting Interstitial Therapy, ICRU Report 58.* Bethesda, Maryland, USA.

Report of American Association of Physicists in Medicine Radiation Therapy Committee Task Group 43 (1995). *Med Phys* **22**: 209–35.

www.oxfordjournals.org/jicru/backissues/reports.html. Reports 50, 62 and 71.

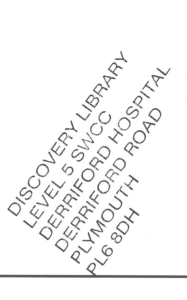

6 Emergency and palliative radiotherapy

Indications for radiotherapy

Emergency radiotherapy, which should be given within 24 h of diagnosis, is only indicated for selected patients with spinal cord compression. Urgent palliative radiotherapy, used to treat various other symptoms from primary disease or metastases, should be given as soon as possible. The set-up and planning are kept as simple as possible for palliative treatments, but they have to be individualised for each patient. Palliation requires as much skill as radical treatment. Accurate definition of the tumour causing the symptom is important and side effects of treatment must be minimised to ensure overall benefit to the patient.

Spinal cord compression

This is a medical emergency. The spinal cord is compressed most commonly by metastatic tumour involving the vertebrae, or less commonly by a benign cause such as a vertebral fracture, abscess or ruptured intervertebral disc. The spinal cord ends at approximately L1 and compression below this level causes the cauda equina syndrome.

Spinal cord compression (SCC) occurs in approximately 5 per cent of patients with cancer, most commonly with primary tumours of the lung, prostate, breast, kidney and thyroid, and lymphoma and multiple myeloma.

The most important determinant of outcome is the severity of neurological damage at the time treatment is initiated which is why treatment must be considered as an emergency. Of patients without significant neurological deficit, 80 per cent remain ambulant or regain the ability to walk, whereas only 50 per cent of those with even a mild transverse myelopathy and 5 per cent of those with paraplegia, do so. The prognosis is dependent on the type and extent of the primary malignancy. Untreated patients with SCC often die within a month. With treatment, the median overall survival ranges from 3 to 16 months.

■ Clinical features

A high index of suspicion is needed to detect cases early while neurological function is still intact. Common features of SCC in the thoracic area are back pain (typically radicular), sensory disturbance in the lower limbs, bladder or bowel dysfunction and leg weakness. The neurological signs are of bilateral upper motor neurone lesions in the legs and a sensory level. Cervical cord involvement may be suspected if there are signs and symptoms in the arms. In the lumbar spine area, compression may be of the cauda equina, causing nerve root pain in the back and legs, urinary disturbance, signs of a lower motor neurone lesion in the legs and patchy asymmetrical sensory loss. Nerve root irritation may be shown by limitation of straight leg raising. Onset of symptoms may be insidious, or occasionally paraplegia may develop rapidly with few preceding symptoms. Any delay in diagnosis and treatment will impact on functional outcome. Complete sudden paraplegia is usually associated with vascular damage and is commonly irreversible.

■ Investigations

A patient with suspected SCC needs an emergency MR scan of the whole spine, which is the most informative and least invasive technique. There are frequently multiple levels involved and clinical signs can appear to be out of keeping with the vertebral level involved (Fig. 6.1).

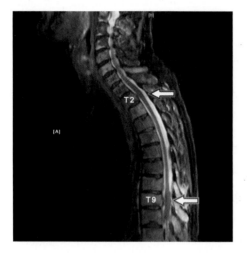

Figure 6.1 MRI of spine showing spinal cord compression at T2 and T9.

A diagnosis of malignancy may already be known. If not, a good history and general examination should be undertaken to search for a primary tumour. Investigations such as a chest X-ray, tumour marker estimations, biopsy or fine needle aspiration and cytology should be performed.

■ Treatment

At presentation, all patients suspected to have SCC should be given high dose steroids (e.g. dexamethasone 16 mg daily).

■ Sequencing of multimodality treatment

When planning treatment, the overall picture of the patient's health status, neurological function, site and histology of the primary, sites of metastases, prognosis and further treatment options, performance status and previous treatments, especially with radiotherapy, need to be taken into account. In patients who are not known to have malignancy, surgical decompression should be the first consideration; or if malignancy is highly suspected and the patient is not fit for surgery, an image guided vertebral biopsy can be performed.

A neurosurgeon should urgently assess all patients who are fit for surgery, reviewing clinical features and MRI to assess whether there is a place for multimodality treatment. Immediate consultation is made possible with remote image viewing. Surgery for SCC involves an anterior decompression and stabilisation of the spine. The indications for surgery are:

- unknown primary tumour
- unstable spine or vertebral displacement
- relapse following spinal radiotherapy
- neurological symptoms which progress during radiotherapy
- relatively radio-resistant tumour
- paralysis of rapid onset.

There is evidence that some patients have a better functional outcome if treated with emergency spinal decompressive surgery followed by postoperative radiotherapy.

Some patients have very chemo-sensitive tumours such as lymphoma or small cell carcinoma of the lung, and chemotherapy can be started urgently before radiotherapy.

If surgery or chemotherapy are not appropriate, EBRT is given immediately to prevent further neurological damage, to improve function and for pain relief.

■ Clinical and radiological anatomy

A full neurological examination should include search for motor impairment, sensory levels, and local pain and tenderness. These symptoms and signs should be correlated with MRI appearances in consultation with a radiologist. Metastases may be lytic or sclerotic, and collapse, compression laterally or posteriorly, and any paravertebral soft tissue mass should be noted. The sensory level detected in a skin dermatome arises from compression of the corresponding cord segment, which lies at a higher level than the vertebral body of the same number, e.g. a sensory level at T10 on the skin arises from compression of its cord segment at the level of the T8 vertebra.

■ Data acquisition

The patient is planned and treated ideally in the prone position using a direct posterior beam to avoid increased skin dose from treatment through the couch top. However, the supine position using an undercouch beam may be easier and more comfortable for the patient. Treatment should be planned using a CT scanner for virtual simulation or a simulator. Information from clinical examination and the MR scan is used to design the target volume.

Three reference tattoos are placed at the isocentre and bilaterally.

■ Target volume definition

The GTV includes vertebral and soft tissue tumour as seen on CT planning scan and diagnostic MRI. The CTV includes the spinal canal, the width of the vertebra and one vertebra above and below the SCC if the planning is based on MRI, or two vertebrae above and below if based on X-ray or CT to allow for uncertainty about extent of microscopic disease. The CTV to PTV margin is 1 cm.

In patients who have had surgery, the CTV will also include any metal that has been used to stabilise the spine.

■ Dose solutions

3D CT planning or virtual simulation may be used (Fig. 6.2). To treat the PTV adequately at depth, a direct 6 MV photon beam may be used. For lumbosacral lesions, a better dose distribution may be obtained with opposing beams. If treatment is delivered with a cobalt-60 source, an extra margin for the penumbra should be added according to departmental protocol. The field edge defined at the simulator to cover the PTV represents the 50 per cent isodose.

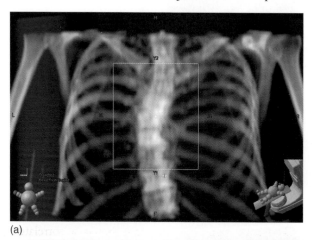

(a)

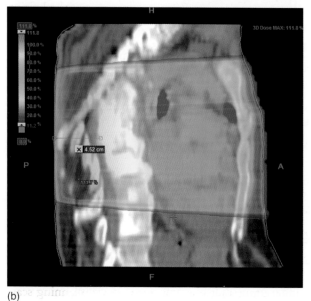

(b)

Figure 6.2 Virtual simulation for treatment of spinal cord compression showing (a) posterior beam arrangement, and (b) sagittal dose distribution from 6 MV beam. (Depth to anterior spinal canal 4.52 cm.)

The dose prescription point is the depth of the anterior spinal canal. This can be assessed from axial imaging and usually at 5–7 cm in the cervical and thoracic region, and at 7–8 cm in the lumbar region.

Occasionally SCC is caused by a primary tumour such as a plasmacytoma, and radical radiotherapy can produce permanent local control or even cure. In this situation, a planned homogeneous dose distribution with wedged posterior oblique beams with or without a direct posterior beam (Fig. 6.3), or electron therapy can be used.

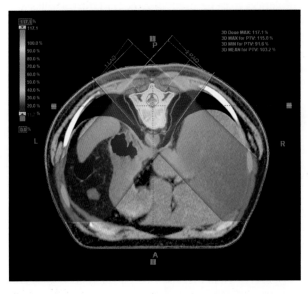

Figure 6.3 CT plan (with dose colourwash) to treat tumour of vertebral body using 6 MV posterior oblique wedged beams.

■ Dose fractionation

Palliation for good prognosis disease where radiotherapy is the first definitive treatment and postoperatively

20 Gy in 5 daily fractions of 4 Gy given in 1 week.
30 Gy in 10 daily fractions of 3 Gy given in 2 weeks.

A single dose of 8 Gy may be used for palliation of pain in patients with established paraplegia for >24 h.

Radical doses

Solitary plasmacytoma: 45 Gy in 25 daily fractions of 1.8 Gy given in 5 weeks.
Lymphoma: 30–36 Gy in 15–18 daily fractions given in 3–3½ weeks.

■ Treatment delivery and patient care

An experienced multidisciplinary team should care for a patient during treatment. A patient with an unstable spine or undergoing surgery needs specialist nursing and physiotherapy. Those undergoing radiotherapy need specialist input from experienced radiographers, nurses and physiotherapists to help them to rehabilitate and regain neurological function. Ongoing oncological management needs to be planned and the palliative care team involved for symptom control and support. Doses of dexamethasone should be reduced gradually after completion of radiotherapy.

Superior vena caval obstruction

■ Indications for radiotherapy

Over 90 per cent of cases of superior vena caval obstruction (SVCO) have a malignant cause. Although uncommon in patients with lung cancer, the commonest cause of SVCO is nevertheless small cell and non-small cell lung cancer. Other malignant causes are lymphoma and metastasis from mesothelioma, thymoma or any tumour that spreads to mediastinal lymph nodes.

The obstruction arises from compression of the SVC by tumour at the right main or upper lobe bronchus or by large volume mediastinal lymphadenopathy. Symptoms may be severe when the obstruction is below the entry of the azygous vein. The clinical features are neck swelling and distended veins over the chest. There may be swelling of one or both arms, shortness of breath, hoarse voice and headaches. The diagnosis is made on contrast-enhanced spiral or multi-slice CT scans, which can accurately identify the site of occlusion or stenosis and the presence of intravascular thrombus. Impending SVCO may also be diagnosed on CT scans.

SVCO is no longer considered a radiotherapy emergency, as outcome is not related to the duration of symptoms. Urgent action may be needed to prevent SVCO leading to airway obstruction from laryngeal or bronchial oedema, or coma from cerebral oedema.

Confirmation of histology is important and can be obtained by biopsy of the primary tumour at bronchoscopy or mediastinoscopy, by percutaneous CT-guided biopsy, or by biopsy of an involved cervical lymph node. Tumour markers such as α-fetoprotein (AFP) and β-hCG for germ cell tumours, lactic dehydrogenase for lymphoma, and prostate-specific antigen (PSA) for prostate cancer may be helpful.

■ Sequencing of multimodality treatment

Steroids such as high dose dexamethasone are traditionally given as part of SVCO management. Their use should be of short duration.

SVC stenting has been shown to be the most effective treatment with rapid relief of symptoms and should be considered first wherever available or for patients who fail to respond to chemotherapy or radiotherapy.

Chemotherapy should be considered in chemo-sensitive tumours such as small cell lung cancer, lymphoma, leukaemia and germ cell tumours. Radiotherapy should be considered in non-small cell lung cancer and other less chemo-sensitive tumours and when SVC stenting is not available.

■ Data acquisition

Where patients cannot lie down, they may be treated sitting upright using a direct anterior beam with margins determined from clinical examination, chest X-ray or CT appearances mapped on the patient by reference to landmarks such as the suprasternal notch. Beam sizes of 12×12 cm are usually adequate.

Ideally, patients should be treated supine with 3D conformal CT planning, virtual CT simulation or simulator planning. The CT scans are taken with 3–5 mm slices from the lower neck to the diaphragm.

■ Target volume definition

The GTV is defined on the contrast-enhanced CT scans, including any mediastinal mass and the site of SVCO (Fig. 6.4).

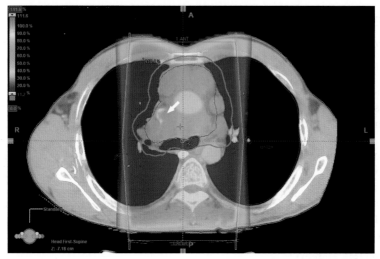

Figure 6.4 Axial CT slice showing anterior and posterior opposing beams created with virtual simulation to treat SVCO (arrowed).

The CTV is chosen according to tumour type and patterns of spread. The CTV-PTV margin is 1–2 cm. The margin is modified to spare normal lung tissue if possible.

■ Dose solutions

3D conformal planning can be used to treat the PTV and spare as much normal lung and spinal cord as possible. Conventionally, treatment is given with anterior and posterior beams with MLC or lead shielding.

■ Dose fractionation

20 Gy in 5 daily fractions of 4 Gy given in 1 week.
30 Gy in 10 daily fractions of 3 Gy given in 2 weeks.

For some chemo-sensitive tumours, a single fraction of 4 Gy in conjunction with chemotherapy may give adequate immediate palliation.

Bone pain

■ Indications for radiotherapy

Pain from bone metastases which persists in spite of analgesia can be successfully treated by radiotherapy with good relief in 80 per cent of cases. The commonest tumours to metastasise to bone are prostate, breast and lung cancers, but bone metastases may occur from any primary tumour site. Assessment of metastatic bone pain requires a full evaluation of the sites of metastases by isotope bone scanning or

MRI to determine whether local or systemic therapy is appropriate. If the cortex of the bone is eroded and there is risk of fracture, or if the bone has already fractured, surgical stabilisation should be performed followed by postoperative radiotherapy. Isotope therapy of diffuse prostatic cancer bone metastases may be considered.

■ Data acquisition

Immobilisation is individualised to the patient and the site of the bone metastases to be treated. Most sites can be treated with the patient supine, except vertebral lesions which are ideally treated with the patient prone. This is especially relevant for cancers with a long natural history where a possible need for re-treatment makes skin sparing desirable, particularly over the sacrum. Ankle stocks and head rests can be used to aid immobilisation. Lesions in the upper cervical spine are best treated with the patient supine, immobilised in a thermoplastic shell so that opposing lateral beams can be used to avoid irradiating the oral cavity and pharynx. Patients who are to be treated with electron or orthovoltage applicators can be immobilised supine, prone or on their side.

The area to be treated is planned using a virtual CT or conventional simulation with reference to diagnostic X-rays, bone scans, CT, MRI and sites of symptoms.

■ Target volume definition

The origin of the pain must be ascertained to ensure the correct site is treated. For example knee pain may radiate from the hip, femur or spine, and rib pain may radiate from the vertebral body. The volume chosen must balance symptom relief with sparing of normal tissues to minimise side effects (e.g. small bowel with pelvic treatments).

Where possible, the whole structure should be treated, e.g. a whole vertebra with consideration for matching adjacent fields that may be required with subsequent treatments. It is usual to include one or two vertebrae above and below the site of involvement.

When treating a bone postoperatively, the entire prosthesis or intramedullary nail should be covered with a margin of normal bone. This is the area most at risk of residual tumour. In patients with multiple painful bone metastases, wide field half-body volumes can be treated. Treatment portals are marked on the patient with reference tattoos as a permanent record. Photographs, DRRs or simulator films should be taken as a record and for reference for future treatment planning.

When planning the treatment volume, it is important to remember that the beam edge represents the 50 per cent isodose and a margin must be added to ensure the target volume is covered by the 90–95 per cent isodose.

■ Dose solutions

The majority of treatments are given with a single direct photon beam, for example to the spine, or as opposing anterior and posterior beams, e.g. pelvis. Sites such as the ribs can be treated with direct electron or orthovoltage beams. A single fraction of 8 Gy has been shown overall to be equivalent to higher doses. For large volumes, situations where long-term survival is expected, or where long segments of spinal cord are included, a fractionated course of treatment may reduce acute and late morbidity.

Anterior and posterior opposing beams are used for half body radiotherapy. A lower dose is used for upper half body radiotherapy to keep lung dose within tolerance. The prescription point for a single beam, e.g. spine, should be the depth of the vertebral body taken from imaging and is usually between 5 cm and 7 cm in the cervical and thoracic region and 7–8 cm in the lumbar region. The prescription point for opposing anterior and posterior beams is the MPD. The prescription point for electron therapy is 100 per cent on the central axis and the energy is chosen to cover the target volume at depth by the 90 per cent isodose.

Orthovoltage beams are prescribed to D_{max} at 100 per cent. A 250–500 kV beam will give an 80 per cent isodose at a depth of 3–3.5 cm, with a relative increase in the dose to bone compared with megavoltage and electron beams.

■ Dose-fractionation

8 Gy single fraction.
20 Gy in 5 daily fractions of 4 Gy given in 1 week.
30 Gy in 10 daily fractions of 3 Gy given in 2 weeks.

Half body EBRT

Lower 8 Gy single fraction.
Upper 6 Gy single fraction.

Haemorrhage

Bleeding from advanced tumours of the breast, bladder, bronchus and other sites can be effectively palliated with radiotherapy. Simple arrangements such as opposing anterior and posterior beams for treatment of the bronchus or bladder, or small tangential beams for breast tumours, are used. The size is chosen clinically as the smallest needed to palliate the bleeding effectively with the fewest side effects, and may not include the whole tumour.

The following dose fractionations can be used:

Single 8 Gy fraction.
20 Gy in 5 daily fractions given in 1 week.
30 Gy in 5 fractions given in 6 weeks (6 Gy once weekly) can be used for patient convenience where higher doses are needed.

Information sources

NICE (2008) *Metastatic Spinal Cord Compression*. Guideline 75. www.nice.org.uk/guidance/index (accessed 4 December 2008).

Patchell RA, Tibbs PA, Regine WF *et al.* (2005) Direct decompressive surgical resection in the treatment of spinal cord compression caused by metastatic cancer. A randomised trial. *Lancet* Aug 20–26, **336**: 643–8.

Rowell NP, Gleeson FV (2002) Steroids, radiotherapy, chemotherapy and stents for superior vena caval obstruction in carcinoma of the bronchus: a systematic review. *Clin Oncol* **14**: 338–51.

Sze WM, Shelley MD, Held I *et al.* (2003) Palliation of metastatic bone pain: single fraction versus multifraction radiotherapy – a systematic review of randomised trials. *Clin Oncol* **15**: 345–52.

Skin

Each cell type in the skin can give rise to a different type of cancer. It is convenient to classify skin tumours into non-melanoma skin cancers (NMSC) and malignant melanoma (MM). Secondary deposits from other cancers can also present in the skin. This chapter covers the role of radiotherapy for NMSC (basal and squamous cell carcinomas), MM and other rare tumours such as cutaneous lymphoma, Kaposi's sarcoma, angiosarcoma, and Merkel cell tumours. Radiotherapy is also used for benign conditions such as keloids.

Non-melanoma skin cancer

Basal cell carcinoma

■ Indications for radiotherapy

Radiotherapy gives cure rates for primary or recurrent basal cell carcinoma (BCC) of >90 per cent. BCCs are defined as low and high risk:

- Low risk BCCs are generally small (<2 cm), well defined in a non-critical site with non-aggressive histology. Only 5 per cent of well-defined BCCs <2 cm show subclinical spread beyond 5 mm.
- High risk BCCs are generally large (>2 cm), indistinct or morphoeic, in a critical site (eyes, ears, lips, nose and nasolabial folds), and show aggressive histology such as morphoeic, infiltrative, micronodular or perineural spread.

In many cases BCCs can be managed equally effectively by surgery or radiotherapy. Indications for radiotherapy include:

- large superficial lesions where a better cosmetic result can be obtained with radiotherapy
- large lesions where surgery would cause major loss of function such as paralysis, numbness, dribbling, or ectropion
- extensive lesions where surgery may require nasectomy, ear amputation or eye enucleation
- older patients in whom long-term skin atrophy caused by radiotherapy may not be relevant
- multiple superficial lesions where surgery would be onerous for the patient
- patients who are unfit for, or refuse, surgery
- selected tumours of the eyelids and canthi of the eyes
- selected tumours on the nose, ears and lips; larger lesions overlying cartilage are best treated with electron rather than superficial radiotherapy

- large lesions on the cheek which often respond with minimum scarring
- recurrent lesions after surgery, or with incomplete excision or perineural invasion.

Relative contraindications are:

- patients under 45 years: there is potential for deterioration of the cosmetic outcome over time (>5–10 years) and risk of second malignancy
- large lesions involving cartilage, bone, tendons or joints: the risk of radionecrosis is high, and cure rates are lower
- lesions where there is uncertainty over the histology
- lesions that recur after radiotherapy
- hair-bearing skin such as scalp, eyebrow and eyelashes: risk of permanent epilation
- lesions around the upper eyelid: risk of lacrimal gland dryness and upper lid conjunctival keratinisation
- inner canthus lesions: risk of nasolacrimal duct stenosis
- lesions on the lower leg, back and dorsum of the hand: poor healing and radiation sequelae, particularly telangiectasia, pigmentation, ulceration, and atrophic scarring.

These relative contraindications need to be reviewed in each individual case because alternative treatments may produce even more problems.

Mohs' micrographic surgery can be used in selected patients with BCCs in critical sites such as the eyelids, ears, lips, nose, and nasolabial folds, or morphoeic or infiltrative histological subtype, as well as in patients with recurrent BCC, especially after radiotherapy. Incompletely excised high risk BCCs may be treated by re-excision, or by postoperative radiotherapy.

Not all BCCs require treatment. Aggressive treatment might be inappropriate for patients of advanced age or poor general health, especially for asymptomatic low risk lesions that are unlikely to cause significant morbidity. Some elderly or frail patients with symptomatic or high risk tumours prefer treatments designed to palliate rather than cure.

■ Assessment of primary disease

A biopsy is essential to obtain a histological diagnosis. The six clinicopathological subtypes of BCC are: nodular, pigmented, cystic, morphoeic, superficial and linear. BCC rarely metastasises, and a staging work-up is not necessary. However the extent of recurrent aggressive and neglected BCCs may be delineated by MRI.

The primary tumour should be examined under a bright light. By palpation and using a magnifying glass, the edges and depth of the tumour are defined. Edges of morphoeic lesions are difficult to define due to their wide area of spread. Deep penetration may occur at the inner canthus where tumour may infiltrate along the medial border of the orbit and also at the nasolabial fold, ala nasi, tragus and post auricular areas. MRI may be useful to define extensive lesions.

■ Data acquisition

The majority of skin radiotherapy is based on clinical definition of the treatment volumes and the use of single superficial X-ray or electron beams. In very advanced cases with deep infiltration, a CT-planned photon or electron treatment may be needed.

Immobilisation

The patient is positioned supine, prone or semi-prone so that the tumour to be treated can be accessed by the superficial X-ray machine or electron applicators. Head rests, pillows, sandbags and other supports are used to aid immobilisation as necessary. If the patient requires a plan to treat an extensive tumour, immobilisation will be similar to that for a head and neck cancer using a Perspex shell.

■ Target volume definition

The GTV is defined clinically as described above and marked on the skin. The margin added to the GTV to create the CTV depends on the clinicopathological type of BCC, the site and size of the lesion being treated, and organs at risk. A further margin for set-up error is added to create the PTV. The field size is chosen to ensure the PTV receives 95 per cent of prescribed dose and will vary between superficial and electron beam radiotherapy.

- For a low risk small BCC with a well-defined GTV, a margin of 5–8 mm to create the treatment field using superficial radiotherapy is appropriate.
- For high risk, larger or poorly defined lesions such morphoeic BCCs, a margin of 1–1.5 cm may be necessary to create the treatment field using superficial radiotherapy.

This margin needs to be increased when electron therapy is used to allow for the shape of the isodoses. This will depend on the size of the lesion and the energy of the electron beam. For a 6 MeV electron beam treating a 5 cm circle, an extra 1 cm should be added to the margins above to define the field size with an electron applicator.

Shielding

Superficial radiotherapy

Lead shielding is used to define the treatment field and protect surrounding structures. The superficial machine applicators are applied directly to the skin or standard lead cut-outs may be used. Irregular lesions need individualised lead cut-outs which on the face can be made into lead masks (Fig. 7.1). The thickness of lead depends on the energy of the beam used: 1.5 mm is adequate for 90–150 kV.

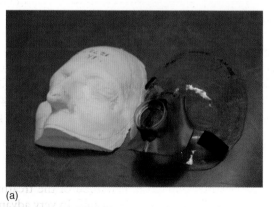
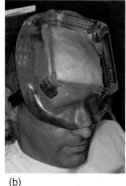

(a)   (b)

Figure 7.1 Lead mask with area cut out for treatment of (a) BCC of nose for superficial radiotherapy and (b) squamous cell carcinoma of the scalp with wax bolus for electron treatment.

When treating lesions of the eyelids a lead shield must be used to protect the eye. Internal lead contact lenses are available in various sizes and shapes (Fig. 7.2a). They are inserted after instillation of local anaesthetic eye drops. The eye must be protected following treatment until the local anaesthetic wears off and the corneal reflex returns. Alternatively, a spade-shaped eye shield may be used under the lower or upper eyelid (Fig 7.2b). An intranasal shield is used to protect the mucosa and cartilage of the nasal septum. The gums can be protected with an internal lead shield when lesions on the skin above the upper lip are treated, but it is important to ensure the shield does not alter the shape of the area, causing stand-off.

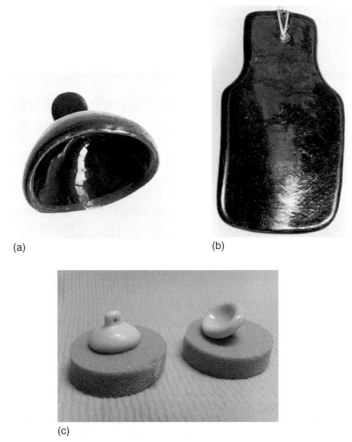

(a)

(b)

(c)

Figure 7.2 (a) Internal lead eye shield. (b) Spade-shaped eye shield. (c) Electron eye shield.

Electron beam radiotherapy

Electron beams may be defined by an electron endplate cut-out inserted into the electron applicator or by shaped lead placed on the skin. 4 mm of lead is adequate for electrons up to 10 MeV. The lead shields for electrons need to be lined with wax or plastic on the inner surface to absorb secondary electrons. Internal eye contact lenses have been designed for use with electron beam therapy around the eye and are made of 3–4 mm lead with a 2–3 mm silicon lining depending on the electron energy used (Fig. 7.2c).

■ Dose solutions

Superficial radiotherapy

Most superficial lesions are treated with 80–150 kV with appropriate filtration which defines the beam characteristics. Percentage DDs for different field diameters and energies are obtained from tables drawn up for each therapy unit, and an appropriate energy is selected to encompass the target volume within the 90 per cent isodose (Table 7.1).

Table 7.1 Sample percentage depth dose data for 80 kV (HVL = 2.0 mm aluminium)

15-cm SSD									
Applicator (cm)	1.0	1.5	2.0	2.5	3.0	3.5	4.0	4.5	5.0
Equivalent diameter (cm)*	1.0	1.5	2.0	2.5	3.0	3.5	4.0	4.5	5.0
BSF†	1.06	1.09	1.11	1.12	1.14	1.15	1.16	1.17	1.18
Depth (cm)									
0	100	100	100	100	100	100	100	100	100
0.5	76	78	80	81	82	83	84	84	85
1.0	58	61	64	66	68	69	71	71	72
2.0	37	40	42	44	46	48	49	50	51
3.0	24	26	28	30	32	33	34	35	36
4.0	16	18	19	21	22	23	23	24	25
5.0	11	12	13	14	15	16	17	17	18
6.0	8	9	10	10	11	12	12	13	13
7.0	6	6	7	7	8	8	9	9	10
8.0	4	5	5	5	6	6	7	7	7
9.0	3	3	4	4	4	5	5	5	6
10.0	2	2	3	3	3	4	4	4	4

25-cm SSD							
Applicator (cm)	6.0	8.0	10.0	12.0	15.0	8 × 10	10 × 15
Equivalent diameter (cm)*	6.0	8.0	10.0	12.0	15.0	9.9	13.3
BSF†	1.20	1.22	1.24	1.25	1.26	1.24	1.26
Depth (cm)							
0	100	100	100	100	100	100	100
0.5	87	88	89	90	90	89	90
1.0	76	78	79	80	81	79	80
2.0	57	59	60	61	62	60	61
3.0	42	44	45	46	48	45	47
4.0	30	32	34	35	37	34	36
5.0	22	25	26	28	29	26	28
6.0	17	19	21	22	23	21	22
7.0	13	15	16	17	19	16	18
8.0	10	12	13	14	15	13	14
9.0	8	9	10	11	12	10	11
10.0	6	7	8	8	9	8	9

*Equivalent diameter of cut-out treatment area.
†BSF, back scatter factor.

Owing to curving body contours, it may not be possible to appose the applicator of the machine to the lead mask, which will result in positive or negative stand-off (Fig. 7.3). An allowance for this stand-off must be made according to the inverse square law. Tables for superficial X-ray therapy units are available which give multiplication factors to correct for different amounts of both positive and negative stand-off (Table 7.2).

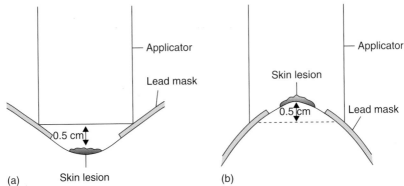

(a) Skin lesion (b)

Figure 7.3 (a) Positive stand-off of 0.5 cm between lesion and applicator. (b) Negative stand-off of 0.5 cm.

Table 7.2 Multiplication correction factors for stand-off calculation

Stand-off distance (cm)	15-cm SSD applicator	25-cm SSD applicator
−1.5	1.23	1.13
−1.0	1.15	1.09
−0.5	1.07	1.04
0.0	1.00	1.00
0.5	0.94	0.96
1.0	0.88	0.92
1.5	0.83	0.89
2.0	0.78	0.86
2.5	0.73	0.83
3.0	0.69	0.80
3.5	0.66	0.77
4.0	0.62	0.74
4.5	0.59	0.72
5.0	0.56	0.69

Sample calculation for superficial radiotherapy

For applicator 3 cm diameter, lead cut-out 2 cm diameter, positive stand-off 0.5 cm treating at 80 kV (HVL = 2.0 mm Al) and 15 cm source skin distance (SSD) with a daily fraction size of 4.5 Gy.

Using data from tables which incorporate back scatter factor (BSF) for size of applicator and treatment area and surface dose rates and treatment times, the treatment time can be calculated.

Beam data
Surface dose rate (SDR) = 2.81 Gy/minute   (Table 7.3)
% DD = 100 per cent   (Table 7.1)
BSF (3 cm) = 1.14   (Table 7.1)
BSF (2 cm) = 1.11   (Table 7.1)
Stand-off correction factor (SOF) = 0.94   (Table 7.2)
 Calculation:

$$\text{Output (Gy/min)} = \text{SDR} \times \frac{\text{BSF (cut out)}}{\text{BSF (applicator)}} \times \text{SOF} \times \frac{\%\ \text{DD}}{100} \quad (7.1)$$

$$\text{Output (Gy/min)} = 2.81 \times \frac{1.11}{1.14} \times 0.94 \times \frac{100\%}{100} \quad (7.2)$$

$$\text{Treatment time per fraction} = \frac{4.5}{2.57} = 1.75\,\text{min} = 1\,\text{min}\,45\,\text{s} \quad (7.3)$$

When there is no stand-off and no cut-out, the treatment time in minutes can be read directly from a table (Table 7.3).

Electron beam therapy

Beam sizes of less than 4 cm diameter should not be used because the advantage of beam flatness is lost. The physical characteristics of electron beams are shown in

Table 7.3 Sample table for calculation of surface dose rate for a given applicator size and treatment time in min (energy = 80 kV, HVL = 2.0 mm, aluminium filtration = 1.7 mm)

Applicator size (cm)	Surface dose rate (Gy/min)	Treatment time (min) for varying doses (Gy)							
		1	4	5	6	6.25	6.3	8	9
15-cm SSD applicators									
1.0 circle	2.46	0.41	1.62	2.03	2.44	2.54	2.56	3.25	3.66
1.5 circle	2.56	0.39	1.56	1.95	2.34	2.44	2.46	3.13	3.52
2.0 circle	2.64	0.38	1.51	1.89	2.27	2.36	2.38	3.03	3.40
2.5 circle	2.75	0.36	1.46	1.82	2.19	2.28	2.29	2.91	3.28
3.0 circle	2.81	0.36	1.42	1.78	2.14	2.22	2.24	2.85	3.20
3.5 circle	2.84	0.35	1.41	1.76	2.12	2.20	2.22	2.82	3.17
4.0 circle	2.87	0.35	1.39	1.74	2.09	2.18	2.19	2.79	3.13
4.5 circle	2.91	0.34	1.37	1.72	2.06	2.14	2.16	2.75	3.09
5.0 circle	2.93	0.34	1.37	1.71	2.05	2.14	2.15	2.73	3.07
25-cm SSD applicators									
6.0 circle	1.03	0.97	3.89	4.87	5.84	6.08	6.13	7.79	8.76
8.0 circle	1.06	0.95	3.78	4.73	5.67	5.91	5.96	7.56	8.51
10.0 circle	1.09	0.92	3.68	4.60	5.51	5.74	5.79	7.35	8.27
12.0 circle	1.10	0.90	3.62	4.52	5.43	5.65	5.70	7.24	8.14
15.0 circle	1.11	0.90	3.59	4.48	5.38	5.61	5.65	7.18	8.07

Figure 2.6 (p. 22). The energy of the electron beam is chosen so that the deep surface of the target volume is encompassed by the 90 per cent isodose with a sharp fall in dose beyond. This spares the underlying tissues. The effective treatment depth expressed in centimetres is about one-third of the beam energy in MeV but depends on the beam size and depth dose data for any particular machine. Bolus is placed on the skin surface to increase dose to 100 per cent and to compensate for irregular surfaces (see Fig. 7.1b, p. 73). This reduces the depth of the 90 per cent isodose which must be taken into account when choosing the electron energy. A correction for any stand-off between the applicator and skin surface can be made using the inverse square law and effective SSD. Tables for varying electron energy and applicator size should be used.

■ Dose-fractionation

The daily dose and fractionation scheme depend on the site and size of the lesion, and the age and performance status of the patient. The convenience of shorter regimens must be balanced against risks of normal tissue damage.

For superficial radiotherapy, the dose is specified at D_{max} and for electrons at 100 per cent on the central axis, ensuring a minimum dose of 90–95 per cent to the whole target volume. Many different regimens have been shown to be effective and are in widespread use.

Lesions <3 cm diameter (superficial radiotherapy [SRT] 80–140 kV)
36 Gy in 8 fractions of 4.5 Gy given in 17 days treating M/W/F.
30–32 Gy in 4 fractions of 7.5–8 Gy given in 2–4 weeks (one or two fractions/week).
18 Gy in a single fraction.

Lesions >3 cm diameter or nose/pinna/poorly vascularised skin (SRT or consider EBRT*)
45 Gy in 9 fractions of 5 Gy given in 21 days treating on alternate weekdays.

Lesions >5 cm diameter (EBRT* or megavoltage radiotherapy)
50–54 Gy in 20 daily fractions of 2.5–2.7 Gy given in 4 weeks.
For SCC use 54 Gy (see below).
60 Gy in 30 daily fractions given in 6 weeks.
(*Consider increasing dose by 10 per cent to account for the reduced relative biological dose of electrons.)

■ Treatment delivery and patient care

The patient lies on the treatment couch with lead mask, cut-out and other shielding such as internal eye shields in place. Any bolus required is applied and the treatment applicator positioned over the target volume. Skin marks, tattoos if appropriate, and photographs of the planned treatment position are used to ensure the correct set-up each day.

Scabs over lesions may need to be removed before treatment to ensure adequate depth dose. Skin should be kept dry, and shaving or the application of make up and chemicals to the area should be avoided. Erythema usually develops in the first week of treatment followed by an exudative reaction. Acute erythema is treated with aqueous cream or soft paraffin. If the skin becomes broken, paraffin gauze or hydrogel is applied with a dry dressing. Vaseline can be used inside the nostril to help prevent scabbing and nose bleeds. If the dose to the lacrimal gland is kept below 35 Gy, the risk of the late complication of dry eye may be minimised.

Long-term side effects include atrophy, hyper- and hypopigmentation, telangiectasia and alopecia. Non-healing skin ulceration, persistent pain and secondary skin cancers are more serious late side effects. Patients should be advised to avoid exposure to cold winds and sun, to use ultraviolet sun barrier cream, and to wear a hat.

Squamous cell carcinoma

Cutaneous squamous cell carcinoma (SCC) is the second most common skin cancer after BCC. Treatments are highly effective and can achieve cure rates of 90 per cent. In the head and neck area, 20 per cent of NMSC are cutaneous SCC, but this rises to 43 per cent in sites such as the pinna. The common premalignant lesion is actinic keratosis.

Primary cutaneous SCCs may grow slowly or rapidly. They may metastasise initially to regional lymph nodes, and later to viscera, with an overall mortality of 3 per cent. Cutaneous SCCs of the head and neck can spread haematogenously to the CNS, or via the perineural space.

Overall, lesions recur locally in 25 per cent. Risk factors for local or nodal recurrence include site (lip and ear SCCs have a higher recurrence rate and are discussed in Chapter 9), size (tumours >2 cm diameter), depth of invasion (>4 mm), cellular differentiation, perineural involvement, host immune status and previous treatment. Tumours arising in non sun-exposed sites, and areas of previous radiation, thermal injury, scarring or chronic ulceration, have higher risk of recurrence and metastases. Poorly differentiated and anaplastic SCCs metastasise more frequently than well-differentiated SCCs. Those on the mid-face and lip are especially prone to neural involvement. Careful follow-up of patients with these high-risk features is essential.

■ Indications for radiotherapy

Treatment of SCC is similar to that described for BCC. However, more radical surgery is required because of the greater metastatic potential. Patients with high risk SCC presenting with involved lymph nodes should be reviewed by a multidisciplinary oncology team including a dermatologist, pathologist, plastic or maxillofacial surgeon, oncologist and clinical nurse specialist.

Radiotherapy is generally reserved for patients over 45 years because of the theoretical risk of inducing further malignancies. It is not suitable for tumours invading underlying cartilage where the risk of radiochondritis is high and cure rates are lower. There is a relative contraindication to treating SCCs in cardiac or renal transplant patients as they may be particularly susceptible to further cutaneous malignancies. The 5-year cure rate for NMSC with radiotherapy is as high as 90 per cent and the cosmetic results are good or acceptable in 84 per cent. The early and late complication rates are low. Radiotherapy is often used as an adjuvant modality for high risk SCC, e.g. lesions over 2 cm with perineural invasion in a high risk site. Radiotherapy may also be used palliatively for patients with lymph node metastases.

Afterloading brachytherapy can be used for SCCs on the dorsum of the hand, lower limb or curved surfaces such as the scalp. A mould of the area to be treated is made and catheters distributed over the area to be treated following the Manchester or Paris rules for an interstitial implant.

Methods of assessment and target volume definition are similar to those described for BCC. However, a larger margin of 1–2 cm is added to the GTV to create the PTV according to risk factors. Dose-fractionation regimens are similar to those described for BCC, but for larger lesions, longer dose-fractionation schedules are preferred.

■ Dose-fractionation

Lesions <5 cm diameter (see also dose-fractionation regimens for BCC)
45 Gy in 9 fractions of 5 Gy given in 21 days treating on alternate weekdays.
54 Gy in 20 fractions of 2.7 Gy given in 4 weeks.

Lesions >5 cm diameter (EBRT* or megavoltage radiotherapy)
54 Gy in 20 daily fractions of 2.7 Gy given in 4 weeks.
66 Gy in 33 daily fractions given in 6 ½ weeks.

Postoperative radiotherapy (EBRT* or megavoltage radiotherapy)
50 Gy in 20 daily fractions of 2.5 Gy given in 4 weeks.
60 Gy in 30 daily fractions given in 6 weeks.

HDR brachytherapy

A typical fractionation is 45 Gy in 10 fractions. A more prolonged fractionation may be advisable in the lower limb.

Palliative radiotherapy

8 Gy in a single fraction.
20 Gy in 5 daily fractions of 4 Gy given in 1 week.
36 Gy in 6 fractions of 6 Gy once weekly given in 6 weeks.
(*Consider increasing dose by 10 per cent to account for the reduced relative biological dose of electrons.)

Malignant melanoma

The primary treatment of melanoma is surgery. Radiotherapy has a primary role in treating *in situ* lentigo maligna, an adjuvant role for postoperative lymph node areas and a palliative role for skin, nodal and visceral metastases. *In vitro* studies have shown a wide shoulder to the cell survival curve for melanoma cell lines suggesting a possible advantage for hypofractionation. This has to be balanced against the risk of increased normal tissue reactions with larger fractions.

Lentigo maligna is the superficial *in situ* phase that progresses to lentigo maligna melanoma in 30–40 per cent of cases. It is typically a large flat, pigmented area most commonly on the face. The treatment is surgical excision or radiotherapy. Radiotherapy is very effective with a recurrence rate of 7 per cent and is a good option for older patients. The lesions may be treated with superficial or electron beam radiotherapy as described for NMSC. The margins need to be carefully defined, as there is often a large area of subclinical disease requiring a margin of up to 2 cm from GTV to PTV. The dose used is the same as for NMSC described above.

There is a 30–50 per cent risk of recurrence following lymph node dissection for melanoma where there is extracapsular extension, three or more involved lymph nodes, lymph node size >3 cm, cervical neck location or recurrence after previous excision. Adjuvant radiotherapy can reduce the risk of local recurrence by over 50 per cent in these high risk cases, but has not been shown to improve survival. There is a high risk of lymphoedema when treating the axillae and groins adjuvantly and radiotherapy is usually avoided in these sites. Radiotherapy to the nodal regions is planned as described in Figure 23.2 (p. 288).

Radiotherapy may be used palliatively to relieve pain and bleeding from skin, nodal, bone and visceral metastases. Brain metastases can be palliated in patients with a good performance status. The recursive partitioning analysis (RPA) classification is helpful in selecting patients for treatment.

- RPA class 1: age <65, Karnovsky performance status (PS) >70, controlled primary, no extracranial metastases
- RPA class 2: all others
- RPA class 3: Karnovsky PS <70

Patients in RPA class 1 may benefit from surgical excision and postoperative whole brain radiotherapy, or focal stereotactic radiotherapy. Patients in RPA class 3 and those with meningeal involvement have such a poor survival that they are best managed with palliative care only. Patients in RPA class 2 may benefit from palliative whole brain radiotherapy.

■ Dose-fractionation

Lentigo maligna

See dose-fractionation regimens for NMSC above. Adjuvant radiotherapy after lymph node dissection:

50 Gy in 20 fractions of 2.5 Gy given in 4 weeks.
60 Gy in 30 fractions given in 6 weeks.

Palliative radiotherapy

8 Gy in a single fraction.
20 Gy in 5 daily fractions of 4 Gy given in 1 week.
36 Gy in 6 fractions of 6 Gy once weekly given in 6 weeks.

Whole brain radiotherapy

12 Gy in 2 daily fractions given on consecutive days.
20 Gy in 5 daily fractions of 4 Gy given in 1 week.

Cutaneous lymphoma

Primary cutaneous lymphomas are rare with an incidence of 0.4 per 100 000, but most are low grade with long survival and therefore the prevalence is much higher. Two thirds are T cell in origin, the majority of which are mycosis fungoides (MF). The WHO/EORTC (Willemze *et al.* 2005) classification is now used and specialist multidisciplinary teams should manage these patients.

■ T cell

Radiotherapy is a very effective single agent for the treatment of MF. It is used in every stage to treat patches and plaques, tumours, and lymph nodes. MF is extremely sensitive to radiotherapy and low doses can be used, allowing adjacent areas to be treated, and recurrences can be retreated safely.

In early stage IA–IIB MF, radiotherapy is used with skin directed therapy such as psoralen ultraviolet A (PUVA) to treat patches and plaques which are planned for treatment in a similar way to NMSC as described above. The margins from GTV to field edge depend on the area being treated and are usually 0.5–1.0 cm.

In stage IIB–IVB MF, radiotherapy can be used alone or with systemic therapies to treat skin patches, plaques and tumours, nodal and visceral metastases. Mucosal involvement of the nasopharynx or pharynx responds well to radiotherapy, which is fractionated to reduce normal tissue toxicity.

Total skin electron beam therapy

Total skin electron beam therapy (TSEBT) can be used to treat the whole skin in any stage of MF. It is used in stage IB disease that is becoming resistant to skin directed treatment such as PUVA, in stage IIB disease to debulk tumours, in stage III disease to treat erythroderma, and palliatively in stage IV disease where patients have good PS. The current standard is the modified Stanford technique (Fig. 7.4) using a conventional linear accelerator in high dose rate electron mode to deliver matched dual fields at a distance of 3.5–4.5 m. A Perspex screen is placed close to the patient to degrade the beam to meet the EORTC consensus of dose maximum at 1 mm depth, 80 per cent isodose at 9 mm depth and 20 per cent isodose at <20 mm. The patient is treated standing and rotates through the six positions shown to maximise unfolding of the skin. On days 1 and 5 TLD measurements are taken from various sites on the skin to map dosimetry accurately. Areas of low dose and inherently shielded areas such as the scalp and soles of the feet are treated separately. Using modern techniques, the whole body photon contamination dose is less than 2.3 per cent (<0.7 Gy). Acute adverse effects of TSEBT are usually minor with attention to care of the patient's skin. The adverse effects include fatigue, temporary alopecia, nail loss, leg swelling and blisters, minor nose bleeds (1 in 30), reduced sweating (1 in 30), minor parotitis (1 in 30), gynaecomastia (1 in 30), and skin infection, which is rare (<1 in 100) but must be treated aggressively. Late effects include skin atrophy, hypothyroidism, nail and finger changes, sun sensitivity and infertility in men. Combined with PUVA, TSEBT adds to the patient's risk of other cutaneous malignancies.

There are other non-MF cutaneous T cell lymphomas that can be effectively treated with radiotherapy using similar doses to MF.

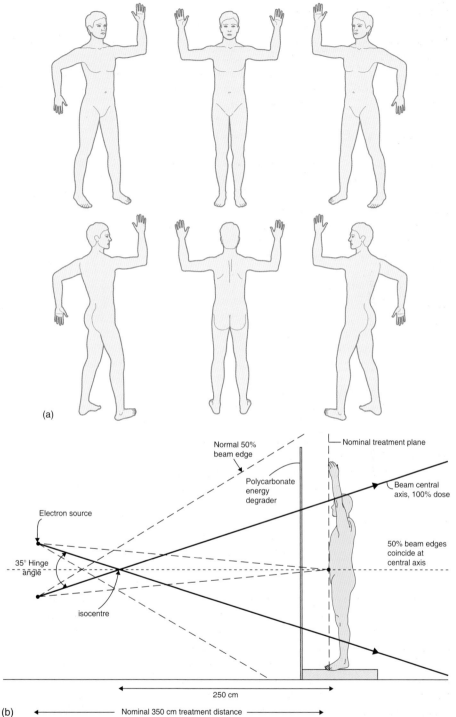

(a)

(b)

Figure 7.4 TSEBT technique used at Guy's and St Thomas' Hospital modified from the Stanford technique: (a) six standing positions and (b) dual field arrangement. Courtesy of Dr P Rudd.

Dose-fractionation

Patch and plaque
8 Gy in 2 fractions of 4 Gy given in 2–4 days.

Tumour
12 Gy in 3 fractions of 4 Gy given in 3–5 days.

Mucosal disease
20 Gy in 10 daily fractions given in 2 weeks.

Lymph nodes
30 Gy in 15 daily fractions given in 3 weeks.

TSEBT
30 Gy in 20 fractions of 1.5 Gy given in 5 weeks.

■ B cell

Primary cutaneous B cell lymphomas (PCBCL) are a heterogeneous group that present in the skin without evidence of extracutaneous disease at diagnosis. The EORTC WHO classification describes two indolent types: primary cutaneous marginal zone lymphoma (PCMZL), primary cutaneous follicle centre lymphoma (PCFCL) and two more aggressive types: primary cutaneous diffuse large B cell lymphoma leg type (PCLBCL LT) and non-leg type. The indolent PCMZL and PCFCL are treated with radiotherapy alone with an excellent 5-year disease-specific survival of over 95 per cent. The more aggressive PCLBCL LT has a 5-year disease-specific survival of 50 per cent and is best treated with CHOP-R (cyclophosphamide, vincristine, doxorubicin and prednisolone, and rituximab) chemotherapy followed by involved field radiotherapy to the primary skin lesions and regional lymph nodes.

If radiotherapy planning margins are inadequate, the relapse rate is much higher. It is currently recommended that margins of 2–3 cm are added to the GTV to form the treatment field when planning superficial radiotherapy, and margins of 3–5 cm are added to the GTV when planning electron beam radiotherapy. Lymph node regions are treated in the same way as nodal lymphoma.

Dose-fractionation

PCMZL and PCFCL
15 Gy in 5 daily fractions of 3 Gy given in 1 week.

PCLBCL LT
30 Gy in 15 daily fractions given in 3 weeks.

Kaposi's sarcoma

Radiotherapy can be used for classical Kaposi's sarcoma and as hyperfractionated accelerated adjuvant radiotherapy (HAART) with chemotherapy for human immunodeficiency virus (HIV)-associated Kaposi's sarcoma. It is very useful for treatment of localised lesions and for the palliation of pain, bleeding and oedema. Nodular localised disease can be treated with superficial or electron therapy with a 0.5–1 cm margin. More widespread lower limb skin involvement can be treated by covering the limb in bolus (or placing it in a water bath) to deliver opposing photon beams. Mucosal lesions (such as the mouth and conjunctiva) are best treated with fractionated courses to avoid the severe mucosal reactions to radiotherapy seen in patients with HIV.

■ Dose-fractionation

Skin
8 Gy in a single fraction.
15 Gy in 3 fractions of 5 Gy given in 1 week.

Mucosal
20 Gy in 10 daily fractions given in 2 weeks.

Cutaneous angiosarcoma

Cutaneous angiosarcoma of the scalp and face is a rare condition that primarily affects elderly patients. The tumours have ill-defined margins, are often multifocal and the scalp and face location makes complete resection difficult. It is biologically aggressive with a high risk of metastases and the 5-year survival is 15 per cent with a 50 per cent mortality rate at 15 months.

The primary treatment is surgical excision if possible. In cases with involved or close margins, postoperative adjuvant radiotherapy is advised. For inoperable disease, high dose palliative electron therapy with large margins around the tumour produces local control and palliation. Radiotherapy has been combined with liposomal daunorubicin and with adjuvant recombinant interleukin 2 (rIL2) with reported success. Lesions on the scalp need to be treated with wide margins and often require several electron fields with moving match lines to avoid overdose when matching fields. Lesions involving the face require large electron fields with electron eye shielding.

■ Dose-fractionation

Adjuvant
50 Gy in 25 fractions given in 5 weeks.

Palliative
44 Gy in 11 fractions of 4 Gy given in 3 ½ weeks
   or
60 Gy in 30 daily fractions given in 6 weeks.

Merkel cell carcinoma

Merkel cell carcinoma is a rare primary dermal tumour that is known to have a high local recurrence rate, frequent nodal involvement and high risk of metastases. It most commonly occurs on the head and neck and extremities. The overall 3-year survival is reported as 31–62 per cent. A multidisciplinary approach to treatment is advised. Wide local excision (WLE) of the primary tumour with a 2–3 cm margin is the initial treatment. When the margins are not clear or the tumour is larger than 2 cm in diameter, postoperative adjuvant radiotherapy to the tumour bed and scar using electrons with a 3–5 cm margin should be considered. In patients unfit for surgery or where the tumour is inoperable, radiotherapy can be used as the primary treatment. Chemoradiotherapy gives similar local control and survival results to surgery.

The regional lymph nodes should be managed by sentinel node biopsy followed by a completion lymph node dissection (CLND). For patients with extensive lymph node disease, adjuvant radiotherapy following the CLND can be considered. This is planned in the same way as regional lymph nodes for lymphoma. Locally advanced and metastatic Merkel cell tumours can be treated with standard palliative radiotherapy doses and chemotherapy.

■ Dose-fractionation

Radical radiotherapy
60 Gy in 30 daily fractions given in 6 weeks.

Radical chemoradiotherapy
50 Gy in 25 daily fractions given in 5 weeks.

Adjuvant tumour bed
50 Gy in 20 daily fractions of 2.5 Gy given in 4 weeks.
45 Gy in 15 daily fractions of 3 Gy given in 3 weeks.

Adjuvant lymph nodes
50 Gy in 25 daily fractions given in 5 weeks.

Keloids

Following surgical excision of keloid scars, radiotherapy can be used to prevent the reformation of scar tissue. Superficial radiotherapy (50–80 kV) is used to treat the surgical scar with a narrow margin. The treatment should be planned to minimise any scatter of radiation to normal tissues and a customised lead cut-out made. The use of radiotherapy for benign conditions such as keloids requires caution, especially in children and young adults given the risk of carcinogenesis. This is particularly true for keloids overlying areas that have been shown to be at increased risk such as the breast and thyroid.

■ Dose-fractionation

9 Gy in a single fraction 24–72 hours after surgery.

Information sources

Bichakjian C K, Lowe L, Lao CD *et al.* (2007) Merkel cell carcinoma: critical review with guidelines for multidisciplinary management. *Cancer* **110**: 1–12.

Botwood N, Lewanski C, Lowdell C (1999) The risks of treating keloids with radiotherapy. *Br J Radiol* **72**: 1222–4.

British Association of Dermatology. Patient information and clinical guidelines. www.bad.org.uk.

Derm IS. Dermatology Information System. www.dermis.net.

Holden CA, Spittle MF, Jones EW (1987) Angiosarcoma of the face and scalp, prognosis and treatment. *Cancer* **59**: 1046–57.

Motley R, Kersey P, Lawrence C (2002) Multiprofessional guidelines for the management of the patient with primary cutaneous squamous cell carcinoma. *Br J Dermatol* **146**: 18–25.

Schlienger P, Brunin F, Desjardins L *et al.* (1996) External radiotherapy for carcinoma of the eyelid. Report of 850 cases treated. *Int J Radiat Oncol Biol Phys* **34**: 277–87.

Senff NJ, Hoefnagel JJ, Neelis KJ *et al.* (2007) Results of radiotherapy in 153 primary cutaneous B cell lymphomas classified according to the WHO-EORTC classification. *Arch Dermatol* **143**: 1520–6.

Telfer NR, Colver G, Bowers PW (1999) Guidelines for the management of basal cell carcinoma. *Br J Dermatol* **141**: 415–23.

Whittaker SJ, Marsden JR, Spittle M *et al.* (2003) Joint British Association of Dermatologists and UK Cutaneous Lymphoma Group guidelines for the management of primary cutaneous T-cell lymphomas. *Br J Dermatol* **149**: 1095–107.

Willemze R, Jaffe ES, Burg G *et al.* (2005) WHO-EORTC classification for cutaneous lymphomas. *Blood* **105**: 3768–85.

8 Head and neck: general considerations

Conformal volume-based radiotherapy of head and neck cancers requires knowledge of anatomy and patterns of spread of disease, which are often specific to each tumour site. This chapter explains the common principles of treatment of these tumours.

Radiotherapy alone with daily 2 Gy fractions is no longer regarded as standard for locally advanced head and neck cancer. Altered fractionation or the addition of chemotherapy or targeted agents improves outcomes in patients able to tolerate a more intensive approach.

Initial patient assessment

Head and neck tumours and their treatments can cause complex anatomical and functional deficits. A thorough initial assessment of tumour and patient factors including function, comorbidity and personal preference is essential to choose the optimal treatment pathway. The ideal forum for this assessment is a multidisciplinary clinic where surgeon and oncologist assess the patient together with input from a clinical nurse specialist, dietician, speech and language therapist and restorative dentist.

The extent of the primary tumour should be clearly recorded in the patient record with the aid of diagrams and photographs. This can be especially useful if postoperative radiotherapy is later recommended. Both sides of the neck should be examined and any palpable lymph nodes recorded with a measurement of their size and position.

Assessments by a dietician and a speech and language therapist are important to document initial functional problems and to plan support through radiotherapy and surgery.

Smoking and alcohol abuse are the two principal causes of head and neck tumours, and their role in cardiovascular and respiratory diseases means patients often have comorbidity.

Cross-sectional imaging to document local tumour extent and assess nodes is recommended in all but very early vocal cord tumours. Histological confirmation should be obtained by fine needle aspiration of lymph nodes or by incisional biopsy of the primary tumour or nodes. Tissue samples should be reviewed by a specialist head and neck pathologist.

Indications for radiotherapy including sequencing with surgery

Although the primary site and involved or at-risk cervical lymph nodes are usually treated with the same modality, it is useful to consider the indications for radiotherapy for the primary site and nodes separately.

■ Primary tumour – curative treatment

If a tumour is technically resectable with clear margins, local control rates with non-surgical therapy can never exceed those with surgery. However, it is important to consider not only tumour control but also long-term function – particularly swallowing and speech. A radiotherapy-based approach can provide equivalent local control rates but better long-term function, as long as there is careful follow-up, so that salvage surgery can be used if tumours recur. Improvements in radiotherapy with more conformal treatments, altered fractionation and the addition of chemotherapy or molecular agents mean that radiotherapy is the treatment of choice for many patients with head and neck cancer. The indications for primary radiotherapy as opposed to primary surgery are considered in site-specific chapters.

■ Primary tumour – adjuvant treatment

After a curative resection the surgeon, pathologist and oncologist should meet to discuss the role and extent of adjuvant radiotherapy. For each patient, the most likely sites of residual disease or recurrence can be specifically targeted with modern radiotherapy techniques. The clearest indication for adjuvant radiotherapy is where resection margins are positive and further surgery is not possible. It should also be considered when factors predicting local recurrence after surgery are present, including locally advanced tumours (usually T 3/4), close resection margins (<5 mm), high grade and perineural or vascular invasion. A clinicopathological discussion is especially important when a laser excision has been carried out. The piecemeal excision of a tumour and frozen section analysis of radial margins will preclude measurement of margins of excision, which is the most useful indicator of the need for adjuvant radiotherapy.

■ Cervical nodes – prophylactic treatment

Historical series of neck dissections or observational follow-up provide the best evidence for estimating the risk of recurrence in clinically negative neck nodes. If the risk is ≥20 per cent the relevant nodal levels should be removed surgically or irradiated prophylactically. Modern imaging techniques are more likely to discover enlarged nodes and stage patients N+ so patients may be upstaged when compared with historical controls. The AJCC TNM (6th edition, 2002) staging for head and neck nodes – excluding nasopharyngeal and thyroid cancer – is shown in Table 8.1.

Selecting the appropriate nodal levels depends on a thorough knowledge of lymph node drainage pathways of the head and neck as well as data from previous series of patients found to have nodal metastases when clinically N0.

The choice of surgery or radiotherapy to treat the N0 neck usually depends on the treatment of the primary tumour.

Table 8.1 AJCC TNM (6th edn, 2002*) nodal staging for head and neck cancer except nasopharynx and thyroid

Nx	Regional lymph nodes cannot be assessed
N0	No regional lymph node metastasis
N1	Metastasis in a single ipsilateral lymph node, ≤3 cm in greatest dimension
N2a	Metastasis in a single ipsilateral lymph node >3 cm and ≤6 cm in greatest dimension
N2b	Metastasis in multiple ipsilateral lymph nodes, all ≤6 cm in greatest dimension
N2c	Metastasis in bilateral or contralateral lymph nodes, all ≤6 cm in greatest dimension
N3	Metastasis in a lymph node >6 cm in greatest dimension

*With permission.

■ Cervical nodes – curative treatment

When staging indicates lymph node involvement the neck is treated with a neck dissection, radiotherapy or a combination of the two. Radical dissection of the neck, where all nodal levels are resected with removal of the internal jugular vein, accessory nerve and sternocleidomastoid muscle, is being replaced by more selective approaches sparing these structures and removing nodal levels at high risk of containing tumour. Surgical and CT-based descriptions of lymph node levels are similar though not identical.

If radiotherapy is to be used as treatment of the primary tumour where there is N1 neck disease, radiotherapy alone to selected nodal levels is adequate. For N2 and N3 disease, particularly where nodes are >3 cm in diameter, a combination of surgery and radiotherapy has been recommended. Surgery followed by radiotherapy has the advantages of quickly obtaining local control of disease (useful if there is a rapidly growing mass or skin involvement) and providing definitive staging information. But radiotherapy volumes are more difficult to define with certainty postoperatively than in the unoperated neck and there is increasing evidence that (chemo)radiation alone can control neck disease, particularly when involved nodes are smaller than 3 cm at diagnosis. We recommend initial radiotherapy to selected nodal levels in the neck with consideration of a selective neck dissection 3 months after radiation if there is evidence of residual nodal disease. There is increasing data that PET-CT is most useful in providing this evidence as pathological data have shown that residual lymphadenopathy clinically or on CT or MRI may not contain viable tumour.

■ Cervical nodes – adjuvant treatment

If an initial neck dissection is carried out adjuvant radiotherapy is recommended if there is macroscopic residual disease (e.g. nodes dissected off the carotid artery), microscopic extracapsular nodal spread or if two or more nodes contain tumour. Adjuvant radiotherapy should also be considered if a single involved node is >3 cm in greatest diameter.

■ Palliative treatment

It is often challenging to select patients for a palliative approach when they present with locally advanced disease that is theoretically curable with surgery and or radiation. When the chance of cure is low or potential cure would entail significant morbidity – for example when a total glossectomy or laryngopharyngectomy is proposed or when comorbidity precludes optimal curative approaches – palliative radiotherapy may provide control of local symptoms such as pain and airways obstruction. Palliative radiotherapy to the primary site can also be useful when metastases are present at diagnosis, or in locally recurrent disease to ameliorate fungating tumour or reduce bleeding.

Dose-fractionation

For many years, daily 2 Gy fractions, 5 days a week, have been regarded as the standard of care in curative radiotherapy for head and neck cancer. In the UK, 66 Gy has often been prescribed to the primary and involved nodes but 70 Gy is the standard dose in most clinical trials and international centres and is recommended here.

In adjuvant radiotherapy 60 Gy has been the standard dose with 66 Gy if there are positive resection margins or extranodal spread.

The prophylactic dose to uninvolved nodal levels has often been 50 Gy. We recommend 44 Gy, as supported by the control arm of the CHART trial and other clinical series, because recurrence rates are equally low and there is no need to match a posterior electron field.

There is now good evidence that improved local control and cure rates can be achieved by using altered fractionation regimens, by combining drugs with radiation, or possibly by a combination of these approaches. The choice depends on the resources and philosophy of the treating clinician, but for locally advanced (T3/4 or N+) head and neck cancer in patients able to tolerate more aggressive therapy, one of these methods should be used.

Each of these approaches not only improves local control but also increases acute and/or late side effects, suggesting that they make dose escalation possible rather than improving the therapeutic ratio. Careful collection of data on side effects is as important as local control rates in assessing outcomes.

Refining target volumes in the context of increasingly conformal radiotherapy will, on the other hand, improve the therapeutic ratio. Better imaging techniques and clinical expertise lead to more accurate selection and definition of target volumes, and improvements in treatment delivery such as IMRT lead to more conformal dose solutions. This allows the same dose to be delivered to the tumour with reduced side effects or may make dose escalation possible without increasing side effects.

■ Accelerated radiotherapy

Accelerated radiation schedules shorten the overall treatment time to reduce tumour repopulation during a course of radiotherapy and theoretically increase local control or cure. Examples of pure accelerated techniques include using 6 fractions per week (DAHANCA) or a concomitant boost schedule where the smaller second phase volume is treated at the same time as the larger prophylactic volume rather than after it (Fig. 8.1). Between fractions given on the same day there should be a gap of at least 6 hours to allow normal tissues to repair sublethal damage.

Individual trials and meta-analyses have shown an improvement in local control with accelerated regimens of 7–10 per cent but an absolute survival benefit has been harder to demonstrate. Acute effects are increased so careful support through radiotherapy is necessary. There is also evidence that late effects are increased.

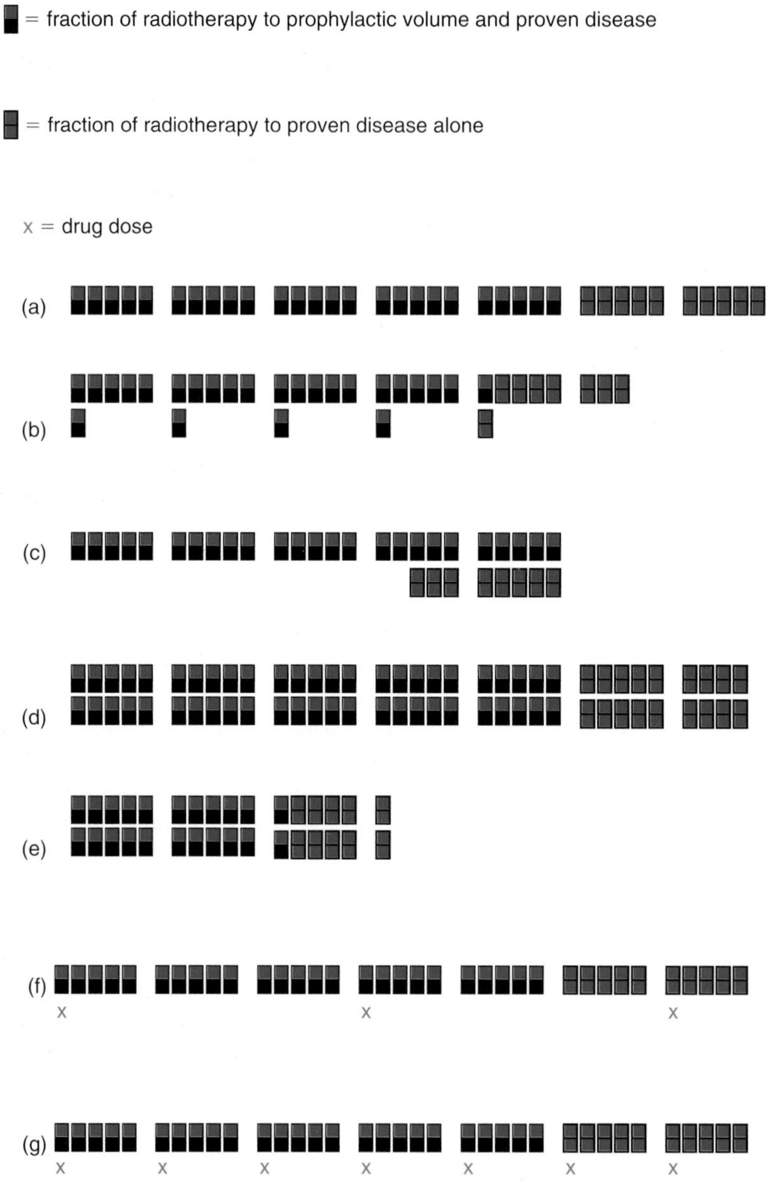

■ = fraction of radiotherapy to prophylactic volume and proven disease

▤ = fraction of radiotherapy to proven disease alone

x = drug dose

Figure 8.1 Schematic examples of fractionation and radiochemotherapy schedules for head and neck cancer. (a) Conventional 2 Gy/fraction. (b) Accelerated DAHANCA – 6 fractions/week. (c) Concomitant boost. (d) Hyperfractionation (1.2 Gy/fraction). (e) GORTEC very accelerated regimen (2 Gy/fraction). (f) Radiochemotherapy with 3 weekly cisplatin. (g) Radiochemotherapy with weekly cisplatin or cetuximab.

The GORTEC group has used a very accelerated regimen of twice daily 2 Gy fractions throughout a course of treatment and shown that 62–64 Gy over 32–33 days produces better local control and equivalent survival to 70 Gy in 35 daily fractions but with more acute toxicity.

■ Hyperfractionation

Reducing the dose per fraction (usually 1.0–1.2 Gy) and using two fractions per day should, according to radiobiological principles, reduce the risk of late effects for the same dose and allow dose escalation with an improved therapeutic ratio. An example is the RTOG 9003 schedule of 1.2 Gy given twice daily to a total dose of 81.6 Gy in 68 fractions. A meta-analysis suggests improvement in local control and overall survival of 8 per cent at 5 years with hyperfractionation. Again, acute effects are increased with hyperfractionated regimens.

■ Altered fractionation – hyperfractionation and acceleration

Many altered fractionation regimens are both accelerated and hyperfractionated. The CHART protocol uses 54 Gy in 36 fractions of 1.5 Gy over 12 days and has been shown to produce equivalent local control to 66 Gy in 33 daily fractions. The benefit of altering fractionation needs to outweigh the total dose reduction necessary to make acute side effects tolerable.

■ Hypofractionation

There is evidence that more hypofractionated regimens can produce local control and survival rates comparable with the regimens described above but there are few RCT data to support this. Examples are: 50 Gy in 16 fractions, 55 Gy in 20 fractions and 60 Gy in 25 fractions. A shorter overall treatment time will reduce the risk of tumour repopulation at the cost of a theoretical increase in late effects due to the higher dose per fraction. The small volumes in early laryngeal cancer make this less of a concern and 55 Gy in 20 fractions is used for T1/2 N0 laryngeal tumours in many centres.

■ Palliative

When the goal of treatment is to improve symptoms and quality of life, a short course of radiotherapy with minimal side effects is ideal. Several regimens have been advocated including 20 Gy in 5 daily fractions and 30 Gy in 5 fractions (treating twice a week). Such regimens improve symptoms in between 50 and 70 per cent of patients and responses typically last for some months.

Radiotherapy with chemotherapy

■ Concomitant radiotherapy and chemotherapy

Chemotherapy given during a course of conventionally fractionated radiation improves survival compared with radiation alone. A meta-analysis confirms an absolute improvement in survival of 8 per cent with various chemotherapy regimens in the curative setting. Cisplatin-based chemotherapy is particularly effective. Carboplatin is substituted in renal impairment or if cisplatin is not tolerated. Concomitant chemotherapy increases the acute side effects of radiation – particularly the intensity and duration of mucositis. There is less good evidence to quantify late effects of combined regimens.

Cisplatin-based chemotherapy is most commonly used with a small weekly dose (30–$40\,mg/m^2$) or larger dose every 3 weeks ($100\,mg/m^2$). Regimens including 5-fluorouracil may increase mucositis. There are theoretical and practical advantages to a weekly schedule: the chemotherapy is present for more fractions, there are fewer side effects, and it is easier to omit chemotherapy if acute toxicity is a problem. The chemotherapy is usually given early in the week and before that day's fraction of radiotherapy, but there is no evidence that the timing of chemotherapy is critical.

■ Concomitant radiotherapy with cetuximab

Cetuximab is a humanised monoclonal antibody against the epidermal growth factor receptor (EGFR) which is overexpressed in many head and neck cancers. An RCT adding cetuximab to conventional radiotherapy showed improvements in overall survival and local control comparable with that obtained with radiochemotherapy. Mucositis is not increased but cetuximab does cause an acneiform rash which can be severe.

■ Concomitant radiotherapy and hypoxic sensitisers

Hypoxic cell sensitisers attempt to mimic the effects of oxygen in fixing radiation-induced DNA damage in tissues thereby increasing cell kill. The DAHANCA 5-85 trial combined EBRT with nimorazole, and showed an improvement in local control compared with EBRT alone.

■ Altered fractionation with concomitant chemotherapy

Altering fractionation or adding cisplatin or cetuximab to conventional EBRT gives similar improvements in local control and overall survival with increased acute toxicity and no good evidence of worsening late toxicity. Radiochemotherapy is the most frequently used of these strategies as it requires less resource, at least for the delivery of EBRT. The next step is to see if these approaches can be combined to improve the therapeutic ratio and therefore local control and cure rates.

■ Induction chemotherapy

The excellent (50–70 per cent) response rate of head and neck cancers to cisplatin-based chemotherapy makes the idea of induction chemotherapy, given before radiation, attractive but the evidence shows only a non-significant 2 per cent improvement in overall survival. Chemotherapy can be started quickly, can reduce the volume of disease and theoretically make curative EBRT more likely to succeed, and may reduce the rate of distant metastases.

The side effects of induction chemotherapy mean that a proportion of patients will be less well equipped to deal with the toxicity of subsequent radiochemotherapy. There is also a concern that increasing the overall duration of anticancer therapy may lead to tumour repopulation and may negate any benefit of smaller treatment volumes. Radiochemotherapy as the gold standard for definitive treatment must not be compromised by induction chemotherapy.

Brachytherapy

Brachytherapy can be used as definitive treatment for small tumours of the lip, oral tongue, floor of mouth and buccal mucosa, when expertise is available. It can also be used to boost dose to primary tumour after EBRT. Treatment with intraluminal catheters can increase dose to the primary site in nasopharyngeal cancer. Interstitial brachytherapy can be used to aid local control in the neck where there is extracapsular spread.

Re-irradiation

Potentially curative re-irradiation can be given in highly selected patients with unresectable local recurrence after previous radiotherapy or for an adjacent unresectable second primary tumour. The disease-free interval should be at least 2 years, and the volume as small as possible. The patient should have excellent performance status and be fully aware of the increased risk of potentially serious late effects. IMRT can be useful to conform dose more closely to target volumes and to minimise the volume treated to a high dose. In some cases, though, it may be preferable to use a simpler solution, as IMRT will irradiate a greater volume of tissue, albeit to a lower dose, and therefore overlap more with previously irradiated volumes.

3D data acquisition

■ Immobilisation

The proximity of tumour to critical normal tissues in head and neck cancer with relatively limited intra-fractional motion of organs means that good immobilisation will enable smaller treatment margins and reduce side effects.

A Perspex shell constructed from a plaster cast of the patient has been regarded as the most accurate way of immobilising the patient. This is usually constructed with the patient supine with their head on a customised head rest and as flat as possible to maintain the spinal cord parallel to the couch top. Some patients, particularly those with excessive secretions, need to have their head more elevated. The shell should be fixed to the couch top in at least five places to reduce movement (Fig. 8.2). A mouth bite can be used to push the hard palate away from the treated volume in oral cavity tumours or to depress the tongue when sinonasal tissues are treated. Grip bars at the side of the couch may help to pull the shoulders inferiorly. Once anterior and lateral reference marks have been made on the shell, selected parts can be cut out to reduce skin dose in regions where full dose to the skin is not required. An anterior midline tattoo below the inferior extent of the shell is useful to improve shoulder alignment. Modern thermoplastic materials can immobilise patients to a similar degree of accuracy and have a skin-sparing effect.

All immobilisation solutions can induce anxiety in patients prone to claustrophobia. The skill of the radiographers and technicians can help alleviate this but some patients need benzodiazepines or hypnotherapy to relax them in order to construct a mask that will be tolerable and practical.

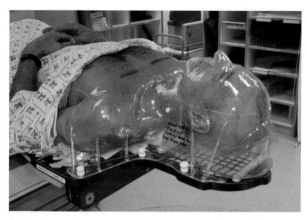

Figure 8.2 Perspex immobilisation shell fixed to the couch top in six places.

Each department should assess the random and systematic errors of their immobilisation system to determine the margin to be added from the CTV to the PTV. A margin of 3 mm should be achievable with high quality immobilisation.

■ CT scanning

Ideally, CT slices should be 3 mm (but no more than 5 mm) thick to aid accurate target volume definition and to produce good quality DRRs for verification. Intravenous contrast will highlight the internal jugular vein and may help to define involved lymph nodes more accurately but is not essential when diagnostic imaging is available. Lateral and midline reference marks are drawn on the shell.

Fusing MRI and CT scans can help to define both tumour volumes and critical normal tissues (e.g. optic chiasm, lacrimal glands) particularly in sinonasal (Fig. 8.3) and oropharyngeal tumours or those involving the skull base.

Target volume definition

General principles for target volume definition which can be applied throughout the head and neck are defined here.

■ GTV

The GTV is defined as the primary tumour and any lymph nodes over 10 mm in short axis dimension or smaller nodes with necrotic centres or rounded contours thought to contain tumour. If induction chemotherapy has been used, the post-chemotherapy GTV is contoured, but the pre-chemotherapy extent of tumour should be included in the CTV70.

The diagnostic images and records and photographs of initial evaluation (in clinic or at examination under anaesthesia [EUA]) are critical to assess the extent of the primary tumour and the exact site of involved lymph nodes. Discussion with the surgeon performing the endoscopic assessment and with an experienced radiologist will enable GTV to be defined as accurately as possible. A planning CT scan done at an interval after the diagnostic one should be carefully reviewed for evidence of residual local disease after surgery or unexpected new cervical

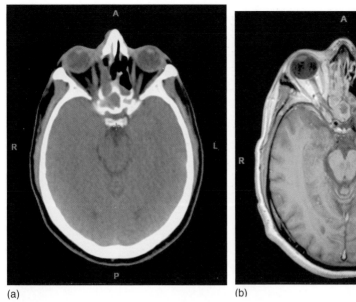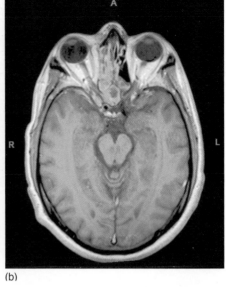

(a)   (b)

Figure 8.3 Adjuvant radiotherapy of an ethmoid tumour. (a) Planning CT. (b) Fused MRI–CT of the same axial slice to help to define volumes and critical normal structures. Note ethmoid opacities seen on CT are shown to be postoperative secretions on MRI.

lymphadenopathy. We recommend reviewing the planning system settings with a radiologist and defining optimal settings for each region of the body, always using these settings when defining volumes.

Starting on a central slice of the primary tumour, the GTV is defined on each axial CT image moving superiorly and then inferiorly. Involved nodes can then be defined in the same way. Viewing the GTV on coronal and sagittal DRRs ensures consistency of definition between slices so that no artificial steps in the volume are created. A volume should not be cut and pasted onto sequential slices for risk of pasting an error: it is more accurate to redraw the GTV on each slice. If there are slices where the GTV cannot be defined – for example due to dental artefact – the planning software will usually allow the missing contours to be interpolated from those either side.

■ Primary tumour CTV (CTV-T)

We recommend growing the GTV by an isotropic margin of 10 mm except where there are natural tissue barriers on the basis that a surgical margin of 10 mm is considered adequate for local excision. The CTV is then edited slice by slice – again starting in the centre of the volume – to subtract air and adjacent structures such as bone which are definitely not involved. The CTV margin can be locally expanded by more than 10 mm if local structures such as muscle or soft tissue are at risk of involvement (Fig. 8.4).

■ Postoperative primary tumour CTV

It is more difficult to specify guidance for CTV definition postoperatively as the anatomy is distorted by the resection and by any reconstructive myocutaneous flaps. A discussion between surgeon, pathologist and oncologist is important to

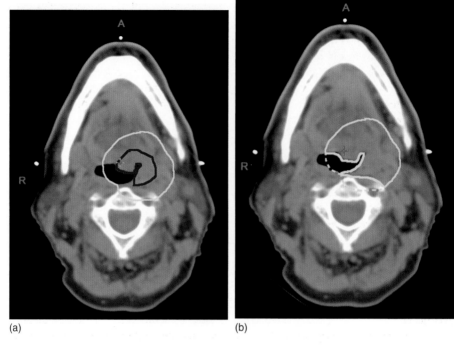

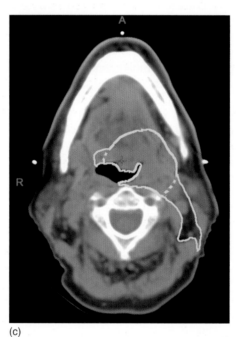

Figure 8.4 Step-wise CTV definition for a left tonsillar cancer invading the base of tongue. (a) GTV is grown isotropically by 10 mm to produce a CTV. (b) CTV is edited off uninvolved bone and air. (c) CTV is expanded to cover possible invasion of the contralateral base of tongue and to include adjacent level II nodes.

define the exact anatomical sites at risk of residual disease. Radio-opaque clips used to mark close or involved margins can be helpful but should not be confused with vascular ligation clips which may be distant to the original tumour. It is not known whether the whole operative field should be included in the CTV but a more individualised, selective approach seems reasonable. It is sometimes useful to define the site of the preoperative GTV on the planning CT to orientate the possible sites of microscopic disease but this is less helpful when the anatomy is very different following a major resection. If there is bulky residual disease a GTV can be defined and expanded to form the CTV as above.

■ Cervical lymph node CTV (CTV-N)

In previous decades head and neck radiation fields included all lymph nodes on both sides of the neck for all but small or well-lateralised tumours. Surgical evidence that a selective approach to neck dissection is as effective as more radical operations, and the ability to create and treat relevant smaller nodal volumes, has changed this approach.

Defining nodal CTVs requires both selection of appropriate nodal levels and delineation of those levels on the CT dataset. Selection is covered in individual tumour chapters as it will necessarily differ for each site and stage of disease. Often two nodal CTVs are selected – a high risk volume containing involved nodes or those close to the primary site and a lower risk volume containing levels thought to be at risk of microscopic disease. These are labelled according to dose, e.g. CTV44.

■ Lymph node delineation

There are published guidelines for delineation of nodal CTVs in the node-negative, node-positive and postoperative neck. It is very useful to have these guidelines available when defining nodal CTVs. The consensus guidelines for the node-negative neck are available as an online atlas and specify CT anatomy of nodal levels in the neck. The retropharyngeal nodes, levels Ia, Ib and II–V, are defined according to CT-based anatomical criteria which correspond closely to the surgical definitions of nodal levels (Table 8.2; Fig. 8.5).

In the node-positive neck, two further volumes are defined. When level II nodes contain tumour, the fatty retrostyloid space around the jugulo-carotid vessels between the superior portion of level II and the skull base should be outlined. A nodal space corresponding to the supraclavicular fossa is contoured when level IV or lower level V nodes contain tumour (Table 8.3).

The nodal volumes in the positive neck are adjusted from the guidelines for the node-negative neck to take account of the risk of extracapsular spread, usually into adjacent muscles. Nodal size is related to the risk of extracapsular spread with 25 per cent of 10 mm nodes and 80 per cent of 30 mm nodes having breached the capsule. Where involved nodes are large or where adjacent structures look involved on imaging, that structure should be included in the nodal CTV. Muscle fascia provides a barrier to tumour invasion but once breached, tumour can spread longitudinally along muscle fibres. It is not known whether part or all of an involved muscle should be included in the CTV (Fig. 8.6).

It should be remembered that the division into nodal levels is on anatomical and not functional grounds. Where a low level II node contains tumour it is appropriate

Table 8.2 CT-based anatomical guidelines for the delineation of nodal volumes in the N0 neck (from Gregoire et al. 2003*)

Level	Cranial	Caudal	Anterior	Posterior	Lateral	Medial
	Anatomical boundaries					
RP	Base of skull	Cranial edge of body of hyoid bone	Fascia under the pharyngeal mucosa	Prevertebral muscles	Medial edge of internal carotid artery	Midline
Ia	Geniohyoid muscle, plane tangential to basilar edge of mandible	Plane tangential to body of hyoid bone	Symphysis menti, platysma muscle	Body of hyoid bone	Medial edge of anterior belly of digastric muscle	N/A
Ib	Mylohyoid muscle, cranial edge of submandibular gland	Plane through central part of hyoid bone	Symphysis menti, platysma muscle	Posterior edge of submandibular gland	Basilar edge/inner side of mandible, platysma muscle, skin	Lateral edge of anterior belly of digastric muscle
II	Caudal edge of lateral process of C1	Caudal edge of body of hyoid bone	Posterior edge of submandibular gland, anterior edge of internal carotid artery, posterior edge of posterior belly of digastric muscle	Posterior edge of sternocleidomastoid muscle	Medial edge of sternocleidomastoid	Medial edge of internal carotid artery, paraspinal muscles
III	Caudal edge of body of hyoid bone	Caudal edge of cricoid cartilage	Posterolateral edge of sternohyoid muscle, anterior edge of sternocleidomastoid muscle	Posterior edge of sternocleidomastoid	Medial edge of sternocleidomastoid	Medial edge of internal carotid artery, paraspinal muscles
IV	Caudal edge of cricoid cartilage	2 cm cranial to sternoclavicular joint	Anteromedial edge of sternocleidomastoid	Posterior edge of sternocleidomastoid	Medial edge of sternocleidomastoid	Medial edge of internal carotid artery, paraspinal muscles
V	Cranial edge of body of hyoid bone	CT slice including the transverse cervical vessels	Posterior edge of sternocleidomastoid	Anterior border of trapezius muscle	Platysma muscle, skin	Paraspinal muscles
VI	Caudal edge of body of thyroid cartilage	Sternal manubrium	Platysma muscle, skin	Separation between trachea and oesophagus	Medial edges of thyroid gland, skin and anteromedial edge of sternocleidomastoid	N/A

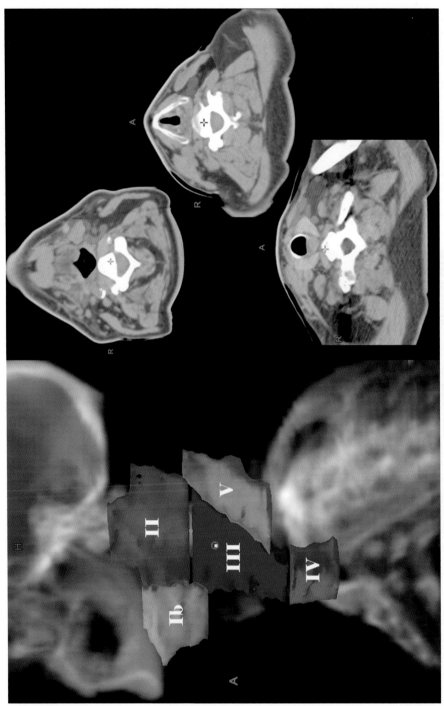

Figure 8.5 Lateral DRR and corresponding axial planning CT slices to illustrate cervical lymph node levels Ib and II, levels III and V, and level IV.

Table 8.3 CT-based anatomical guidelines for delineation of the retrostyloid space and supraclavicular fossa (from Gregoire *et al.* 2006*)

Level	Anatomical boundaries					
	Cranial	Caudal	Anterior	Posterior	Lateral	Medial
Retrostyloid	Base of skull (jugular foramen)	Upper limit of level II	Parapharyngeal space	Vertebral body/base of skull	Parotid space	Lateral edge of RP nodes
Supraclavicular fossa	Lower border of level IV/V	Sternoclavicular joint	Sternocleidomastoid muscle, skin, clavicle	Anterior edge of posterior scalenus muscle	Lateral edge of posterior scalenus muscle	Thyroid gland/ trachea

*With permission.

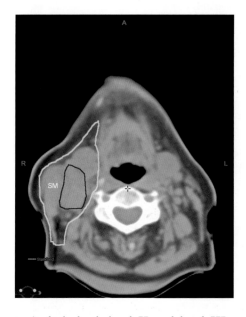

Figure 8.6 Level II node with possible extracapsular spread into sternocleidomastoid muscle (SM). Nodal clinical target volume is therefore extended to cover the whole muscle.

to include both level II and level III nodes within the high dose CTV. When a matched anterior neck field is used to treat the uninvolved low neck, nodal volumes need not be defined. If there are involved nodes in the low neck, nodal GTV and CTV should be contoured to ensure adequate coverage (see below).

For postoperative neck irradiation, the whole operative field is usually defined in the CTV, particularly when there was extracapsular spread. Where nodes abutted muscles or other structures not removed at operation, those structures should be included in the CTV.

■ PTV

Each CTV is grown isotropically to create a PTV. By recording and analysing systematic and random errors in a series of patients, CTV-PTV margins for each centre can be defined, with the assumption that there is no intra-fractional organ motion in the head and neck. Such margins are usually 3–5 mm.

■ OAR and PVR

OAR are outlined in a similar fashion to the GTV – on serial axial CT slices. Ideally, the tumour volumes should be hidden or turned off so that they do not compromise OAR definition. Depending on the location of the PTV, OAR contours will include the spinal cord, parotid glands, optic nerves and chiasm, lacrimal glands and lenses. With more information on how DVHs relate to side effects, contouring of other structures such as the pharyngeal constrictor muscles may be useful in the future.

Owing to the catastrophic effect of late spinal cord damage, the spinal cord PRV is usually defined either by adding an isotropic 5 mm margin round the cord or by contouring the bony spinal canal as a surrogate for the cord PRV. Some centres also recommend adding a 3–5 mm margin to the optic nerves and chiasm to create PRVs.

Dose solutions

Dose solutions for tumour subtypes will be covered in the relevant chapters but general principles are covered here.

■ Conventional/conformal

Anterior neck field

The standard conventional beam arrangement of opposing lateral beams or a unilateral plan to treat the primary site and involved nodes is matched to an anterior neck beam. With this arrangement recurrences in the low neck are uncommon but if nodal volumes are delineated as described above, a 6 MV anterior photon beam will not provide adequate coverage of nodal volumes (Fig. 8.7). In most patients the risk of recurrence in the low neck is low, and we recommend continuing with an anterior beam. The lateral border is 1 cm lateral to the intersection of the first rib and clavicle on a posteroanterior radiograph and the inferior border is at the inferior head of the clavicle. If the target volume is unilateral the medial border is 1 cm from midline to avoid the cord, pharynx and larynx. If it is bilateral, 2 cm midline shielding is added. MLC shielding is used inferior to the clavicle to spare the apex of the lung (Fig. 8.8).

When the low neck is included in the high risk volume (e.g. involved level IV nodes or in the high risk postoperative neck) the nodal CTV should be formally delineated. Either anteroposterior opposing photon beams can be used (which will increase dose to the posterior neck) or an anterior beam with dose prescribed at 3 cm depth is used to improve coverage at the expense of a hot-spot underneath the skin surface.

Matching techniques

The common practice of using an anterior beam to treat the low neck nodes necessitates matching at the junction with superior fields. The problems are the divergent edges of the photon beams in different planes and the beam penumbra.

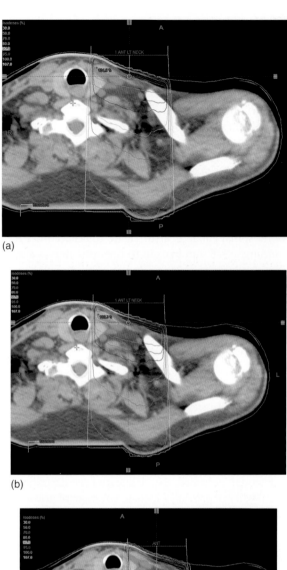

(a)

(b)

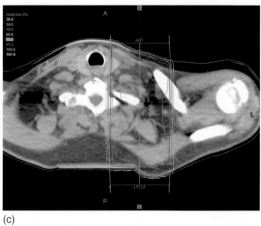

(c)

Figure 8.7 Possible beam arrangements for prophylactic treatment of low neck (level IV) nodes. Beam edges are chosen as described in the text. (a) Anterior beam prescribed to D_{max}. (b) Anterior beam prescribed to 3 cm. (c) Anterior and posterior opposing beams.

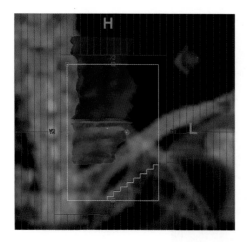

Figure 8.8 Standard borders of an anterior neck beam to treat the low neck prophylactically. The superior border is determined by the inferior extent of the high dose planning target volume. Sites of normal level III (blue) and IV (pink) nodal volumes are shown for illustration.

The most elegant solution – which deals with both problems – is to use a single isocentre technique. Both the anterior neck beam and the plan superior to it use only half the beam (the other half shielded by an asymmetric jaw) so that they match at the isocentre without penumbra or beam divergence.

Another technique is to calculate angles required so that both beam edges diverge perpendicular to the match plane. This will result in slight overlap at depth as the width of the penumbra increases. Simpler solutions are to match the beams at the 50 per cent (light beam) isodose or to leave a gap of 5–10 mm on the skin surface. Both will produce a perfect match at one depth but underdose anterior to this and overdose posteriorly where the divergent beams overlap.

The level at which the anterior beam is matched depends on the PTV. Ideally it should be below the high dose PTV or in between nodal CTVs as matches overlying the PTV risk underdosing disease at the match plane. If this is unavoidable the junction can be moved by 1 cm half way through the course of treatment to blur this match.

Electron therapy

If IMRT is not available, electron beams of 9–12 MeV may be used to treat posterior nodes overlying the spinal cord, especially if the prescribed dose would exceed spinal cord tolerance, i.e. if 50 Gy in 25 fractions is chosen as the prophylactic dose rather than 44 Gy in 22 fractions. The lateral 'bowing' of electron isodoses at depth means perfect matching with the photon beam is not possible so a compromise of matching the 50 per cent photon surface isodose with the 50 per cent electron surface isodose is usually chosen (Fig. 8.9). This is achieved by matching the edges of the two light beams on the surface of the shell. With CT algorithms for electron beams it is possible to view electron isodoses on a three-dimensional plan so that underdosing at areas of high risk (e.g. involved nodes) can be avoided if possible.

Tissue equivalent bolus

When volumes are defined as described above, the nodal PTV often comes close to the skin surface. Unless there is felt to be a risk of tumour in the epidermis or dermis, it is preferable to accept a slight underdosing of this part of the volume rather than use tissue equivalent bolus which will increase skin reactions significantly.

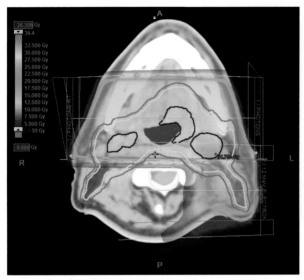

Figure 8.9 Treatment of a high dose planning target volume extending posterior to the spinal cord. Opposing photon beams are matched to 12 MeV electrons. Note the hot-spot created by the lateral bowing of electron isodoses at depth and the unavoidable matching close to the GTV. Only the left electron beam is shown for illustration purposes.

■ Complex

IMRT is particularly useful for head and neck tumours, given the concave PTVs and their proximity to critical structures. IMRT offers parotid sparing in oropharyngeal and some nasopharyngeal cancers to reduce the risk of xerostomia, avoids the risk of underdosing or overdosing at photon–electron junctions and provides a more uniform dose distribution in sinonasal and nasopharyngeal tumours.

In the future, careful mapping of recurrent disease and improved knowledge of the relationship between toxicity and critical organ doses should allow volume definition to be refined so that increased dose can be given to the tumour with tolerable side effects – thereby improving cure. This will be enhanced by the ability to paint dose to areas of highest risk of recurrence as identified by functional imaging or radiogenomics.

Treatment delivery and verification

■ Gaps in treatment delivery

Squamous cell cancers of the head and neck are particularly sensitive to prolongation of a course of treatment so gaps in therapy should be avoided whenever possible. If an unintended gap occurs, hyperfractionation is used, avoiding days when chemotherapy is also given.

■ Verification

Several off-line and online strategies for verification and correction are described. A commonly used protocol is for the treatment isocentre on lateral and anterior DRRs from the CT simulation to be compared with EPIs from the treatment machine taken on days 1–3 and weekly thereafter. An off-line correction is made relative to the isocentre position if the mean error in any one plane is >3 mm. If there is a >5 mm error on any one day the patient should not be treated until the error has been corrected. Re-verification in the simulator or a repeat planning CT scan may be required.

■ Inter-fractional motion

During a course of head and neck radiotherapy, tumour shrinkage or unintentional weight loss can occur leading to two problems.

First, immobilisation may become less effective introducing error into treatment delivery. The mould room technician may be able to adjust the immobilisation but if there is concern that subsequent changes in the set-up are significant (i.e. outside the margin allowed for systematic and random errors), the planning CT should be repeated. The original beam arrangement is then overlaid onto the new CT dataset and corrections made as necessary. If the immobilisation cannot be corrected either a new plan must be created with a larger CTV-PTV margin to account for the increased motion or a new shell must be constructed. Either runs the risk of introducing a gap in the course of treatment.

Second, a reduction in tissue volume (usually manifest as a gap between the shell and the skin) may mean the beam penetrates more deeply towards critical normal tissues, increasing the risk of damage. In these cases repeating a planning or cone-beam CT can provide reassurance or enable the plan to be changed.

Patient care before and during radiotherapy

The severity of acute side effects of head and neck radiotherapy mandates meticulous assessment and support before, during and after radiotherapy. This is particularly important where dose escalation with altered fractionation and/or concomitant drugs are used. Those most at risk of nutritional problems are single men and this should be taken into account when supporting them through treatment or even when deciding on dose-escalation approaches.

■ Dental assessment

Before radiotherapy commences, a thorough dental assessment should be carried out and an orthopantomogram (OPG) performed to look for signs of decay in teeth likely to be within the treated volume. Any teeth at risk of decay should be removed to avoid the potential for radionecrosis and chronic infection that can occur when dental work is carried out in a previously irradiated mouth or in patients with xerostomia. Patients should be given advice about maintaining good oral hygiene.

■ Smoking

Continued smoking increases the severity of mucositis, and patients still smoking should be offered formal cessation advice.

■ Haemoglobin

There is evidence that low haemoglobin predicts poor outcomes in head and neck cancer. There is less good evidence that maintaining haemoglobin above 12 g/dL with transfusions improves survival. Erythropoietin is ineffective. Anaemia may therefore be a marker of poor prognosis rather than a correctable influence of survival.

■ Weight loss

The common acute side effects of mucositis, pain, altered taste and altered saliva all contribute to a reduction in calorie intake during radiotherapy. Patients with pre-existing swallowing problems (e.g. tongue base or hypopharyngeal tumours or significant oral or pharyngeal pain) should be assessed by a specialist dietician before radiotherapy. Losing more than 10 per cent weight during treatment is associated with delayed recovery and increased complications as well as making immobilisation more difficult. When a patient is felt to be at risk of losing more than 10 per cent weight during treatment a prophylactic enteral feeding tube is recommended.

During treatment patients should be seen weekly by a dietician as part of a multidisciplinary assessment team (with doctor or specialist radiographer and speech and language therapist) and weighed each week. Soft and high calorie diets and high energy protein-based supplement drinks can be useful to maintain oral intake when it is limited by pain or dysphagia.

Speech and language therapy can be valuable during treatment to maintain effective swallowing, to assess aspiration risk and to advise on vocal care. When swallowing stops completely, rehabilitation after treatment is more difficult and therefore only patients with risk of aspiration should be denied oral intake.

Patients in whom treatment includes part of the eyes (e.g. sinonasal tumours) should be seen regularly throughout treatment by an ophthalmologist for advice on preventing corneal damage with lubricating drops and to treat corneal abrasions or infections promptly.

As mucosal reactions peak up to 2 weeks after therapy, particularly with accelerated fractionation or hypofractionation, careful weekly assessment should continue until acute effects are subsiding.

■ Pain and mucositis

Mucositis and the consequent pain is the principal side effect for most patients having head and neck radiotherapy. Benzydamine hydrochloride (Difflam) is the only substance shown to delay the onset of mucositis in an RCT and should be used four to eight times a day from the start of treatment, diluted with water if necessary. No other topical mouthwashes are of proven value and alcohol-based washes should be avoided. Topical anaesthetic agents such as lidocaine (Xylocaine) can be helpful if used before eating, but they have a short duration of action. *Candida* infections are common and should be treated with fluconazole, or nystatin if not severe.

Pain should be managed proactively with systemic analgesia to avoid a reduction in oral intake as much as possible. Many patients having significant portions of their oral cavity or pharynx irradiated require opioids. Transdermal patches can be especially effective when oral intake is difficult.

Systemic steroids can occasionally be useful if pharyngeal or laryngeal oedema is severe.

■ Saliva and taste

The combination of dysphagia and the build up of thick, sticky saliva is a major problem during treatment. Good oral hygiene is important while a humid atmosphere helps keep secretions moist and easier to swallow. Nausea caused by secretions stimulating the soft palate is best managed with 5-hydroxytryptamine antagonists. Taste is commonly affected by radiotherapy but the mechanisms of dysgeusia are complex and poorly understood.

■ Skin

Skin reactions can be minimised by applying aqueous cream topically four times daily to treated areas. Tight collars should be avoided and men should avoid wet shaving.

key trials

Adelstein DJ, Li Y, Adams GL *et al.* (2003) An Intergroup phase III comparison of standard radiation therapy and two schedules of concurrent chemoradiotherapy in patients with unresectable squamous cell head and neck cancer. *J Clin Oncol* **21**: 92–8.

Bonner JA, Harari PM, Giralt J *et al.* (2006) Radiotherapy plus cetuximab for squamous-cell carcinoma of the head and neck. *N Engl J Med* **354**: 567–78.

Bourhis J, Lapeyre M, Tortochaux J *et al.* (2006) Phase III randomized trial of very accelerated radiation therapy compared with conventional radiation therapy in squamous cell head and neck cancer: a GORTEC trial. *J Clin Oncol* **24**: 2873–8.

Bourhis J, Overgaard J, Audry H *et al.* (2006) Hyperfractionated or accelerated radiotherapy in head and neck cancer: a meta-analysis. *Lancet* **368**: 843–54.

Fu KK, Pajak TF, Trotti A *et al.* (2000) A radiation therapy oncology group (RTOG) phase III randomized study to compare hyperfractionation and two variants of accelerated fractionation to standard fractionated radiotherapy for head and neck squamous cell carcinomas: first report of RTOG 9003. *Int J Radiat Oncol Biol Phys* **48**: 7–16.

Overgaard J, Hansen HS, Sprecht L *et al.* (2003) Five compared with six fractions per week of conventional radiotherapy of squamous-cell carcinoma of head and neck: DAHNACA 6&7 randomised controlled trial. *Lancet* **362**: 933–40.

RTOG 0129: A phase III trial of concurrent radiation and chemotherapy (followed by surgery for residual primary/N2–3 nodal disease) for advanced head and neck carcinomas (standard fractionation v concomitant boost). In progress.

RTOG 0421: A phase III trial for locally recurrent, previously irradiated head and neck cancer: concurrent re-irradiation and chemotherapy versus chemotherapy alone. In progress.

RTOG 0522: A randomised phase III trial of concurrent accelerated radiation and cisplatin versus concurrent accelerated radiation, cisplatin, and cetuximab (C225) (followed by surgery for selected patients) or stage III and IV head and neck carcinomas. In progress.

Information sources

Bernier J, Bentzen SM (2006) Radiotherapy for head and neck cancer: latest developments and future perspectives. *Curr Opin Oncol* **18**: 240–6.

Bernier J, Cooper JS, Pajak TF *et al.* (2005) Defining risk levels in locally advanced head and neck cancers: a comparative analysis of concurrent postoperative radiation plus chemotherapy – trials of the EORTC (#22931) and RTOG (# 9501). *Head Neck* **27**: 843–50.

Cancer Care Ontario Head and Neck Cancer Evidence-based Series and Practice Guidelines [online] (2008). Available at: www.cancercare.on.ca/english/home/toolbox/qualityguidelines/diseasesite/head-neck-ebs/ (accessed 6 October 2008).

Corvo R (2007) Evidence-based radiation oncology in head and neck squamous cell carcinoma. *Radiother Oncol* **85**: 156–70.

Fowler JF (2007) Is there an optimum overall time for head and neck radiotherapy? A review with new modelling. *Clin Oncol* **19**: 8–22.

Gregoire V, Levendag P, Ang KK *et al.* (2003) CT-based delineation of lymph node levels and related CTVs in the node-negative neck: DAHANCA, EORTC, GORTEC, NCIC, RTOG consensus guidelines. *Radiother Oncol* **69**: 227–36.

Gregoire V, Coche E, Gosnard G *et al.* (2004) Selection and delineation of lymph node target volumes in head and neck conformal and intensity-modulated radiation therapy. In: Gregoire V, Scalliet P, Ang KK (eds) *Clinical Target Volumes in Conformal and Intensity-modulated Radiation Therapy*. Springer, Berlin, pp. 69–90.

Gregoire V, Eisbruch A, Hamoir M *et al.* (2006) Proposal for the delineation of the nodal CTV in the node-positive and the post-operative neck. *Radiother Oncol* **79**: 15–20.

Gregoire V, Levendag P. DAHANCA, EORTC, GORTEC, NCIC and RTOG endorsed consensus guidelines for the delineation of the CTV in the N0 neck of patients with head & neck squamous cell carcinoma. [online] Available at: www.rtog.org/hnatlas/main.html (accessed 14 July 2008).

J Clin Oncol (2006) **24** – series of review articles covering controversies in head and neck cancer.

Lengele B, Hamoir M, Scalliet P *et al.* (2007) Anatomical bases for the radiological delineation of lymph node areas. Major collecting trunks, head and neck. *Radiother Oncol* **85**: 146–55.

Pignon JP, Bourhis J, Domenge C *et al.* (2000) Chemotherapy added to locoregional treatment for head and neck squamous-cell carcinoma: three meta-analyses of updated individual data. MACH-NC Collaborative Group. Meta-Analysis of Chemotherapy on Head and Neck Cancer. *Lancet* **355**: 949–55.

Scottish Intercollegiate Guidelines Network Guideline 90 (2006) *Diagnosis and Management of Head and Neck Cancer. A National Clinical Guideline*. Available at: www.sign.ac.uk/guidelines/fulltext/90/index.html.

Lip, ear, nose and treatment of the neck in skin cancer

This chapter describes radiotherapy for squamous cell cancers of the lip, external ear canal and middle ear and nasal vestibule, as well as management of the neck in skin cancers of the head and neck. Superficial skin tumours of the nose and pinna are considered in Chapter 7.

Lip

■ Indications for radiotherapy

Most lip cancers arise on the vermillion border of the lower lip – the junction between the skin and the lip itself – and are diagnosed at an early stage because they are visible. They are usually superficial squamous cell tumours linked to long-term sun exposure and smoking. Surgery, EBRT and brachytherapy all give local control rates of 90 per cent or higher at 5 years. The choice of treatment depends on the expertise available, the likely cosmetic and functional outcomes and patient choice. Radiotherapy is particularly appropriate when the commissure of the lip is involved (as function may not be as good after surgery), and for larger tumours where more extensive resection and reconstruction would be required. Commissure tumours have higher rates of local recurrence than lower lip cancers.

If excision margins are positive or close (<3 mm), adjuvant radiotherapy should be considered if it would result in better function and cosmesis than a further excision. In elderly patients with significant comorbidity it may be appropriate to observe clinically rather than treat with adjuvant radiotherapy, even if margins are close. Involved neck nodes are usually managed with a neck dissection and postoperative radiotherapy if required (see below).

■ Sequencing of multimodality therapy

When adjuvant radiotherapy is indicated it should ideally commence within 6 weeks of surgery but a longer gap may be required to allow adequate recovery from a major resection.

■ Clinical and radiological anatomy

Most lip cancers are superficial and have a low risk of lymph node spread. The relevant nodes should be assessed clinically and with imaging (CT or MRI) of the neck if there is palpable lymphadenopathy. The lymphatic drainage of the lower lip is to ipsilateral level Ib and then level II nodes. The midline portion drains to level Ia and then to bilateral levels Ib and II but there can be direct drainage to level III. The upper lip drains to level Ib, sometimes via the buccal nodes, which lie under the superficial muscle layer of the face (Fig. 9.1).

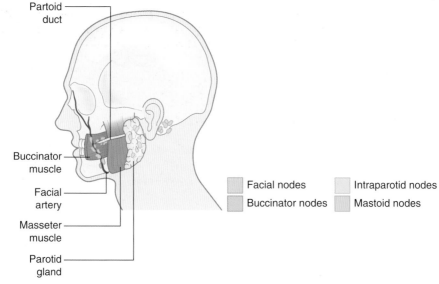

Figure 9.1 Superficial lymph nodes of the head and neck.

■ Assessment of primary disease

Careful clinical examination with a strong light and magnifying lens is essential to define the extent of the tumour. Palpation is used to assess thickness. An OPG and cross-sectional imaging are recommended if bony erosion is suspected.

■ Target volume definition

For small (<2 cm diameter) well-defined tumours, a 3–5 mm margin can be added to the GTV to produce a CTV with a further 5 mm CTV to PTV margin. In practice, the PTV is drawn on the surface of the skin and lip with a fine marker pen using a strong light, magnifying lens and a ruler to measure the margin from the visible GTV. Larger tumours or those with indistinct edges need a larger GTV-CTV margin of 5–10 mm.

When adjuvant radiotherapy is used a 5 mm margin from the resection edge is used to define the CTV.

■ Dose solutions

Most tumours are treated with electrons or superficial X-rays. The PTV should be covered by the 90 per cent isodose of the electron or superficial X-ray beam. Once the PTV has been defined and marked as above, isodose charts are used to select the required energy to give 90 per cent coverage from the surface to the deep margin. Tissue equivalent bolus is used as required either to increase the surface dose or to reduce unwanted deep penetration. The applicator size can then be calculated. If electrons are used, the 90 per cent isodose in the lateral plane is 3–5 mm inside the edge of the applicator, which represents the 50 per cent dose. Electrons bow inwards at depth at higher energies, so if a high energy is chosen the applicator size will need to be correspondingly larger to avoid underdosing the deep lateral margin.

A 3–4 mm thick lead mask is then constructed with a cut-out area over the target volume. An intraoral lead shield is used to protect the gums and teeth from the exit beam. It is lined with wax to absorb secondary electrons.

■ Dose-fractionation

55 Gy in 20 daily fractions of 2.75 Gy given in 4 weeks.

■ Treatment delivery and patient care

Mucositis of the outer and inner lip occurs from the third week of treatment. White soft paraffin is used to keep the lips moisturised and systemic analgesics should be prescribed if necessary. Sunburn and smoking should be avoided.

■ Verification

Verification is by daily inspection of the set-up compared with photographs taken at planning.

■ Other points

Brachytherapy for lip squamous cell cancer

Where technical expertise exists, brachytherapy can produce excellent local control rates, cosmesis and function. The target volume is defined as above. Rigid needles are implanted horizontally along the axis of the lip, using either a single plane for superficial lesions, or three or more sources distributed in a equilateral triangle or square in the cross-sectional plane for deeper tumours. A plastic template can be used to provide stability. Sources are usually 10 mm apart and 5–8 cm long which inevitably means treating most of the lip, making this a useful technique in more extensive tumours or those with indistinct margins (Fig. 9.2).

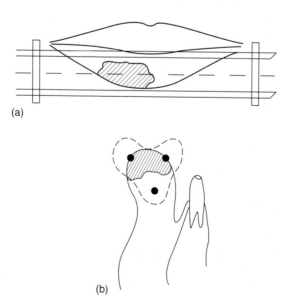

(a)

(b)

Figure 9.2 Three-source implant for carcinoma of the lip. (a) Anterior view. (b) Sagittal view showing arrangement of sources in an equilateral triangle.

Ear

■ Indications for radiotherapy

Cancers of the external auditory canal and middle ear are rare. There is no agreed staging system but most tumours present when locally advanced with bone erosion or cranial nerve palsies. Local invasion and the complexity of a temporal bone resection mean that close or positive resection margins are common. For these patients, surgery and postoperative radiotherapy are recommended and can produce 5-year survival rates of 40–60 per cent. Early tumours confined to the external ear canal without soft tissue or bone involvement can be treated with either primary radiotherapy or surgery.

■ Sequencing of multimodality therapy

When adjuvant radiotherapy is indicated it should ideally commence within 6 weeks of surgery but a longer gap may be required to allow adequate recovery from a major resection.

■ Clinical and radiological anatomy

The external ear canal is a 25 mm long tube with an outer cartilaginous portion and an inner bony segment lined with mucosa. The middle ear contains the ossicles and semicircular canals and communicates posteriorly with the mastoid air cells.

Ulceration and submucosal spread in the ear canal is best assessed by otoscopy. Medially, tumour can spread into the temporal bone (causing VII nerve palsy), around the internal carotid artery and through the Eustachian tube into the nasopharynx. Anterior extension into the temporomandibular joint, parotid gland and masticator space can cause trismus. Posterior spread occurs into the mastoid air cells and thence to the posterior cranial fossa. Superiorly, tumour can invade into the middle cranial fossa and inferiorly into the jugular foramen, causing IX, X and XI cranial nerve palsies, or into the cervical vertebrae.

Lymph node spread at presentation is uncommon. Tumour can spread to the parotid nodes (sometimes divided into the preauricular, subparotid and superficial and deep intraparotid). The posterior part of the external canal drains to the mastoid nodes. Further spread to level II can occur. If tumour reaches the nasopharynx, it can spread to the retropharyngeal nodes.

■ Assessment of primary disease

A combination of clinical examination to look for cranial nerve palsies, MRI for soft tissue extent and CT to evaluate bone destruction is most useful to assess local spread.

■ Data acquisition

Immobilisation

The patient is immobilised lying supine in a custom-made shell with the neck extended to move the orbit superiorly out of the treated volume.

CT scanning

CT slices are obtained from the skull base to the hyoid bone. Slices should be no more than 5 mm thick and ideally 3 mm. Fusion of MR and CT planning images can be particularly helpful to define skull base anatomy.

Simulator

3D conformal planning is recommended in all patients because of the complex anatomy and proximity of critical structures.

■ Target volume definition

Discussion with the surgeon and pathologist is critical to establish the sites at highest risk of recurrence after a temporal bone resection. Preoperative imaging should be available during planning. If there is macroscopic residual disease or positive resection margins can be defined, these sites are contoured as a GTV, ideally with the surgeon. The GTV is expanded isotropically by 10 mm and then edited depending on natural tumour barriers to form a CTV66.

For adjuvant treatment, the CTV60 is contoured on each axial CT slice with the aid of the corresponding slices on preoperative imaging and the operation details, aiming to encompass all resection margins in the CTV60 and to have a 10 mm margin from the resection edge at high risk sites. This 10 mm margin should be individualised depending on natural tumour barriers and possible routes of spread. Though the risk of involvement is low, adjacent parotid, mastoid and high level II nodes are included in the CTV60 as they tend to be superficial to the resection margins and can be treated without an increase in morbidity. The CTV is expanded isotropically to form the PTV by a margin determined for each department by the observed random and systematic errors – usually 3–5 mm.

The brainstem, spinal cord and adjacent temporal lobe should be contoured as organs at risk. The CTV and PTV should be defined without reference to the organs at risk and vice versa. The PTV may end up overlapping a critical structure but the dosimetrist and oncologist can then evaluate the beam arrangements and MLC shielding to balance the risks and benefits. If the CTV or PTV is edited away from an organ at risk to protect that organ, the opportunity to deliver dose to the whole target by an innovative beam arrangement may be lost and the good coverage of the PTV will be falsely reassuring. It is better to accept a compromise in dose to the PTV when the plan is produced, than to guess where this compromise needs to be made at the volume definition stage.

For early external ear canal tumours confined to the mucosa, the GTV as defined by clinical examination is outlined on a planning CT. A 10 mm isotropic margin is added to produce a CTV but this is expanded to include the adjacent temporal bone.

■ Dose solutions

The photon beam arrangement is individualised depending on the PTV, but usually anterior and posterior oblique wedged beams are used, often with an additional lateral beam. The angle of the posterior oblique beam is chosen to avoid the brainstem and spinal cord. Where the PTV comes close to these structures or to the temporal lobe, the risk of late radiation damage must be weighed against the risk of tumour recurrence. The oncologist should take this decision but must inform the patient of the possible risks of late effects and possible benefits of giving more dose to high risk sites.

If a compromise is needed it is better to use two phases of treatment rather than underdose the PTV throughout the whole course. The whole PTV should be included in the phase 1 volume (usually for 20–25 fractions), with a smaller phase 2 shaped with MLCs to protect critical structures. A summated plan is created from the two phases to allow evaluation of DVHs. Numbers of fractions for each phase can be varied so that the best compromise can be achieved for individual patients. It may also be necessary to reduce the total dose to protect OAR (Fig. 9.3).

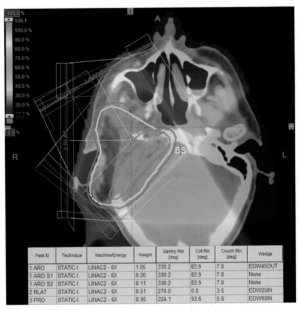

Field ID	Technique	Machine/Energy	Weight	Gantry Rtn [deg]	Coll Rtn [deg]	Couch Rtn [deg]	Wedge
1 ARO	STATIC-I	LINAC2 - 6X	1.05	330.2	83.9	7.0	EDW45OUT
1 ARO S1	STATIC-I	LINAC2 - 6X	0.20	330.2	83.9	7.0	None
1 ARO S2	STATIC-I	LINAC2 - 6X	0.11	330.2	83.9	7.0	None
2 RLAT	STATIC-I	LINAC2 - 6X	0.51	270.0	0.0	3.5	EDW25IN
3 PRO	STATIC-I	LINAC2 - 6X	0.95	224.1	93.6	5.0	EDW60IN

Figure 9.3 Beam arrangement for postoperative external beam radiotherapy of a middle ear tumour with skull base invasion. The PTV60 is covered by the 95 per cent isodose but prescribing 60 Gy would exceed tolerance of the brainstem (BS). The prescribed dose must be reduced or the PTV coverage compromised for at least some of the treatment. A PTV66 (purple) has also been defined to include known positive resection margins.

■ Dose-fractionation

60 Gy in 30 daily fractions given in 6 weeks to PTV60.
66 Gy in 33 daily fractions given in 6½ weeks to PTV66.

Higher doses are associated with an increased risk of osteoradionecrosis of the temporal bone.

■ Treatment delivery and patient care

After a temporal bone resection patients usually have considerable morbidity with cranial nerve palsies affecting swallowing and speech, and a feeding gastrostomy tube is often in place. A dietician and speech and language therapist should assess patients weekly. Although the local acute effects of radiotherapy are limited to skin erythema and localised mucositis, lethargy and anorexia can be debilitating when radiotherapy follows such major surgery. The shell can be cut out over the treated volume to reduce skin reaction if the PTV is not close to the skin surface.

■ Verification

Portal images are compared with DRRs as for other head and neck tumours with *in vivo* dosimetry on the first day of treatment.

Nose

■ Indications for radiotherapy

Cancers of the nasal vestibule behave like skin tumours, are usually diagnosed when small and have a 90 per cent local control rate with radiotherapy or surgery. Radiation gives better cosmesis except for very small lesions. External beam radiotherapy can be combined with brachytherapy. Larger tumours with bone involvement are rare but have a low chance of cure by radiation alone. Resection may be followed by adjuvant radiotherapy.

■ Sequencing of multimodality therapy

When adjuvant radiotherapy is indicated it should ideally commence within 6 weeks of surgery but a longer gap may be required to allow adequate recovery from a major resection.

■ Clinical and radiological anatomy

The nasal vestibule is the entrance to the nasal cavity, lined by squamous epithelium. Tumours of the proximal nasal cavity lined by respiratory epithelium are covered in Chapter 16. The columella is the midline, medial wall of the vestibule and tumours arising here can spread submucosally onto the upper lip or posteriorly along the roof of the hard palate. Cross-sectional imaging with MR or CT is important to define their extent.

Lymph node spread is uncommon at diagnosis but the vestibule drains to levels Ia and Ib or to the buccinator node overlying the buccinator muscle and then to level II.

■ Assessment of primary disease

Careful clinical examination with a strong light and magnifying lens is essential to define the extent of the tumour. Palpation is used to assess thickness.

■ Data acquisition

Immobilisation

The patient is immobilised in a thermoplastic or Perspex shell with wax nostril plugs to help produce a more homogeneous dose distribution.

CT scanning

Slices 3 mm thick are obtained from the inferior orbit to the hyoid bone to include level I nodes.

Simulator

3D conformal therapy is recommended given the small fields required and possible dose inhomogeneities created by adjacent air spaces.

■ Target volume definition

The GTV is outlined on the planning CT scan with the help of clinical examination and diagnostic imaging. To produce the CTV it is easiest to add a 10 mm isotropic margin to the GTV and edit this to take account of natural tumour barriers, air and possible submucosal spread into the lower lip. The CTV-PTV margin is determined by local audit but ideally should be no more than 3 mm.

■ Dose solutions

Two lateral oblique photon beams provide the most conformal coverage plan for the PTV. The angle of the beams is chosen to ensure adequate dose to any posterior extension along the roof of the hard palate. Wax is applied on the external surface of the nose and upper lip as needed to increase the surface dose. The epithelial surface thus becomes encased in wax internally and externally to allow the hollow vestibule to be treated as a block, producing a more homogeneous dose distribution (Fig. 9.4).

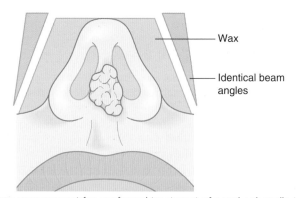

Figure 9.4 Beam arrangement for conformal treatment of nasal columella tumour. Note beams are angled posteriorly to cover possible tumour extension along the roof of the hard palate.

Electrons can also be used for superficial lesions but the contour of the nose, small field sizes and underlying cartilage make conformal photons the preferred solution.

■ Dose-fractionation

55 Gy in 20 daily fractions of 2.75 Gy given in 4 weeks.

Longer fractionation is not necessary given the small volumes treated.

■ Treatment delivery and patient care

The inside of the nasal cavity can become especially sore and topical local anaesthetic or steroid creams as well as systemic analgesics are often needed to enable the patient to tolerate insertion of the wax plugs throughout treatment.

■ Verification

Portal images are compared with DRRs as for other head and neck tumours with *in vivo* dosimetry on the first day of treatment.

Postoperative neck irradiation

■ Indications for radiotherapy

Squamous cell skin cancers of the head and neck may recur in the regional lymph nodes, with a median interval to recurrence of 12 months. Treatment at this time is usually surgical with postoperative radiotherapy indicated unless a neck dissection only reveals a solitary level II–V node without extracapsular spread.

It is possible to identify head and neck skin tumours at higher risk of having occult metastases with size, depth of invasion, high grade and perineural or vascular invasion all increasing the risk. Tumours on or near the external ear are at higher risk of spread to the intraparotid nodes. There is, however, no consensus on the role of prophylactic nodal radiotherapy (or neck dissection) in these tumours.

■ Sequencing of multimodality therapy

Ideally radiotherapy should commence within 6 weeks of surgery, as long as there is adequate healing.

■ Clinical and radiological anatomy

The commonest sites for skin cancers (ear, temple, forehead, anterior scalp and cheek) drain to the intraparotid nodes and thence to level II and on to levels Ib and III–V. Many patients therefore present with a parotid mass. In 25 per cent of patients a primary skin tumour is not identified and a mucosal head and neck tumour should be excluded. The pattern of lymph node spread (intraparotid nodes), immunohistochemistry and the presence of sun-damaged skin may point to the skin as the likely primary source.

■ Assessment of nodal disease

The intraparotid nodes and levels Ib–V should be assessed by clinical examination with MR preferred to CT for imaging the parotid. Surgery usually involves a superficial parotidectomy if there are intraparotid nodes and a neck dissection of levels Ib–III in the clinically negative lower neck. If there are enlarged level Ib–V nodes an appropriate neck dissection is performed.

Discussion with the surgeon and pathologist is important to determine which nodal levels require radiotherapy because of microscopic residual disease or for prophylaxis.

■ Dose solutions

The radiotherapy technique is a combination of that described in Chapter 15 for parotid tumours and in Chapter 8 for the neck. Examples of nodal levels to be covered in the CTV60 and CTV44 are shown in Table 9.1. If the CTV60 includes the parotid bed and low neck, it will be difficult to provide adequate coverage with one plan owing to the change in neck contour. A planned volume superiorly should then be matched to an anterior photon field treating the lower neck with the match plane at a level at relatively low risk of harbouring disease.

Table 9.1 Examples of CTV60 and CTV44 for the neck nodes in head and neck skin squamous cell depending on clinical and pathological findings

Clinically involved nodes	Surgery and pathology	CTV60	CTV44
Intraparotid only	Superficial parotidectomy alone	Parotid bed	Levels Ib, II, III
Intraparotid only	Superficial parotidectomy and level Ib–III dissection. Involved intraparotid nodes only	Parotid bed	Not defined
Intraparotid only	Superficial parotidectomy and level Ib–III dissection. Involved intraparotid and level II nodes*	Parotid bed and level II	Levels Ib, III–V
Intraparotid and neck	Superficial parotidectomy and level Ib–V dissection. Involved intraparotid and level Ib–V nodes*	Parotid bed and levels Ib–V	Not defined

*Neck irradiation can be omitted if there is only one level Ib–V node involved without extracapsular spread.

■ Dose-fractionation

60 Gy in 30 daily fractions given in 6 weeks to PTV60.
66 Gy in 33 daily fractions to sites of positive margins or extracapsular nodal spread.
44 Gy in 22 daily fractions given in 4 ½ weeks to PTV44.

■ Treatment delivery and patient care

See Chapters 8 and 15.

■ Verification

See Chapter 8.

---

key trials

Trans-Tasman Radiation Oncology Group (TROG) trial 05.01. Post-operative concurrent chemo-radiotherapy versus post-operative radiotherapy in high-risk cutaneous squamous cell carcinoma of the head and neck. In progress.

Information sources

De Visscher JGAM, Grond AJK, Botke G *et al.* (1996) Results of radiotherapy for squamous cell carcinoma of the vermilion border of the lower lip. A retrospective analysis of 108 patients. *Radiother Oncol* **39**: 9–14.

Mendenhall WM, Stringer SP, Cassisi NJ *et al.* (1999) Squamous cell carcinoma of the nasal vestibule. *Head Neck* **21**: 385–93.

Ogawa K, Nakamura K, Hatano K *et al.* (2007) Treatment and prognosis of squamous cell carcinoma of the external auditory canal and middle ear: a multi-institutional retrospective review of 87 patients. *Int J Radiat Oncol Biol Phys* **68**: 1326–34.

Veness MJ, Porceddu S, Palme CE *et al.* (2007) Cutaneous head and neck squamous cell carcinoma metastatic to parotid and cervical lymph nodes. *Head Neck* **29**: 621–31.

10 Oral cavity

The oral cavity comprises the anterior two-thirds of the tongue, the floor of mouth, buccal mucosa, hard palate and gingivae (Fig. 10.1). Tumours of the lip are discussed in Chapter 9.

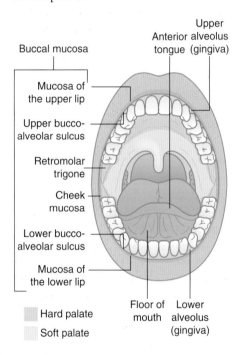

Buccal mucosa

Upper
Anterior alveolus
tongue (gingiva)

Mucosa of
the upper lip

Upper bucco-
alveolar sulcus

Retromolar
trigone

Cheek
mucosa

Lower bucco-
alveolar sulcus

Mucosa of
the lower lip

Hard palate

Soft palate

Floor of   Lower
mouth   alveolus
(gingiva)

Figure 10.1 Subsites of the oral cavity.

Indications for radiotherapy

■ Curative radiotherapy for local disease

For T1 and early T2 tumours, surgery and radiotherapy give equivalent local control rates but only if some or the entire radiation dose is given by brachytherapy. Five-year local control rates for T1 and T2 tumours are 75–95 per cent and 50–85 per cent, respectively. However, brachytherapy is often technically impossible (tumour is close to bone) or the necessary expertise unavailable. Therefore most T1 and T2 tumours of the oral cavity are treated with surgical excision as long as clear margins and good functional outcome can reasonably be expected. Where surgical excision is unlikely to achieve these outcomes, external beam radiation alone is used, most often in the case of a second primary tumour close to a previous resection site. For T1 and T2 cancers of the retromolar trigone, radiotherapy alone can be used if a good functional outcome after surgery is unlikely. There is no proven role for radiotherapy for carcinoma *in situ* of the oral cavity. For tumours of the hard palate, brachytherapy is not technically possible and relative hypoxia in bone may reduce cure rates.

■ Adjuvant radiotherapy for local disease

For larger T2 (>3 cm), T3 and T4 tumours, local control is best achieved by surgery and adjuvant radiotherapy. Adjuvant local radiotherapy is also indicated where a smaller primary tumour is excised with positive margins and the preferred option of further excision is not possible. Where a small primary tumour has been excised with close (<5 mm) margins, a discussion with the surgeon is important to assess the risk of microscopic residual disease. The measured margin must be considered in the context of adjacent structures (whether the margin is adjacent to bone), possible specimen shrinkage, and how easy it may be to detect local recurrence early. Single modality treatment should be the goal for early oral cavity cancer as the best way to maintain function and reduce complications such as osteoradionecrosis. In addition, second primary oral cancers are relatively common and once part of the oral cavity has been irradiated, further surgery or radiation may be difficult. Overall survival rates in locally advanced disease are 40 per cent at best.

■ Radiotherapy to the N0 neck

The clinically and radiologically node negative neck should be treated where the risk of nodal metastases is thought to be ≥20 per cent. Tumours of the floor of mouth or midline tongue or hard palate are at risk of bilateral neck metastases and both sides of the neck should be treated. Several factors increase the risk of occult nodal metastases including depth of primary tumour invasion (≥4 mm), larger primary tumour and site (tongue and floor of mouth tumours are at higher risk owing to richer lymphatic drainage). At risk nodal levels can be treated by a selective neck dissection or radiotherapy.

When surgery is the initial treatment for the primary cancer, a selective neck dissection is usually performed if access to the neck is required for reconstruction, or if the preoperative risk of occult neck metastases is ≥20 per cent. Radiotherapy to the neck is used if histological features of the primary tumour indicate a higher risk of occult metastases than was thought preoperatively, or if radiation is used to treat the primary site. If brachytherapy alone is used to treat the primary it is usually followed by radiation or surgery to the N0 neck (if indicated).

■ Radiotherapy to the N+ neck

When tumour is found in lymph nodes from a neck dissection, adjuvant radiotherapy is recommended unless there is only a solitary positive node ≤3 cm in diameter without extracapsular spread.

If radiation is used to treat the primary disease in a patient with clinically involved lymph nodes, the neck should also be irradiated. Tumours of the floor of mouth or midline tongue or hard palate are at risk of bilateral neck metastases and both sides of the neck should be treated.

■ Palliative radiotherapy

T3 and T4 tumours are best managed by a combination of surgery and adjuvant (chemo) radiation. However, surgery may be inappropriate for locally advanced cancer where clear resection margins are not possible, if the expected functional outcome after surgery is not acceptable to the patient, or if comorbidity precludes surgery. In these cases, radiotherapy alone can be the best method of palliation and may provide a small chance of long-term cure, especially if combined with concomitant chemotherapy.

Sequencing of multimodality therapy

Where EBRT is followed by brachytherapy the overall treatment time should be kept as short as possible to avoid tumour repopulation. A 1-week gap is recommended.

If adjuvant radiotherapy is indicated it should ideally commence 4–6 weeks after surgery but after adequate wound healing has occurred. If radiotherapy is delayed to more than 3 months after surgery because of surgical complications, the potential risks of EBRT may outweigh the benefits.

Concomitant chemotherapy with adjuvant radiotherapy improves local control and disease free survival when there is a high risk of local recurrence, especially if excision margins are positive or there is extracapsular nodal spread.

Clinical and radiological anatomy

Anterior tongue tumours usually present as ulcers, which can spread radially or invade deeply into the tongue muscles or as an exophytic mass. The lateral tongue drains to ipsilateral level Ib nodes. Whilst the level Ib nodes have efferent lymphatic connections to level II and thence to levels III and IV, there are also direct lymphatic connections from the tongue and floor of mouth to level II and level III nodes and occasionally to level IV. This explains the relatively high incidence of skip metastases in oral cavity tumours (10–15 per cent) (Fig. 10.2).

Lymphatics from the floor of mouth and the tip of the tongue drain to level Ia nodes and thence to bilateral Ib nodes, but there can again be direct spread to level III nodes. Floor of mouth tumours are often infiltrative and invade the mandible anteriorly, tongue posteriorly and deep muscles of the floor inferiorly. They commonly present late so surgery and radiotherapy are often both required for local control.

Primary tumours of buccal mucosa can invade deep structures including the mandible and cheek and spread initially to ipsilateral level Ib nodes. Retromolar trigone cancers can spread inferiorly to the mandible and posteriorly to invade the pterygoid muscles causing trismus.

The mucosa of the upper and lower alveolus and hard palate is fixed to the underlying periosteum so invasion of the adjacent bone occurs relatively early making these tumours less suitable for primary radiotherapy. Hard palate tumours may originate from minor salivary glands and spread via the nerve roots towards the skull base. They spread first to ipsilateral level Ib nodes. Midline tumours of the hard palate can spread bilaterally to level Ib. Hard palate tumours invading the

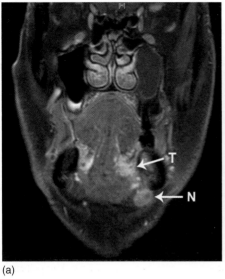
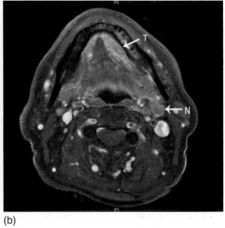

(a)   (b)

Figure 10.2 Primary floor of mouth tumour and lymphadenopathy. (a) Coronal T1-weighted contrast-enhanced MRI with tumour (T) and level Ib node (N) arrowed. (b) Axial T1-weighted contrast-enhanced MRI with tumour (T) and level II node (N) arrowed.

soft palate posteriorly can also spread to level II or retropharyngeal nodes which should be specifically evaluated by cross-sectional imaging.

T staging of oral cavity tumours is shown in Table 10.1.

Table 10.1 UICC TNM (6th edn, 2002*) tumour staging for oral cavity cancer

T1	Tumour ≤2 cm in greatest dimension
T2	Tumour >2 cm but ≤4 cm in greatest dimension
T3	Tumour >4 cm in greatest dimension
T4a	Tumour invades through cortical bone, into deep (extrinsic) muscles of the tongue (genioglossus, hyoglossus, palatoglossus and styloglossus), maxillary sinus or skin of face (i.e. considered resectable)
T4b	Tumour invades masticator space, pterygoid plates or skull base and/or encases internal carotid artery (i.e. considered unresectable)

*With permission.

Assessment of primary disease

The oncologist and maxillofacial surgeon should assess primary disease by careful examination using bimanual palpation to assess tumour thickness when possible as this predicts for occult metastases. EUA should be considered for more extensive tumours to assess local invasion before planning curative treatment.

MRI gives the most accurate information to assess local invasion but a CT scan can also be useful. Superficial mucosal tumours can be difficult to see on cross-sectional imaging. An OPG can help assess invasion of the mandible. Either MRI or CT can be used to stage neck nodes.

Data acquisition

■ Immobilisation

Patients should lie supine with a straight spine, immobilised in a Perspex or thermoplastic shell. A custom-made mouth bite may help to push the tongue inferiorly when irradiating the hard palate or upper alveolus or to separate the roof of the mouth from the inferior oral cavity when irradiating the tongue. Mouth bites can distort the anatomy and make volumes on CT more difficult to define accurately. Some patients find them difficult to tolerate and they may precipitate swallowing and thus cause movement of critical structures.

■ CT scanning

CT slices are obtained from the base of skull to the arch of the aorta with the patient immobilised in the treatment position. Ideally slices should be 3 mm thick to improve volume definition and quality of the DRR but 5 mm thick slices may suffice.

■ Simulator

Where low dose palliative radiotherapy with opposed lateral fields is planned, a lateral simulator radiograph is used to define volumes and field edges after marking any palpable tumour or lymphadenopathy with radio-opaque wires. A midplane separation is taken to calculate the required monitor units.

Target volume definition

When defining volumes, it is important to have all relevant information available including clinical assessments, EUA reports, operation notes, histology results and diagnostic imaging.

■ Curative radiotherapy

The GTV is outlined on a planning computer with window settings adjusted to show soft tissues. There are no studies correlating primary tumour size clinically or on imaging with microscopic spread histologically on which to base GTV-CTV margins. A 10 mm margin from macroscopic tumour edge to surgical resection margin would be regarded as likely to produce local control. We therefore recommend growing GTV isotropically by 10 mm to produce a CTV70.

The CTV70 is edited to take account of local patterns of tumour spread and natural tissue barriers, for example bone can be spared if not clinically involved. The medial pterygoid muscle should be included in the CTV70 if there is local invasion of part of the muscle, for example from a retromolar trigone tumour.

The CTV70 is then further edited to include adjacent positive or high risk nodal volumes. These will depend on the site of the primary tumour but include all levels where there is any lymphadenopathy and levels between the primary site and skip metastases (usually at least levels Ib and II).

The CTV70 is then copied to form the CTV44 which is expanded to include other nodal levels at lower risk of occult nodal metastases. Recommended CTV44 levels depend on the nodal status and whether both sides of the neck are considered to be at risk (Table 10.2).

Table 10.2 Recommendations for the selection of prophylactic nodal levels (CTV44) for oral cavity tumours – anterior two-thirds of the tongue, floor of mouth, buccal mucosa, hard palate and gingivae

Stage	Ipsilateral nodal levels	Contralateral nodal levels
N0/N1 with well-lateralised primary	Ib, II, III; include Ia for tumours involving tip of tongue, floor of mouth or anterior mandible; include IV for tumours of the anterior tongue or involving the oropharynx	Not treated
N0/N1 primary not well lateralised	Ib, II, III; include Ia for tumours involving tip of tongue, floor of mouth or anterior mandible; include IV for tumours of the anterior tongue or involving the oropharynx	Ib, II, III; include Ia for tumours involving tip of tongue, floor of mouth or anterior mandible; include IV for tumours of the anterior tongue or involving the oropharynx
N2a/N2b with well-lateralised primary	Ib, II, III, IV; include Ia for tumours involving tip of tongue, floor of mouth or anterior mandible; include IV for tumours of the anterior tongue or involving the oropharynx; include V if level IV involved	Ib, II, III; consider not treating contralateral neck
N2a/N2b primary not well lateralised	Ib, II, III, IV; include Ia for tumours involving tip of tongue, floor of mouth or anterior mandible; include IV for tumours of the anterior tongue or involving the oropharynx; include V if level IV involved	Ib, II, III; include IV for tumours of the anterior tongue or involving the oropharynx
N2c	Ib, II, III, IV; include Ia for tumours involving tip of tongue, floor of mouth or anterior mandible; include IV for tumours of the anterior tongue or involving the oropharynx; include V if level IV involved	Ib, II, III; include IV if multiple contralateral nodes or for tumours of the anterior tongue or involving the oropharynx; include V if level IV involved
N3	Ib, II, III, IV; include Ia for tumours involving tip of tongue, floor of mouth or anterior mandible; include IV for tumours of the anterior tongue or involving the oropharynx; include V if level IV involved	As for N2a/b (no contralateral nodes) or N2c (contralateral nodes) respectively

■ Adjuvant radiotherapy – primary

The CTV60 is defined using the planning CT scan after discussion with the surgeon and pathologist to define the sites at risk of microscopic residual disease. Postoperative oral cavity CTVs can be difficult to define because oral mucosa is not well defined on CT, dental artefact can obscure the oral anatomy and reconstructive soft tissue flaps can be confused with normal anatomical structures. If there has been reconstructive surgery, the whole flap does not need to be included in the CTV60 but the mucosa adjacent to the primary site should be included with a 10 mm isotropic margin to account for microscopic spread. A CTV66 (which may be equivalent to the CTV60 or smaller) is defined in the case of positive excision margins and includes the sites of incomplete excision.

The CTV-PTV margin should be individualised in each department according to measured random and systematic set-up errors. There should be minimal organ or tumour movement in a head and neck shell with the exception of small tumours of the oral tongue. For these, a separate internal margin may need to be added. Overall CTV-PTV margins should be 3–5 mm in each direction.

■ Adjuvant radiotherapy – neck

If there is an indication to irradiate the neck after a neck dissection (N2/3 disease or extracapsular spread), a CTV60 is defined to include nodal levels where there was tumour at surgery or adjacent levels at high risk of microscopic disease (for example level IV if a selective neck dissection of levels I–III revealed disease in level III). A CTV66 is defined in the case of extracapsular nodal extension.

A CTV44 is defined to include lymph nodes at risk of containing micrometastases in levels not removed at surgery. In the case of a lateral tongue tumour with a heavily node positive ipsilateral neck at neck dissection, levels Ib–III in the contralateral neck could be included in the CTV44.

■ Prophylactic radiotherapy – N0 neck

At risk nodal levels are defined according to patterns of lymphatic drainage from the primary site and outlined as CTV44.

■ Palliative radiotherapy

GTV, CTV and PTV are defined as for curative treatment either on a planning CT scan or lateral simulator radiograph. To minimise normal tissue toxicity (particularly mucositis), smaller margins can be used than for curative treatment – e.g. 5 mm from GTV to CTV.

Dose solutions

■ Conformal

Conformal solutions are preferred because of the complex three-dimensional shape of target volumes in oral cavity tumours and the advantage for the patient of sparing some of the mucosa of the oral cavity and pharynx. The exact multiple beam arrangement will depend on the tumour doses required, the shape of the volumes and consideration of doses to OAR.

In evaluating the plan a careful assessment of mandible dose is essential to reduce the risk of late osteoradionecrosis. Hot-spots of >107 per cent within the mandible should be avoided.

A midline PTV may still need to be treated with lateral opposed beams but MLC shielding will help to spare normal tissues, and wedges can be used to compensate for the change in neck contour and produce a more even dose distribution (Fig. 10.3). When only one side of the neck is treated, an arrangement of three coplanar beams can usually provide good tumour coverage while sparing the contralateral mucosa and parotid gland. At least one of the beams must have no exit dose through the spinal cord for this organ to remain within tolerance. In practice this means the angle of the posterior oblique beam is chosen to provide best coverage of the PTV while avoiding the cord (Fig. 10.4). A matched anterior neck beam is often required to treat low neck nodes (see Chapter 8).

■ Complex

IMRT has the potential to deliver the most conformal radiotherapy to complex target volumes with greater sparing of normal tissues. There are relatively few instances in oral cavity tumours where this is likely to give a therapeutic advantage as PTVs are usually convex and as the contralateral parotid can already be spared if the treated volume is unilateral. Moreover, the extra dose to the oral mucosa and contralateral mandible from IMRT may increase acute and late effects.

IMRT may offer an advantage when both sides of the neck are included in the PTV, both to spare one parotid gland and reduce the risk of xerostomia, and to avoid the uncertainties inherent in a plan with matched posterior electron and anterior neck photon fields. Beam arrangements similar to those chosen for oropharynx IMRT are used.

■ Conventional

Where resources are not available for conformal planning, conventional techniques may be unavoidable. For tumours involving the midline or where bilateral neck nodes require radiotherapy, opposed lateral fields can be used but this does not allow sparing of any adjacent mucosa in the treated volume. If the high dose volume extends posteriorly to the spinal cord, a two phase technique is used with large lateral fields for phase 1 and smaller lateral fields matched to posterior electron fields for phase 2. A matched anterior neck field treats lower neck nodes with midline shielding to reduce dose to the larynx, pharynx and spinal cord.

Where treatment is unilateral, anterior and posterior oblique wedged fields are chosen, with a lateral field sometimes used to improve homogeneity medially in the target volume. An ipsilateral anterior neck field is matched to treat inferior neck nodes if required.

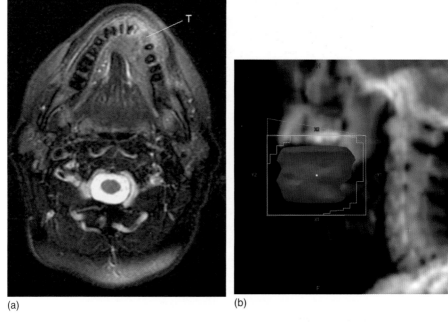

(a)
(b)

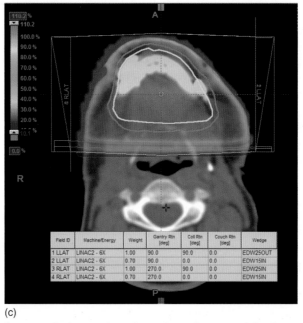

Field ID	Machine/Energy	Weight	Gantry Rtn [deg]	Coll Rtn [deg]	Couch Rtn [deg]	Wedge
1 LLAT	LINAC2 - 6X	1.00	90.0	90.0	0.0	EDW25OUT
2 LLAT	LINAC2 - 6X	0.70	90.0	0.0	0.0	EDW15IN
3 RLAT	LINAC2 - 6X	1.00	270.0	90.0	0.0	EDW25IN
4 RLAT	LINAC2 - 6X	0.70	270.0	0.0	0.0	EDW15IN

(c)

Figure 10.3 Adjuvant radiotherapy for a floor of mouth tumour following excision with close margins and bilateral negative neck dissections (pT4N0). (a) Axial T2-weighted fat-saturated MRI showing primary tumour (T). (b) Lateral DRR showing beam borders and PTV. (c) Axial planning CT slice showing dose distribution.

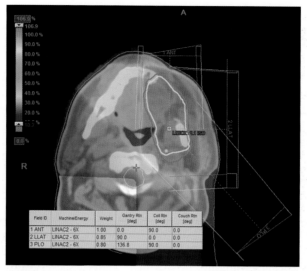

Figure 10.4 Adjuvant radiotherapy for a pT4aN0 buccal mucosa tumour invading the mandible, which has been resected with close margins but no involved lymph nodes.

Dose-fractionation

■ Curative treatment

EBRT with brachytherapy

EBRT

50 Gy in 25 daily fractions given in 5 weeks.

LDR brachytherapy boost

30 Gy to the reference isodose over 3 days.

LDR brachytherapy alone

65 Gy to the reference isodose over 7 days.

EBRT alone

70 Gy in 35 daily fractions given in 7 weeks ± concomitant cisplatin or alternative fractionation, e.g. with concomitant boost.

44 Gy in 22 daily fractions to PTV44 given in 4 ½ weeks.

■ Adjuvant treatment

60 Gy in 30 daily fractions to PTV60 given in 6 weeks ± concomitant cisplatin.

66 Gy in 33 daily fractions given in 6 ½ weeks to high risk sites.

44 Gy in 22 daily fractions to PTV44 given in 4 ½ weeks.

■ Palliative treatment

30 Gy in 5 fractions of 6 Gy given in 3 weeks.

20 Gy in 5 daily fractions of 4 Gy given in 1 week.

Treatment delivery and patient care

See Chapter 8. Excellent oral hygiene is particularly important when part of the oral cavity is being irradiated. Mucositis of the lip can be treated with steroid based paste preparations if there is no concurrent infection. Fungal infections are common and can recur during a course of radiotherapy. The oral cavity should be carefully inspected at least once a week and antifungal agents used as necessary.

Verification

See Chapter 8.

Brachytherapy

Brachytherapy offers excellent conformal radiotherapy to small tumours of the tongue and buccal mucosa that are well demarcated, not close to bone and accessible for implantation. These tumours are usually treated by surgery and the decision to treat with brachytherapy instead is often based on the expertise available. The disadvantages of brachytherapy include the risk of bleeding and infection, the radiation risk to staff and the patient isolation required.

Anterior tongue tumours or small floor of mouth cancers not too close to the mandible are usually treated with iridium-192 hairpins after metal gutters have been inserted. With the patient anaesthetised, the GTV is marked with ink. The depth of tumour infiltration on MRI corresponds accurately with surgical invasion and can be used to assess depth. The CTV is the GTV with a 10 mm margin. There is

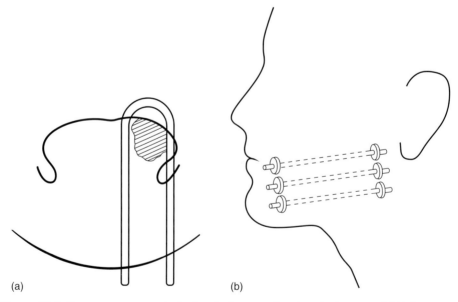

(a)   (b)

Figure 10.5 Source arrangements for brachytherapy of oral cavity tumours. (a) Iridium-192 hairpins for anterior tongue or floor of mouth. (b) Iridium-192 single plane implant for buccal mucosa.

no margin added to form a PTV as there is no daily set-up error or organ motion relative to the radiation. The gutters are inserted 12–15 mm apart according to Paris rules to ensure adequate CTV coverage and their position verified by orthogonal radiographs before the iridium is inserted (Fig. 10.5).

Small buccal mucosa tumours can be treated with a single plane implant using iridium-192 placed in flexible plastic tubes. After the CTV has been defined, hollow needles are placed to provide adequate CTV dose and a guidewire is introduced over which the plastic tubes are placed. Steroids may be required if trauma during the procedure causes enough swelling to compromise the airway. The skin should be cleaned regularly with an antiseptic agent. Analgesia is provided with opiates and non-steroidal anti-inflammatory drugs. The implant is reviewed daily.

key trials	There are no phase III trials evaluating the role of radiotherapy in oral cavity cancers alone, although these patients are often included in studies of head and neck cancer in general (see key trials in Chapter 8).

Information sources

See Chapter 8.

Nag S, Cano ER, Demanes J *et al.* (2001) The American Brachytherapy Society recommendations for high-dose-rate brachytherapy for head-and-neck carcinoma. *Int J Radiat Oncol Biol Phys* **50**: 1190–8.

Parsons JT, Mendenhall WM, Stringer SP *et al.* (1997) An analysis of factors influencing the outcome of postoperative irradiation for squamous cell carcinoma of the oral cavity. *Int J Radiat Oncol Biol Phys* **39**: 137–48.

Shah JP, Candela FC, Poddar AK (1990) The patterns of cervical lymph node metastases from squamous cell carcinoma of the oral cavity. *Cancer* **66**: 109–13.

11 Oropharynx cancer and unknown primary tumour

Indications for radiotherapy

Two approaches can be recommended for curative treatment of oropharyngeal squamous cell cancers: primary radiotherapy ± chemotherapy, or surgery ± postoperative (chemo)radiation. There are no randomised controlled trials comparing these two approaches, although there is indirect evidence suggesting cure rates are similar. The choice depends on likely functional outcomes, particularly with respect to swallowing and speech, local medical expertise, patients' ability to tolerate treatment and individual patient choice. Treatment of the primary site and the neck can be considered separately though one modality is usually used as the initial treatment to all sites of disease. Brachytherapy may have a role in combination with EBRT and is considered in Chapter 5.

Oropharyngeal tumours usually have lymphadenopathy at presentation and thus stage III or IV disease but metastases are uncommon. Patients have often smoked heavily and abused alcohol so assessing functional physiological reserve is important before deciding on a treatment for each patient.

■ Radiation to the primary tumour

Radiation to the primary site is the preferred treatment in oropharyngeal cancer because of the difficulty in obtaining adequate surgical margins while maintaining good swallowing and speech. Target volumes can be defined with greater accuracy if there has been no surgery prior to radiation. The use of concurrent chemotherapy or altered fractionation regimens may improve local control and survival compared with standard radiotherapy in stage III and IV disease. Cure rates vary from 80–90 per cent for early tonsil cancer to 40–50 per cent for larger primary tumours with nodal involvement.

If surgery is used to treat the primary site, adjuvant (chemo)radiation is recommended if surgical margins are positive and should be considered if the margins are close or if there is vascular or perineural invasion.

■ Radiation to the neck N0/N1

The N0 or N1 neck can be managed with either radiation or surgery alone depending on the modality used to treat the primary. If there is no clinical evidence of nodal involvement (N0) prophylactic treatment of the neck is recommended if the risk of occult metastases is over 20 per cent. Because the oropharynx has a rich lymphatic network this is usually the case. In well-lateralised tumours of the soft palate or tonsil, the ipsilateral nodes alone need treatment. The risk of contralateral nodal involvement is higher in T3/4 tumours or any tumour involving the tongue base so prophylactic radiation to the contralateral neck is recommended in these circumstances.

■ Radiation to the neck N2/3

Curative radiotherapy to involved neck nodes is recommended when treatment of the primary site is with radiotherapy. If the risk of nodal metastases at uninvolved nodal levels in the ipsilateral or contralateral neck is greater than 20 per cent, a prophylactic dose is given to these sites. Residual neck disease after radiation requires a neck dissection.

If surgery is used as initial therapy to the primary, a neck dissection is usually performed. Adjuvant radiotherapy is then recommended in the case of N2b/N2c/N3 disease or if there is extracapsular nodal spread. It should be considered in N2a disease particularly if there are poorer prognostic features (see Table 11.1).

Table 11.1 Poor prognostic features after potentially curative surgery

Primary	Nodes
*Positive margins	*Extracapsular spread
Close margins (0–5 mm)	More than one involved node
Perineural invasion	One node >3 cm
Lymphovascular invasion	
Poorly differentiated histology	
T4 tumour (invading local structures)	

*Positive excision margins and extracapsular nodal spread are definite indications for adjuvant radiotherapy.

■ Palliative radiotherapy

In the presence of metastases or if tumour size or comorbidity preclude a curative approach, palliative radiotherapy may improve pain, dysphagia and speech.

■ Unknown primary tumour sites in the head and neck

Patients presenting with a level II/III neck node without a clear primary site often have a primary site in the tonsil, base of tongue, pyriform fossa or nasopharynx. Pathology of the involved nodes obtained by biopsy or excision can suggest a likely primary site as can careful examination of the pharynx. If no primary can be found, radiation is given either to the neck alone or to the neck and possible primary sites, usually encompassing the ipsilateral tonsil, tongue base and pyriform fossa.

■ Oropharyngeal lymphoma

Lymphomas of the oropharynx (usually tonsil) are treated with radiotherapy alone or sequential chemotherapy and radiation to residual disease or high risk sites.

Clinical and radiological anatomy

The oropharynx is the posterior continuation of the oral cavity. Superiorly it joins the nasopharynx at the level of the hard palate and inferiorly it meets the hypopharynx at the level of the hyoid bone. An appreciation of the complex anatomy and physiology of this area is vital in order to understand the mechanisms for local invasion and lymph node spread. The oropharynx has four walls (Fig. 11.1).

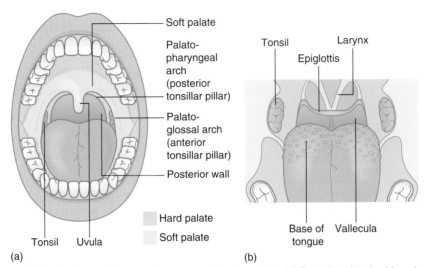

Figure 11.1 Anatomy of the oropharynx. (a) Anterior view. (b) Superior view looking down from the nasopharynx. The valleculae (glossoepiglottic fossae) lie between the base of tongue and the epiglottis.

The commonest site of oropharyngeal tumours is the lateral wall, which is made up of the tonsils, tonsillar fossae and palatoglossal and palatopharyngeal arches. Tonsil cancers tend to be infiltrative and can spread inferiorly to the tongue base or superiorly to the soft palate. The rich lymphatic drainage of the tonsils means spread to ipsilateral lymph nodes is common at presentation. The tonsil is a frequent site for occult primaries to be detected in patients presenting with enlarged neck nodes. Tonsillar tumours extending onto the tongue base have a greater risk of bilateral nodal spread.

The base of tongue and valleculae (glossoepiglottic fossae) comprise the anterior wall and have a rich lymphatic drainage to both sides of the neck. Tumours involving the tongue base are therefore treated with bilateral neck irradiation. The infiltrative nature of most base of tongue tumours in a site critical for swallowing means that patients should be assessed before therapy for evidence of aspiration and a prophylactic feeding tube is advised.

Tumours of the superior wall (soft palate and uvula) and posterior wall are less common. Lateral soft palate tumours spread to ipsilateral lymph nodes while more medial tumours or those arising in the posterior wall have a higher chance of bilateral nodal involvement. The lack of submucosal tissue on the posterior pharyngeal wall means radiation to these tumours often results in a shallow ulcer, which takes many months to heal, can be very painful and can be confused with residual tumour.

Level II nodes are the usual first site of spread. Disease then spreads inferiorly to levels III and IV or superiorly to upper level II (and retrostyloid) or retropharyngeal nodes. Level V involvement is relatively uncommon. Pattern of nodal spread may be less predictable in patients who have had a previous neck dissection.

Assessment of primary disease

The oropharynx, oral cavity and larynx should be carefully examined by the radiation oncologist and ENT surgeon together to assess the mucosal sites of disease. Tonsil and soft palate tumours can be seen by inspection through the oral cavity. The tongue base is best assessed by flexible nasendoscopy or indirect (mirror) examination combined with careful bimanual palpation. EUA may be helpful to define the extent of tumour and to obtain histology.

Investigation of a squamous cell cancer in level II/III nodes without an obvious primary site on examination should include EUA with bilateral tonsillectomies, biopsies of the nasopharynx and pyriform fossae and deep biopsies of the base of tongue.

PET-CT is the most sensitive modality to detect a primary site and can help to direct the biopsies (Fig. 11.2). False positive results may occur if the PET-CT follows the EUA.

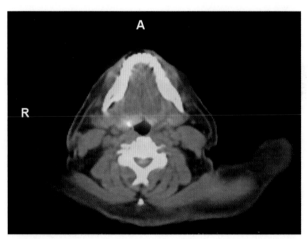

Figure 11.2 PET-CT for an unknown primary head and neck cancer presenting with right level II nodes. Uptake in the right tonsil strongly suggests this is the primary site.

Cross-sectional imaging is essential to define extent of the primary tumour and MRI is preferable to CT in oropharyngeal tumours (Fig. 11.3); however, MRI and CT are equally accurate at assessing neck disease. Cross-sectional imaging should include the whole neck from the skull base to the superior mediastinum to assess retropharyngeal nodes and levels I–V. A node >10 mm is considered pathological but nodes larger than 5 mm should be regarded as suspicious if in a location typical for nodal metastases. In this case ultrasound and fine needle aspiration cytology may be useful to confirm metastases.

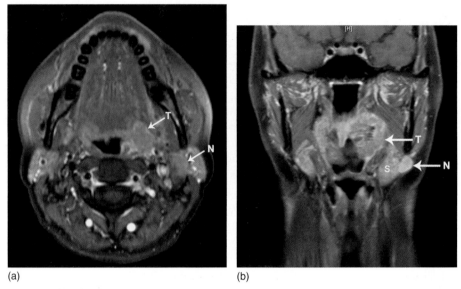

(a) (b)

Figure 11.3 T1-weighted contrast-enhanced MRI of a T2N2b left tonsil cancer. (a) Axial slice showing tumour (T) and level II node (N). (b) Coronal slice showing tumour (T) and level Ib node (N) adjacent to submandibular gland (S).

Data acquisition

■ Immobilisation

The patient lies supine with the spine as straight as possible and no mouth bite, but any dentures should be left in place. A shell with at least five fixation points is constructed to ensure immobilisation (see Chapter 8).

■ CT scanning

CT images – ideally with intravenous contrast – are acquired with 3 mm thick slices from the skull base superiorly to the top of the aortic arch inferiorly. Lateral and midline reference marks are drawn on the mask. The CT dataset is imported into the treatment planning system. Many oropharyngeal tumours are more easily defined with MRI than CT so co-registered images may improve GTV definition.

■ Simulator

If 3D CT-based planning is not available, beam borders can be defined on orthogonal radiographs in the simulator. Lateral and anteroposterior (AP) films are taken when the immobilisation device is fitted. The GTV is drawn on the films with the help of diagnostic clinical information and imaging. The CTVs and PTVs are then defined as for CT planning and beam arrangements chosen.

Target volume definition

■ Curative treatment

The diagnostic images and records and photographs of initial evaluation (in clinic or at EUA) are critical to assess the extent of the primary tumour and the exact site of involved lymph nodes. The GTV is defined as the primary tumour and any lymph nodes over 10 mm in short axis dimension or smaller nodes with necrotic centres or rounded contours thought to contain tumour.

A high dose CTV70 is created to include sites of local and nodal spread and a lower dose CTV44 to include uninvolved nodal levels to receive a prophylactic dose.

The GTV-CTV70 expansion at the primary site is individualised and non-uniform reflecting local barriers to spread and the possible involvement of local structures. For example the CTV70 for a left base of tongue tumour should include the whole tongue base and left tonsillar fossa; the CTV70 for a T1 tonsil cancer is the tonsillar fossa but not tongue base or the nearby medial pterygoid muscle.

For N0 tumours, the CTV70 will include level II nodes adjacent to the primary either ipsilaterally (lateral tonsil or soft palate primary) or bilaterally. In node-positive disease the CTV70 includes all levels with involved lymph nodes and those adjacent to the primary site. If there is involvement of an adjacent muscle due to extracapsular spread, this should be included in the CTV70.

There is no evidence correlating CT data with pathological specimens from which to derive a GTV-CTV margin. In practice, the CTV70 is best achieved by automatically growing the GTV by 10 mm (the pathological margin that a surgeon aims for), and editing it, to include sites of local spread and possible nodal involvement and to exclude soft tissues where there are natural barriers to tumour spread, air spaces and uninvolved bone.

A low dose CTV44 is created from the CTV70 by also including other lymph node sites thought to be at risk of microscopic nodal disease. If this volume is to be treated with a single anterior neck beam, a 3D volume need not be defined.

If the posterior pharyngeal wall is involved the bilateral retropharyngeal nodes should be included in the CTV44. Examples of nodal levels to be included in the CTV44 for different tumours are given in Table 11.2.

Table 11.2 Suggested nodal CTVs for oropharyngeal tumours

Disease site	CTV44
Lateral tonsil or soft palate T1/T2 N0/N1	Ipsilateral levels II–IV (and Ib, RP, retrostyloid if N1)
Lateral tonsil or soft palate T1/T2 N2a,b	Ipsilateral levels Ib–IV, retrostyloid, RP and consider ipsilateral level V
Base of tongue, midline soft palate, posterior pharyngeal wall T1/T2 N0	Bilateral levels II–IV (and RP if posterior pharyngeal wall involved)
Tonsil or soft palate T 3/4 and/or N2c, N3	Consider each hemi-neck separately: N+ neck – levels Ib–IV, retrostyloid and RP nodes and consider level V
Base of tongue, midline soft palate Any T 3/4 and/or N+	N0 neck – levels II–IV (and RP if posterior pharyngeal wall involved)

RP, retropharyngeal.

The CTVs are grown to PTVs by applying a margin which can be determined by the local assessment of random and systematic errors, assuming that tumour movement in head and neck cancer is negligible. This is usually 3–5 mm.

The spinal cord is outlined and grown by 5 mm to produce a PRV. Each parotid gland is contoured where parotid sparing is feasible.

■ CTV for adjuvant radiotherapy

In addition to imaging and clinical information, discussion with the surgeon and pathologist is important in determining the sites at greatest risk of recurrent disease. There is no GTV. If radiation to the primary site is indicated, the CTV60 is the operative tumour bed paying particular attention to sites where excision margins are positive or close. If radiation to the nodes is indicated, the CTV60 includes the nodal levels where there were positive lymph nodes and adjacent structures at sites of extracapsular spread. A CTV44 is only defined if there are nodal levels that were not operated on but have a >20 per cent chance of containing occult metastases (see Table 11.2).

■ CTV for unknown primary

Any macroscopically enlarged nodes are contoured as GTV. The CTV70 is the nodal levels containing tumour with at least a 10 mm margin superiorly and inferiorly and is usually the ipsilateral level II and upper level III nodes. There are two approaches to contouring the CTV.

One is to assume the primary site is in the ipsilateral base of tongue, tonsil or pyriform fossa (and nasopharynx in some parts of the world) and to include these sites in the CTV44 along with their draining lymph nodes. The CTV44 will include levels

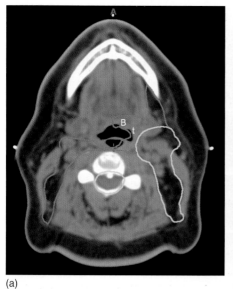 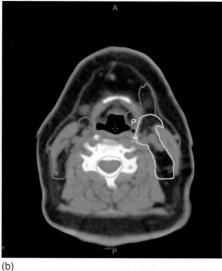

(a) (b)

Figure 11.4 Suggested CTVs for an unknown primary head and neck cancer presenting with a level II node. (a) Axial slice showing the left tonsil (t) and base of tongue (B) in the CTV44 (magenta), CTV70 (cyan). (b) Axial slice showing the left pyriform fossa (P) in the CTV44.

Ib–IV, retropharyngeal and retrostyloid nodes on the involved side and levels II–IV contralaterally (Fig. 11.4). Another approach is to not treat the possible primary sites and only include the ipsilateral levels Ib–IV, retrostyloid and retropharyngeal nodes. This is less toxic as much of the oropharyngeal mucosa can be spared but, if the primary site later becomes apparent it will be very difficult to treat with radiation so close to the original CTV. We recommend the first approach unless comorbidity and performance status suggest such extensive treatment volumes will be poorly tolerated.

Dose solutions

■ Conformal

Phase 1 aims to treat the PTV44 to a dose thought sufficient to eradicate microscopic disease in lymph nodes. Unilateral PTVs are treated with a plan using two or three beams unilaterally to provide dose to the PTV according to ICRU62 (Fig. 11.5). The angle of the posterior oblique beam is chosen so as to avoid the spinal cord PRV which can sometimes mean accepting reduced dose to the most posterior part of the nodal CTV. This is matched to an ipsilateral low neck beam.

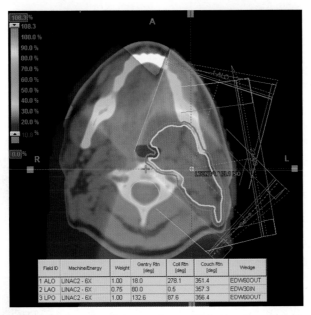

Field ID	Machine/Energy	Weight	Gantry Rtn [deg]	Coll Rtn [deg]	Couch Rtn [deg]	Wedge
1 ALO	LINAC2 - 6X	1.00	18.0	278.1	351.4	EDW60OUT
2 LAO	LINAC2 - 6X	0.75	80.0	0.5	357.3	EDW30IN
3 LPO	LINAC2 - 6X	1.00	132.6	87.6	356.4	EDW60OUT

Figure 11.5 Beam arrangement and dose colourwash for treatment of a tonsillar cancer and ipsilateral neck nodes.

Those PTVs extending to the contralateral side are usually treated with opposing lateral beams with AP wedges and sometimes superior–inferior wedges to compensate for changes in contour. A three-beam arrangement can sometimes be used to try to spare the contralateral parotid gland. Usually the planned superior volume is matched isocentrically to a lower anterior neck beam, with midline shielding to treat more inferior nodes without irradiating midline structures.

Phase 2 aims to treat the PTV70 to a curative dose and the beam arrangements are similar to those in phase 1 but with more shielding if possible. If the PTV70 extends posteriorly to the posterior level II or level V nodes, a matched posterior electron beam (9 MeV or 12 MeV) may be needed. The plans for phase 1 and phase 2 should be reviewed together to ensure PTVs are adequately covered according to ICRU62 and critical structures are not overdosed. Acute side effects will be reduced if the dose to the oral cavity and pharynx outside the PTV is minimised.

■ Complex

IMRT is the ideal treatment for oropharyngeal cancer requiring bilateral neck irradiation as it allows parotid sparing to reduce the risk of xerostomia and obviates the need for matched electron fields (Fig. 11.6). Different PTVs can be treated to different doses within the same plan. If bilateral level II nodes contain tumour, the need to include the retrostyloid nodes in the treated volume may preclude parotid sparing.

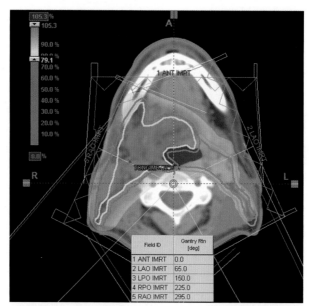

Figure 11.6 Volumes, five beam arrangement, and dose distribution for intensity-modulated radiotherapy of a right base of tongue tumour. Colourwash scale is set from 79 per cent (i.e. 54 Gy) to illustrate the conformality of the plan.

Target volumes are defined as above. Nodal PTVs often come close to the skin surface. To artificially create a skin sparing effect with IMRT the nodal volumes are edited so as to be a minimum of 5 mm from the body contour. The only exception is when an involved node is within 5 mm of the skin surface.

The spinal cord is outlined with a 5 mm isocentric margin as a PRV. Both parotid glands are contoured: they can be difficult to define on a planning CT, particularly when there is dental artefact, though the diagnostic MRI may be helpful. The brainstem is also contoured as an OAR. There is increasing evidence that the dose to the pharyngeal constrictor muscles may relate to the risk of long-term dysphagia. They can be spared inferior to the midline PTV and can either be contoured or can be included as part of an avoidance volume, including the larynx, hypopharynx and trachea, which can help to reduce dose to these midline structures.

When the high dose PTV extends inferiorly below the inferior cricoid cartilage the whole neck is treated in one plan, usually with a seven-beam arrangement of equispaced IMRT beams. If the more inferior nodes only require a prophylactic dose they can be treated with a matched anterior neck beam as for conformal treatment, in which case the superior part of the volume can usually be treated with five equispaced beams.

In practice, the five IMRT beam angles are selected with beam sizes chosen to cover the PTV. The computer software uses an iterative process to try to meet the constraints applied to the target volumes as illustrated in Table 11.3. The operator guides the computer by defining the constraints and weighting them according to their importance. The target constraints and weights are gradually changed until

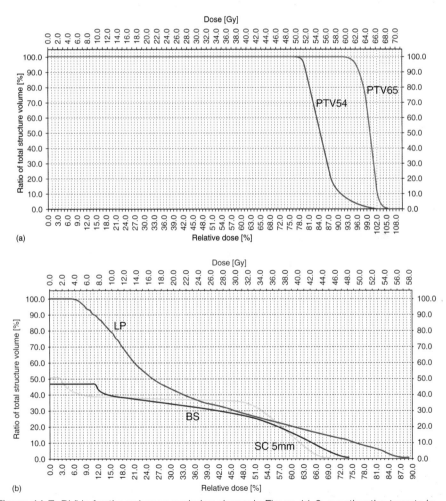

Figure 11.7 DVHs for the volumes and plan shown in Figure 11.6, meeting the targets in Table 11.3. (a) PTV65 (red) and PTV54 (green). (b) Spinal cord PRV (yellow, max dose 45.1 Gy), brainstem (blue, max dose 48.2 Gy), left parotid gland (pink, mean dose 22.6 Gy).

Table 11.3 Suggested targets for PTV and OAR coverage for oropharyngeal IMRT

Structure	Volume	Target dose
PTV65	99 per cent	58.5 Gy (90 per cent)
	95 per cent	61.75 Gy (95 per cent)
	50 per cent	65 Gy (100 per cent)
	≤5 per cent	68.25 Gy (105 per cent)
PTV54	99 per cent	48.6 Gy
	95 per cent	51.3 Gy
	50 per cent	54 Gy
Cord + 5 mm	Any	46 Gy (<1 cm^3 can receive 48 Gy)
Brainstem	Any	54 Gy
Contralateral parotid	Mean dose	<24 Gy
Body – PTVs	<5 per cent	>71.5 Gy (110 per cent)

spinal cord and brainstem are within tolerance, the PTVs are adequately covered and, if possible, the mean contralateral parotid dose is less than 24 Gy (Fig. 11.7).

Dose-fractionation

■ Curative treatment

T1T2N0

70 Gy in 35 daily fractions given in 7 weeks
or
55 Gy in 20 daily fractions of 2.75 Gy given in 4½ weeks.

T 3/4 any N or any T N+

70 Gy in 35 daily fractions given in 7 weeks ± concomitant cisplatin
or
alternative fractionation, e.g. with concomitant boost.
44 Gy in 22 daily fractions to PTV44 given in 4½ weeks.

■ Simultaneous boost IMRT

65 Gy to high dose PTV and 54 Gy to low dose PTV in 30 fractions given in 6 weeks.

■ Adjuvant treatment

60 Gy in 30 daily fractions to PTV60 given in 6 weeks ± concomitant cisplatin.
66 Gy in 33 daily fractions given in 6½ weeks to high risk sites.
44 Gy in 22 daily fractions to PTV44 given in 4½ weeks.

■ Palliative treatment

30 Gy in 5 fractions of 6 Gy twice weekly given in 2½ weeks.
20 Gy in 5 daily fractions of 4 Gy given in 1 week.

Treatment delivery and patient care

Patients are treated daily. Any gap in treatment must be corrected – ideally by treating twice in one day. There must be at least a 6-hour gap between fractions on any day when a patient receives two doses.

Weekly assessment by doctor or radiographer and dietician is important. Regular advice by a speech and language therapist can help maintain safe, functional swallowing. Most patients are at high risk of weight loss and should be considered for a gastric feeding tube inserted for prophylaxis before radiotherapy. Further details are given in Chapter 8.

Verification

See Chapter 8.

---

key trials

See Chapter 8 – most phase III trials in head and neck cancer contain a majority of patients with oropharyngeal cancers.

Calais G, Alfonsi M, Bardet E *et al.* (1999) Randomized trial of radiation therapy versus concomitant chemotherapy and radiation therapy for advanced-stage oropharynx carcinoma. *J Natl Cancer Inst* **9**: 2081–6.

Denis F, Garaud P, Bardet E *et al.* (2004) Final results of the 94–01 French Head and Neck Oncology and Radiotherapy Group randomised trial comparing radiotherapy alone with concomitant radiochemotherapy in advanced-stage oropharynx carcinoma. *J Clin Oncol* **22**: 69 –76.

Information sources

Chao KS, Majhail N, Huang CJ *et al.* (2001) Intensity-modulated radiation therapy reduces late salivary toxicity without compromising tumour control in patients with oropharyngeal carcinoma: a comparison with conventional techniques. *Radiother Oncol* **61**: 275–80.

Eisbruch A, Ten Haken RK, Kim HM *et al.* (1999) Dose, volume, and function relationships in parotid salivary glands following conformal and intensity modulated irradiation of head and neck cancer. *Int J Radiat Oncol Biol Phys* **45**: 577–87.

Jackson SM, Hay JH, Flores AD *et al.* (1999) Cancer of the tonsil: the results of ipsilateral radiation treatment. *Radiother Oncol* **51**: 123–8.

Maes A, Weltens C, Flamen P *et al.* (2002) Preservation of parotid function with uncomplicated conformal radiotherapy. *Radiother Oncol* **63**: 203–11.

12 Hypopharynx

Indications for radiotherapy

■ Curative treatment for T1T2 N0 tumours

Table 12.1 gives tumour staging for hypopharyngeal cancer. Early stage hypopharyngeal tumours are rare but can be treated with curative intent by surgery or radiotherapy. Choice depends on local expertise and patient preference but as clear margins and good pharyngeo-laryngeal function are difficult to achieve surgically, radiotherapy is recommended. There are no RCTs comparing these approaches.

Table 12.1 UICC TNM (6th edn, 2002*) tumour staging for hypopharyngeal cancer

T1	Tumour limited to one subsite (postcricoid, pyriform sinus or posterior pharyngeal wall) and ≤2 cm in greatest dimension
T2	Tumour invades more than one subsite of hypopharynx or an adjacent site, or measures 2 cm but ≤4 cm in greatest dimension, without fixation of the hemilarynx
T3	Tumour >4 cm in greatest dimension, or with fixation of the hemilarynx
T4a	Tumour invades any of the following: thyroid/cricoid cartilage, hyoid bone, thyroid gland, oesophagus, central compartment soft tissue (prelaryngeal strap muscles and subcutaneous fat)
T4b	Tumour invades prevertebral fascia, encases carotid artery, or invades mediastinal structures

*With permission.

Pyriform fossa tumours have the best prognosis – radiotherapy can achieve local control in 90 per cent of T1 tumours and 80 per cent of T2 tumours with a 5-year overall survival of 50–65 per cent. Involvement of the apex of the pyriform fossa (which may imply occult invasion of cartilage) predicts a lower chance of cure. Postcricoid carcinomas have a 20–50 per cent cure rate with radiotherapy which is equivalent to that in surgical series. There are fewer data available for posterior wall tumours but cure rates are similar to those for postcricoid cancer.

■ Curative treatment for T3–4 or N+ tumours

Most hypopharyngeal cancers are locally advanced at presentation and many patients have significant smoking and alcohol exposure and cardiac, respiratory and other comorbidities. Treatment is therefore tailored and options range from pharyngolaryngectomy with adjuvant radiochemotherapy, radiochemotherapy alone to no attempt at cure with palliative care only. Treatment choice depends on the site and stage of disease and patient preference acknowledging the balance between possible cure, treatment morbidity and likely functional outcomes.

There are phase III data to support an organ preserving approach for advanced pyriform fossa cancer. Large volume primary disease, particularly with cartilage destruction, is best treated with surgery and postoperative radiotherapy.

■ Adjuvant radiotherapy

Adjuvant radiotherapy to the site of primary tumour is recommended for all resected T3/T4 tumours and for T1/T2 tumours with positive or close resection margins (usually <5 mm or <10 mm where there is surgical concern). Adjuvant radiotherapy to the involved neck is recommended in N2/3 disease or N1 disease with extracapsular spread.

■ Palliative treatment

Locally advanced hypopharyngeal cancers – particularly those originating in the postcricoid and posterior pharyngeal wall – have a low chance of cure with any approach. Patients' wishes, advanced age and comorbidity mean that palliative treatment should be discussed with all patients with locally advanced disease. Palliative radiotherapy may improve pharyngeal pain and obstructive symptoms and help to control neck disease but hardly ever improves complete dysphagia. Supportive care alone is an option for patients with incurable disease, complete dysphagia and few other symptoms.

Sequencing of multimodality therapy

If primary surgery is used and adjuvant radiotherapy is indicated, radiation should begin 4–6 weeks postoperatively or when adequate healing has taken place. Concomitant cisplatin chemotherapy should be considered, especially when resection margins are positive or there is extracapsular nodal spread.

Radiotherapy following induction chemotherapy in patients with a response should ideally begin 3 weeks after the start of the last chemotherapy cycle. Addition of concomitant chemotherapy to this regimen is recommended if the patient can tolerate such intensive treatment.

Clinical and radiological anatomy

The pyriform fossae are mucosa-lined spaces on either side of the larynx (Fig. 12.1). Each is shaped like an inverted pyramid with the apex between the cricoid cartilage medially and the thyroid cartilage laterally at the level of the cervical oesophagus. The posterior pharyngeal wall is the posterior mucosa in between the pyriform fossae extending from the level of the hyoid bone to the inferior border of the cricoid cartilage. The postcricoid mucosa is the anterior surface of the hypopharynx from the arytenoid cartilages to the inferior border of the cricoid. It is continuous posterolaterally with the inferior portion of the posterior pharyngeal wall (Fig. 12.2).

Tumours can spread mucosally to involve adjacent mucosal sites – other subsites of the hypopharynx, the supraglottic larynx or tongue base. If other sites are invaded, lymph node target volumes should include levels draining these sites. Because the hypopharyngeal mucosa is thin, tumours readily spread into the adjacent

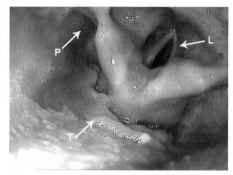

Figure 12.1 Transnasal oesophagoscopic view of the hypopharynx. Note the pyriform fossa (P) and larynx (L). There is a tumour of the posterior pharyngeal wall (T).

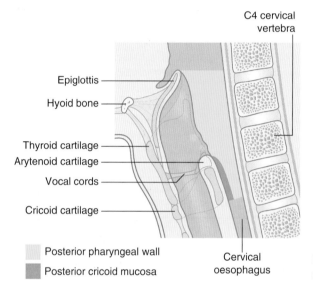

C4 cervical vertebra

Epiglottis

Hyoid bone

Thyroid cartilage

Arytenoid cartilage

Vocal cords

Cricoid cartilage

Posterior pharyngeal wall

Posterior cricoid mucosa

Cervical oesophagus

Figure 12.2 Midline sagittal anatomy of the hypopharynx.

sites – medially from the pyriform fossae to the paraglottic space (and then into the larynx), laterally into the soft tissues of the neck, or posteriorly into the prevertebral fascia. They can also invade the arytenoid, thyroid and cricoid cartilages. Submucosal spread is common and should influence GTV-CTV margins. Postcricoid tumours can spread into the cervical oesophagus.

Lymph node spread is common at presentation and occult disease is found in up to 60 per cent of patients with no lymphadenopathy. The pyriform fossae drain to ipsilateral levels II and III nodes initially, and other sites to levels II, III and IV, usually bilaterally. Tumours involving the posterior pharyngeal wall can also spread directly to the retropharyngeal nodes. If levels II–IV are involved, tumour can spread to level Ib or V or to retropharyngeal nodes. Postcricoid cancers can also spread inferiorly to the paratracheal and paraoesophageal nodes.

Assessment of primary disease

Most pyriform fossa cancers are visible at nasendoscopy during which vocal cord function is assessed. Vocal cord paralysis is a poor prognostic sign. Tumours are more visible if the fossae are distended by the patient performing a Valsalva manoeuvre with the nostrils pinched. Transnasal oesophagoscopy allows other hypopharyngeal sites to be assessed and biopsies to be taken if necessary. Palpable lymphadenopathy should be recorded and fine needle aspiration of lymphadenopathy is often an easier way to confirm the diagnosis histologically.

EUA allows assessment of mucosal extent and deep fixation of the tumour and should be performed if surgery is considered. The EUA should include laryngoscopy, oesophagoscopy and bronchoscopy to assess involvement of adjacent organs.

Cross-sectional imaging with either CT or MRI is performed (Fig. 12.3). Both are equally good at demonstrating lymphadenopathy though MRI may provide slightly better imaging of the primary tumour. CT is preferable for more inferior tumours that may have spread to the superior mediastinal nodes as it allows easy imaging of the head, neck and thorax contiguously. A barium swallow can be helpful to document the superior and inferior extent of the primary tumour as well as to assess aspiration and fixation to the prevertebral muscles.

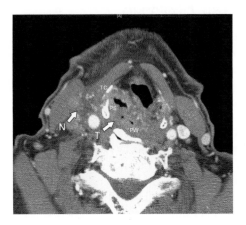

Figure 12.3 Diagnostic CT scan of a right pyriform fossa tumour (T) growing into the paraglottic space (PS), through the thyroid cartilage (TC) and invading onto the posterior pharyngeal wall (PW). (Note the adjacent involved lymph node (N).)

Data acquisition

■ Immobilisation

Patients lie supine on a headrest to keep the spine straight, with a custom-made shell fixed to the couch top in at least five places to reduce movement. The treated volume will usually extend inferior to the level of the shoulders which should be as low as possible to facilitate beam entry. No mouth bite is required.

■ CT scanning

With the patient immobilised, CT images are obtained from the skull base to the carina. The inferior border is at the carina to facilitate planning with lateral beams angled inferiorly if required. Slices should ideally be 3 mm thick. Intravenous contrast may help in the definition of lymph node volumes but is unlikely to add more information than contrast-enhanced diagnostic imaging which must be available at the time of target volume definition. Contrast can be particularly helpful when there has been tumour shrinkage after induction chemotherapy as the residual GTV will differ from that demonstrated on the original diagnostic scan.

There is as yet no proven role for image fusion with MRI or PET in defining tumour volumes. MRI is unlikely to add much to CT-based planning as hypopharyngeal tumours are seen almost as well on CT. The role of PET for target volume definition is evolving and may facilitate dose escalation by identifying a smaller target volume within the GTV which could receive a higher dose.

■ Simulator

Ideally all patients with hypopharyngeal cancer are planned three-dimensionally using CT images in view of the complex volume shape and position. If opposing lateral beams are to be used, the borders can be defined in the simulator on a lateral radiograph.

Target volume definition

■ CTV for curative radiotherapy T1/T2 N0

The GTV is defined using endoscopy, EUA reports and diagrams, and diagnostic imaging. There is no evidence on which to base GTV-CTV margins at the primary site but submucosal spread is common and can extend at least 10 mm from the GTV. We recommend the GTV is grown by the planning computer by a 10 mm axial margin and a 15 mm longitudinal margin to create a CTV70. This is then edited to take account of patterns of spread and natural barriers to tumour progression (e.g. bone). The CTV70 is also edited to include adjacent lymph nodes (usually level III but occasionally part of levels II and IV) on the same axial slices as the CTV70. For lateral pyriform fossa tumours these high risk nodes will be ipsilateral; for other hypopharyngeal tumours they will be bilateral.

The CTV70 is then copied to become the CTV44. The CTV44 is edited to include other lymph node groups at risk of micrometastases. For lateral pyriform fossa tumours this will include ipsilateral levels II–IV. For other tumours with bilateral lymph node drainage, bilateral nodes are included. Retropharyngeal nodes are included for tumours involving the posterior pharyngeal wall.

■ CTV for curative radiotherapy T 3/4 or N+

Some patients in this group will have been treated with and responded to induction chemotherapy. CTVs should therefore be based on the initial pattern of disease as well as on the residual tumour seen on the planning CT. The GTV should be defined on the planning CT from the residual volume but should include any nodes that were involved at diagnosis even if they are not now enlarged.

To allow for submucosal spread, the GTV is enlarged by 10 mm axially and 15 mm longitudinally to form the CTV70. The CTV70 is edited to take account of natural barriers to tumour progression (e.g. bone, air and uninvolved muscle) and to include all sites of primary disease at presentation. For example, a pyriform fossa cancer invading the tongue base at diagnosis may respond to induction chemotherapy to leave residual tumour in the pyriform fossa alone. The tongue base should be included in the CTV70. The CTV is further edited to include sites of high risk nodal disease. For N+ disease the CTV70 includes level II–IV nodes adjacent to the primary GTV, any involved nodes at other levels and any nodes in between.

When the CTV70 has been defined it is copied to become the CTV44. This volume is then edited to include nodal sites at lower risk of containing microscopic disease (Table 12.2; Fig. 12.4).

Table 12.2 Suggested CTVs for hypopharyngeal tumours

Disease site	CTV44
T 1/2 N0 pyriform fossa (confined to lateral wall)	Ipsilateral II–IV
T 1/2 N0 post cricoid /posterior pharyngeal wall	Bilateral II–IV. Include bilateral RP nodes if posterior pharyngeal wall involved
T 3/4 N0 pyriform fossa	Bilateral level II–IV
T 3/4 N0 postcricoid/posterior pharyngeal wall	Bilateral levels II–IV. Include bilateral RP nodes if posterior pharyngeal wall involved. Include level VI nodes if tumour extends into cervical oesophagus
Pyriform fossa N+	Bilateral level II–IV. Level Ib and V nodes on the side of any lymphadenopathy. Bilateral RP nodes if N2b/3 or if posterior pharyngeal wall involved
Postcricoid/posterior pharyngeal wall N+	Bilateral level II–IV, RP nodes. Level Ib and V nodes on the side of any lymphadenopathy. Level VI nodes if tumour extends into the cervical oesophagus

RP, retropharyngeal.

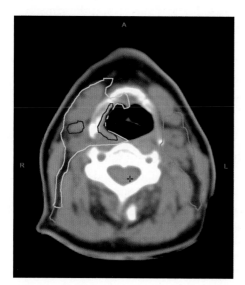

Figure 12.4 GTV, CTV70 and CTV44 for a T1N1 right pyriform fossa tumour.

■ CTV for adjuvant radiotherapy

After careful discussion with the surgeon and pathologist, the CTV60 is defined as sites of possible residual microscopic disease. If a large resection with reconstruction and flaps has been performed, the anatomy visible on the planning CT will be very different from that on the initial diagnostic images.

The CTV60 should include the margins of resection and sites of any dissected nodal levels where there was tumour. Sites of positive resection margins or where there was extracapsular nodal spread should be further defined as CTV66. In practice it can be impossible to accurately define these sites separately from the CTV60, in which case only the CTV66 should be defined. When the patient has had a laryngectomy, the stoma should be included in the CTV60 if subglottic extension was present or if the surgeon is concerned about the risk of parastomal recurrence.

If a clinically node negative tumour has been excised with an elective neck dissection and there is unexpected tumour in the neck nodes, a CTV44 can also be defined. This should ensure that the nodal levels defined in Table 12.2 have been treated either surgically or with radiotherapy. For example if surgery for a T2 pyriform fossa tumour included an ipsilateral level II–IV neck dissection at which multiple involved nodes were identified (pN2b), the CTV44 should include ipsilateral levels Ib and V, contralateral levels II–IV and bilateral retropharyngeal nodes.

■ CTV for palliative radiotherapy

The goal of palliative radiotherapy is to treat all symptomatic disease with minimal toxicity. The GTV is defined from clinical information and imaging. If treatment is planned on the simulator, a 15 mm margin from GTV to beam edge (50 per cent) is recommended. If CT planning is used, the GTV should be expanded by 5 mm to produce the CTV.

■ Planning target volume

CTVs are expanded isotropically to form PTVs by a margin depending on the measured random and systematic errors in the department – usually 3–5 mm.

Dose solutions

■ Conformal

Both PTV44 and high dose volumes often extend bilaterally into the neck. The usual conformal plan for many hypopharyngeal tumours uses opposing lateral photon beams shaped to the PTV with MLCs. Wedges in both the AP and superoinferior planes may be needed to compensate for changes in the contour of the neck.

If the high dose PTV extends posterior to the plane of the spinal cord a two-phase technique will be needed. Opposing lateral beams in phase 1 will include the spinal cord. A second phase using smaller lateral photon beams with posterior border anterior to the spinal cord is then matched to electron beams to the posterior neck. The electron energy is chosen to keep within spinal cord tolerance but cover PTV if possible. Alternatively, the opposing photon beams can be angled to treat the PTV while avoiding the cord (Fig. 12.5).

The PTV usually extends inferiorly to below the level of the shoulders. The inferior part of the volume can be treated with a matched anterior photon beam with midline shielding. The match plane should ideally be inferior to the lower border of the high dose volume to avoid matching through sites of macroscopic or high risk microscopic disease. An alternative is to angle the opposing lateral

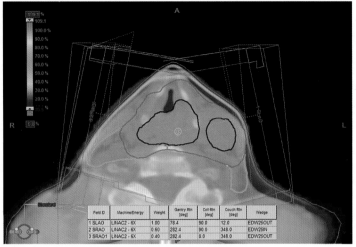

(a)

Field ID	Machine/Energy	Weight	Gantry Rtn [deg]	Coll Rtn [deg]	Couch Rtn [deg]	Wedge
1 SLAO	LINAC2 - 6X	1.00	78.4	90.0	12.0	EDW25OUT
2 SRAO	LINAC2 - 6X	0.60	282.4	90.0	348.0	EDW25IN
3 SRAO1	LINAC2 - 6X	0.40	282.4	0.0	348.0	EDW25OUT

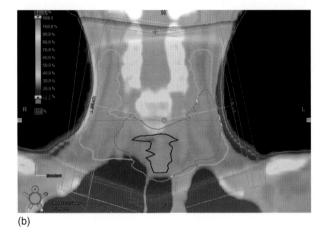

(b)

(c)

Field ID	Machine/Energy	Weight	Gantry Rtn [deg]	Coll Rtn [deg]	Couch Rtn [deg]	Wedge
1 SLPO	LINAC2 - 6X	1.00	99.0	296.8	15.9	EDW25IN
2 SRAO	LINAC2 - 6X	0.60	284.6	70.5	348.0	EDW25IN
3 SRAO1	LINAC2 - 6X	0.50	284.6	366.9	348.2	EDW300UT

Figure 12.5 Treatment of a T4aN1 posterior pharyngeal wall tumour with radiotherapy. In this patient with significant comorbidity, a decision was made not to treat the level II nodes to reduce acute effects.
(a) Axial slice to show phase 1 beams angled posteriorly.
(b) Coronal slice to show phase 1 beams angled inferiorly. (c) Axial slice to show phase 2 beams angled to avoid the spinal cord.

beams caudally by 10–30°. Superoinferior wedges compensate for the change in contour of the neck but it can still be difficult to produce a homogeneous dose distribution for adequate dose to the inferior part of the volume. An anterior neck beam can help to achieve this.

If the volume extends both posterior to the cord and inferior to the shoulders there is no conformal option other than to use opposing photon and posterior electron beams and a matched anterior neck beam. If the match plane is through a high risk site, it should be moved once during the course of treatment to reduce the risk of under- or overdosing at the junction.

If the volume extends unilaterally (e.g. lateral T1/2 N0 pyriform fossa), a unilateral beam arrangement will provide a more conformal dose distribution whilst sparing contralateral pharyngeal mucosa and salivary glands. A plan with three beams can be used with beam angles chosen to avoid the spinal cord with the posterolateral beam and to minimise dose to the uninvolved mucosa.

■ Complex

IMRT has several advantages. No anterior neck beam matching is needed and therefore the risk of under or overdosing at the match plane is reduced. Matched electron beams to treat posteriorly behind the cord will not be needed. It can provide a more even dose distribution if the volume extends inferiorly into the low neck or superior mediastinum. It facilitates dose escalation by allowing smaller, high dose volumes to be treated in one phase with a simultaneous boost technique. It can reduce the risk of xerostomia by sparing salivary glands.

A seven-beam coplanar technique is usually needed to achieve these aims though five beams are sometimes adequate. Spinal cord (with a 5 mm isotropic margin), parotid glands and brainstem are contoured as organs at risk. Oral or pharyngeal mucosa outside the PTV should be contoured to allow these sites to be spared as much as possible.

■ Conventional

Patients having palliative radiotherapy can be treated conventionally with lateral opposing beams chosen in the simulator. If the volume extends inferior to the shoulders or for any curative treatment, a conformal CT based plan is recommended.

Dose-fractionation

■ Curative treatment T1/T2 N0

70 Gy in 35 daily fractions given in 7 weeks.

■ Curative treatment T3/4 or N+

70 Gy in 35 daily fractions given in 7 weeks ± concomitant cisplatin weekly.
or
alternative fractionation, e.g. with concomitant boost.
44 Gy in 22 daily fractions to PTV44 in 4 ½ weeks.

■ Adjuvant treatment

60–66 Gy in 30–33 daily fractions given in 6–6½ weeks ± concomitant chemotherapy.

■ Simultaneous boost IMRT

65 Gy to high dose PTV and 54 Gy to low dose PTV in 30 fractions given in 6 weeks.

■ Palliative treatment

30 Gy in 5 fractions of 6 Gy given in 3 weeks.
or 20 Gy in 5 fractions of 4 Gy given in 1 week.

Treatment delivery and patient care

Weekly assessment by doctor or radiographer and dietician is important. Regular speech and language therapist advice can help maintain safe, functional swallowing. Most patients are at high risk of weight loss and should be considered for a gastric feeding tube inserted for prophylaxis before radiotherapy. Further details are given in Chapter 8.

Verification

See Chapter 8.

---

key trials

See chapter 8 – many phase III trials in head and neck cancer contain patients with hypopharyngeal cancers.

Lefebvre JL, Chevalier D, Lunoinski B *et al.* (1996) Larynx preservation in pyriform sinus cancer: preliminary results of a European Organisation for Research and Treatment of Cancer phase III trial. EORTC Head and Neck Cancer Cooperative Group. *J Natl Cancer Inst* **88:** 890–9.

Information sources

Mendenhall WM, Parsons JT, Stringer SP *et al.* (1993) Radiotherapy alone or combined with neck dissection for T1–T2 carcinoma of the pyriform sinus: an alternative to conservation surgery. *Int J Radiat Oncol Biol Phys* **27:** 1017–27.

Montgomery PQ, Rhys Evans PH, Henk JM (2003) Tumours of the hypopharynx. In: Rhys Evans PH, Montgomery PQ, Gullane PJ (eds) *Principles and Practice of Head and Neck Oncology*. Martin Dunitz, London, pp. 253–78.

13 Nasopharynx

Indications for radiotherapy

■ Curative

Radiotherapy is the principal treatment modality in nasopharyngeal cancer (NPC) and is often combined with chemotherapy in advanced disease (stage IIb, III and IV). The role of surgery is confined to neck dissections for persistent or recurrent lymphadenopathy or, rarely, to salvage recurrent nasopharyngeal disease.

NPC is endemic in southern China, relatively common around the Mediterranean, and uncommon in northern Europe and the USA. The WHO classification identifies three histological subtypes. Type 1 (keratinising squamous cell carcinoma) is more common in the West but less common in endemic areas, and local control is harder to achieve. Because there is a relatively low incidence of occult cervical lymph node involvement in WHO1 disease with no palpable lymphadenopathy, elective neck irradiation can be less extensive. Types 2 (non-keratinising differentiated carcinoma) and 3 (undifferentiated) make up most of endemic cases. While lymphadenopathy at presentation is common, these tumours are relatively sensitive to chemotherapy and radiotherapy, so local control rates are good. Failure, particularly in WHO3 tumours, is often with metastases.

Genetic, environmental and dietary factors may all play a role in the aetiology of NPC. High levels of Epstein–Barr virus antibodies are found in the WHO3 subtype and can correlate with stage and response to treatment.

The most frequently used staging systems are the UICC TNM and Ho's staging. T staging reflects local invasion as described below. N staging criteria in the UICC system are different from those for other head and neck cancers to reflect the high incidence of lymphadenopathy and relative sensitivity to radiation (Table 13.1).

Overall 5-year survival rates are about 50 per cent, but different staging systems and case mix make comparisons between series difficult. T1/2 N0/1 disease (stage I and II in most systems; Table 13.2) has a 5-year local control rate of 70–90 per cent with radiotherapy alone. Chemotherapy is recommended in addition to radiotherapy for stage IIb–IV disease, to achieve 5-year local control rates of 50–70 per cent.

■ Recurrent disease

Local recurrence in the nasopharynx is difficult to treat surgically. Brachytherapy with iodine-125 or gold-198 seeds can be used to treat small volume persistent or recurrent disease, or can be combined with surgery. However, most local recurrences are detected when they are too large to be cured with brachytherapy.

Table 13.1 Comparison of UICC TNM (6th edn, 2002*) and Ho's (1978) staging for nasopharyngeal cancer

Stage	UICC TNM (6th edn, 2002)	Ho's (1978)
T1	Tumour confined to nasopharynx	Tumour confined to nasopharynx
T2	Tumour extends to soft tissues. T2a – extends to oropharynx and/or nasal cavity without parapharyngeal extension. T2b – with parapharyngeal extension	Extension to the nasal fossa, oropharynx, or adjacent muscles or nerves below the base of the skull
T3	Tumour invades bony structures and/or paranasal sinuses	Beyond T2 limits. T3a Bone involvement of the base of the skull – includes floor of the sphenoid sinus. T3b Involvement of the base of the skull. T3c Involvement of the cranial nerve(s). T3d Involvement of the orbits, laryngopharynx, or infratemporal fossa
T4	Tumour with intracranial extension and/or involvement of cranial nerves, infratemporal fossa, hypopharynx, orbit or masticator space	Not defined
N1	Unilateral metastasis in nodes ≤6 cm in greatest dimension, above the supraclavicular fossa	Node(s) wholly in the upper cervical level bounded below by the skin crease extending laterally and backward from or just below the thyroid notch (laryngeal eminence)
N2	Bilateral metastasis in nodes ≤6 cm in greatest dimension, above the supraclavicular fossa	Node(s) palpable between the crease and the supraclavicular fossa
N3	Metastasis in nodes >6 cm in dimension or in the supraclavicular fossa. N3a – >6 cm in dimension. N3b – in the supraclavicular fossa	Supraclavicular fossa nodes and/or skin involvement

*With permission.

Table 13.2 Stage groupings for UICC TNM (6th edn, 2002*) classification

Stage I	T1 N0 M0
Stage IIA	T2a N0 M0
Stage IIB	T1 N1 M0
	T2a N1 M0
	T2b N0–1 M0
Stage III	T1 N2 M0
	T2a–2b N2 M0
	T3 N0–2 M0
Stage IVA	T4 N0–2 M0
Stage IVB	Any T N3 M0
Stage IVC	Any T any N M1

*With permission.

Re-irradiation to a curative dose can be considered. It provides cure in 35 per cent but must be balanced against the high rate (at least 30 per cent) of serious late effects, including bone necrosis and temporal lobe damage. An interval of more than 2 years from first treatment, and highly conformal planning are desirable.

Sequencing of multimodality therapy

The relative chemo-sensitivity of nasopharyngeal tumours has led to the use of chemoradiation to try to improve local control and overall survival. Neoadjuvant or adjuvant chemotherapy, concomitant (usually cisplatin) chemotherapy, and a combination of both have all been reported to improve local control and overall survival rates. The relative chemo-sensitivity of NPC and high rate of distant metastases makes neoadjuvant treatment theoretically attractive, but there is so far no proof of benefit from clinical trials. For stage IIb–IV disease, three cycles of cisplatin-based induction chemotherapy are given initially (except in patients with significant comorbidity), followed by radiation with concomitant cisplatin either weekly or 3-weekly for all patients.

Clinical and radiological anatomy

The nasopharynx is a mucosa-lined space behind the nasal cavities and above the oropharynx. Understanding the anatomy of this region helps correlate presenting symptoms with local invasion and is vital in order to define the CTV accurately (Fig. 13.1). Tumours most commonly arise in the roof or lateral wall – often the fossa of Rosenmüller behind the Eustachian tube orifice. Tumour can spread via the mucosa or submucosa, to invade the nasal cavity anteriorly or the oropharynx inferiorly. The lateral wall is formed by the pharyngeal fascia which offers relatively little resistance to tumour spread. Deep to the fascia is the parapharyngeal space containing the lateral retropharyngeal lymph nodes (nodes of Rouvière), cranial nerves IX–XII, carotid artery and internal jugular vein. Direct extension or nodal involvement can lead to IX–XII cranial nerve palsies. Tumour can grow out of the parapharyngeal space superiorly into the middle cranial fossa, and anteriorly into the pterygopalatine fossa and inferior orbital fissure towards the orbit.

The roof slopes downwards to become the posterior wall. Medially it is formed by the sphenoid sinus and laterally by the foramen lacerum at the skull base. This provides relatively little barrier to local invasion into the cavernous sinus, which contains cranial nerves III–VI and the internal carotid artery. Skull base invasion occurs in 30 per cent of cases.

The nasopharynx drains directly to both the lateral retropharyngeal nodes in the parapharyngeal space and to level II and upper level V nodes. Ipsilateral lymphadenopathy is detected in 60–90 per cent of patients at diagnosis and 50 per cent have involved contralateral nodes. The lateral retropharyngeal nodes lie medial to the internal carotid artery and anterior to the spinal column from the occiput to C3. These nodes are not palpable and should be assessed on MRI or CT, with a node >5 mm considered pathological. Involved cervical nodes are usually palpable but the whole neck and supraclavicular fossae should be imaged.

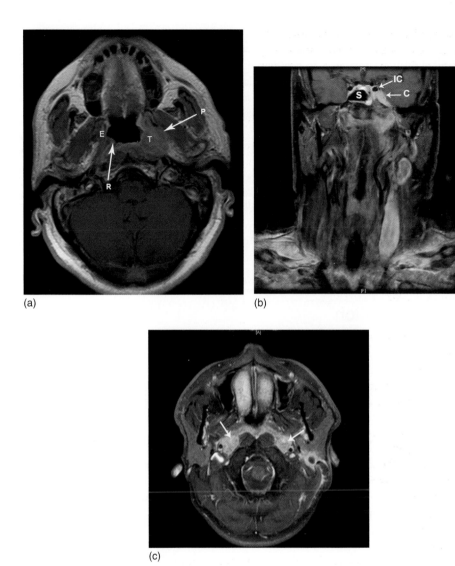

Figure 13.1 Diagnostic MR scans to illustrate nasopharyngeal anatomy and routes of tumour spread. (a) Axial T1-weighted contrast-enhanced MRI showing tumour (T) invading parapharyngeal space (P). The normal contralateral fossa of Rosenmüller (R) and normal Eustachian tube orifice (E) are also shown. (b) Coronal T1-weighted contrast-enhanced MRI showing cavernous sinus invasion (C), the sphenoid sinus (S) and internal carotid artery (IC). (c) Axial T1-weighted contrast-enhanced MRI showing bilateral retropharyngeal nodes (arrowed).

Distant metastases are uncommon at presentation. All patients should have a chest radiograph performed but chest CT, liver imaging and bone scans are only required in the presence of advanced disease (N3) or symptoms and signs suggestive of metastases.

Assessment of primary disease

Careful clinical examination and cross-sectional imaging are required to assess local invasion and lymph node spread. Particular attention should be paid to sites where local invasion is suspected on the basis of clinical symptoms and signs. Clinical examination should include a nasendoscopy or EUA to assess mucosa, submucosa and extent of spread in the nasopharynx. Documentation of cranial neuropathies can direct imaging assessment. MRI is preferred to CT with contrast as it provides better imaging of soft tissue invasion, particularly the parapharyngeal space and retropharyngeal lymph nodes. CT with bone windows is better for detecting bone involvement and may also be required if skull base invasion is suspected.

All patients should have a dental assessment and OPG as xerostomia after treatment is common. A baseline audiogram is useful as tumour, radiotherapy and chemotherapy can all contribute to hearing loss.

Data acquisition

■ Immobilisation

Patients are treated supine with head and shoulders immobilised in a Perspex shell or thermoplastic mask with at least five fixation points. The chin is elevated to spare the oral cavity and orbit, but the spine should be kept as straight as possible if posterior neck nodes are present, to facilitate matching of an electron boost. A mouth bite may be used to depress the tongue away from the treated volume. If IMRT is used, the patient can be immobilised with the chin in a neutral position.

■ CT scanning

CT scan slices measuring 3–5 mm are obtained from 2 cm above the superior orbital ridge (to include the skull base) to the arch of the aorta inferiorly. Intravenous contrast may help definition of cervical nodes. Reference marks are placed on the shell at the CT visit to aid verification.

■ Simulator

3D conformal radiotherapy or an IMRT technique is preferred because local extent of disease can be better determined. However, Ho's technique (modified here slightly) relates likely patterns of spread to bony anatomy, so 2D simulator-based planning with opposing lateral fields can be used.

Target volume definition

The GTV is first contoured on the planning CT using diagnostic images and clinical information. Particular attention should be given to the parapharyngeal space as described above, and to the lateral pharyngeal lymph nodes. Retropharyngeal nodes >5 mm and cervical nodes >10 mm in short axis diameter are contoured as GTV. If induction chemotherapy has been used, the GTV should reflect the initial sites of disease.

Three CTVs are defined: a high dose CTV70 reflecting the clinically apparent disease; a high risk CTV60 reflecting the high risk of local spread in and adjacent to the nasopharynx; and a prophylactic CTV50 to treat at risk but clinically uninvolved nodes.

The GTV is expanded isotropically by 5 mm to form the CTV70 which is then edited to reflect natural tumour barriers. In particular, the posterior margin can be reduced if the vertebral column is not involved, and this will help minimise brainstem dose.

The CTV70 is copied to form the CTV60 which is expanded to reflect possible local spread in the nasopharynx. It should include the whole nasopharynx, adjacent retropharyngeal lymph nodal regions, parapharyngeal space, pterygoid plates, pterygomaxillary fissures, floor of the sphenoid sinus, foramen lacerum and the posterior part of the nasal cavity (5 mm anterior to the GTV) (Fig. 13.2). If a T1 primary tumour is small and well defined on imaging, some of these sites can be excluded from the CTV60 (e.g. contralateral parapharyngeal space).

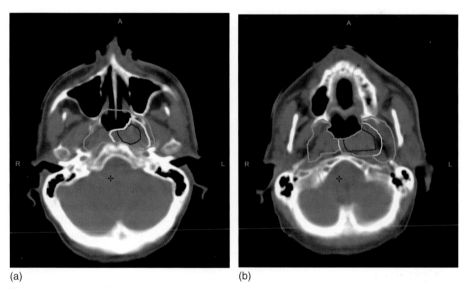

(a) (b)

Figure 13.2 GTV, CTV70 (cyan) and CTV60 (purple) for a T2b nasopharyngeal cancer shown on two axial levels: (a) and (b).

The CTV60 is copied to form the CTV50. This is expanded to include bilateral level Ib and II–V nodes. In N0 disease, level Ib can be omitted bilaterally. In N1 disease, the contralateral level Ib can be omitted. In the rare situation of WHO1 disease that is clinically N0, level IV and inferior level V nodes can also be omitted. If level IV or low level V nodes are involved the supraclavicular nodes on that side should be included in the CTV50. A CTV-PTV margin is applied (usually 3–5 mm) based on measured set-up errors assuming no tumour motion.

The brainstem and spinal cord should always be defined. The parotid glands, pituitary gland, temporomandibular joints (TMJs), optic apparatus, temporal lobes and middle ear apparatus (adjacent to the fossa of Rosenmüller) should also be contoured as critical structures if IMRT is used, as dose sparing may be possible.

Dose solutions

■ Conformal

As the PTV50 includes both a midline tumour and bilateral cervical nodes, it is difficult to obtain adequate coverage conformally with anything other than opposing lateral photon beams. Conformal planning is still preferable as it will allow MLC shielding to shape to PTVs rather than to bony anatomy. Treatment of the PTV60 and PTV70 with a conformal plan will reduce the dose to adjacent critical structures such as the brainstem and temporal lobes.

PTV50 is initially treated to 40 Gy in 20 fractions with opposing lateral photon beams as shown (Fig. 13.3). MLC shielding is applied to oral cavity, orbit and brain. This is matched to a bilateral anterior neck beam with the match plane at least 10 mm below the nodal GTV.

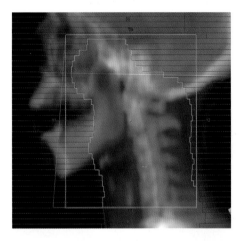

Figure 13.3 BEV of lateral beam for phase 1 treatment of nasopharyngeal cancer.

The second phase treats the nasopharynx (PTV60) with a further 20 Gy in 10 fractions with a three-beam plan using an anterior infraorbital in addition to small lateral beams to reduce temporal lobe and TMJ dose. This arrangement is also used for the final 10 Gy in 5 fractions with additional shielding to reduce the treated volume if possible (Fig. 13.4).

The second phase also includes a matched anterior neck beam covering the elective nodal PTV50 bilaterally. This can be reduced to cover sites of involved nodes only (nodal PTV70) from 50 Gy. If the nodal PTV70 is small, it can be treated with electrons from 50 Gy to 70 Gy.

An anterior neck beam prescribed to D_{max} will not cover all the cervical node PTV with the 95 per cent isodose, but this arrangement has been used for decades without a high incidence of isolated nodal recurrence, so the dose delivered seems to be adequate for tumour control. If a higher dose to the nodes is required, for example when level V nodes are present, either the prescription point can be changed to 3 cm (which will produce a hot-spot of 115 per cent) or opposing anterior and posterior fields weighted anteriorly can be used (which will increase the volume of normal tissue treated to a high dose).

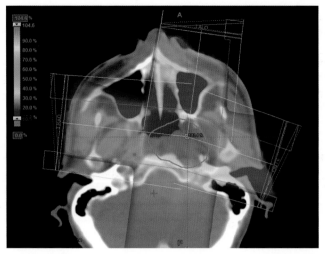

Figure 13.4 Conformal treatment of the PTV70 for phase 3 in nasopharyngeal cancer.

There is evidence that toxicity (especially xerostomia) is reduced using a more complex arrangement of five to six coplanar beams, sometimes with an additional non-coplanar vertex beam.

■ Complex

The complex PTVs and adjacent critical normal structures make IMRT of the nasopharynx a good solution in theory. Five or seven equally spaced coplanar IMRT beams can provide good target volume coverage, keep neural tissues within tolerance and spare parotid function to prevent long-term xerostomia. Several dose levels can be stipulated in the plan so that the three PTVs can be treated to different doses in a single phase. The low neck can be included in the IMRT volume or treated with a matched anterior neck beam as above.

■ Conventional

Where resources are not available for conformal planning, conventional techniques may be unavoidable. Ho's technique describes a similar solution to the conformal one described above with bony landmarks used to define beam edges. For example beam borders for the first phase of treatment are: anterior – bisecting antrum; posterior – 2 cm posterior to nodes; superior – 5 mm above anterior clinoid.

Dose-fractionation

■ Simultaneous boost IMRT

65 Gy to PTV70, 60 Gy to PTV60 and 50.4 Gy to PTV50 in 30 fractions given in 6 weeks.

■ Conformal/conventional

70 Gy in 35 daily fractions given in 7 weeks to PTV70 ± concomitant cisplatin (60 Gy/30fractions and 50 Gy/25 fractions to PTV60 and PTV50, respectively).

Treatment delivery and patient care

A dental assessment is carried out before radiotherapy because of the risk of long-term xerostomia. We recommend that a prophylactic feeding tube is inserted before radiotherapy in all patients with N2/3 disease and is considered for others thought to be at increased risk of weight loss during treatment.

See Chapter 8 for details.

Verification

See Chapter 8.

key trials

Al-Sarraf M, LeBlanc M, Giri PG *et al.* (1998) Chemoradiotherapy versus radiotherapy in patients with advanced nasopharyngeal cancer: Phase III randomised Intergroup study 0099. *J Clin Oncol* **16**: 1310–17.

Information sources

Chau RMC, Teo PML, Choi PHK *et al.* (2001) Three-dimensional dosimetric evaluation of a conventional radiotherapy technique for treatment of nasopharyngeal carcinoma. *Radiother Oncol* **58**: 143–53.

Jen Y-M, Shih R, Lin YS *et al.* (2005) Parotid gland-sparing 3-dimensional conformal radiotherapy results in less severe dry mouth in nasopharyngeal cancer patients: a dosimetric and clinical comparison with conventional radiotherapy. *Radiother Oncol* **75**: 204–9.

Lee AWM, Poon YF, Foo W *et al.* (1992) A retrospective analysis of 5037 patients with nasopharyngeal carcinoma treated during 1976–1985, overall survival and patterns of failure. *Int J Radiat Oncol Biol Phys* **23**: 261–70.

Liu L-Z, Zhang GY, Xie CM *et al.* (2006) Magnetic resonance imaging of retropharyngeal lymph node metastasis in nasopharyngeal carcinoma: patterns of spread. *Int J Radiat Oncol Biol Phys* **66**: 721–30.

Wolden SL, Chen WC, Pfister DH *et al.* (2006) Intensity-modulated radiation therapy (IMRT) for nasopharyngeal cancer: update of the Memorial Sloan-Kettering experience. *Int J Radiat Oncol Biol Phys* **64**: 57–62.

Larynx

14

Indications for radiotherapy

■ Early stage squamous cell cancer of glottic larynx (T1–2, N0)

Squamous cell carcinomas confined to the glottic larynx can be treated with either surgery (often laser excision) or radiotherapy. Large retrospective series suggest equivalent cure rates as long as radiotherapy is followed by close surveillance to detect and treat recurrences. Radiation alone gives 5-year local control rates of 75–90 per cent in T1 tumours. Local surgical and radiotherapeutic expertise, patient choice and likely voice quality all influence the treatment decision. If the anterior commissure is involved, voice quality with surgery may be worse as it can be more difficult to oppose the vocal cords after resection.

■ Early stage squamous cell cancer of supraglottic larynx (T1–2, N0)

The supraglottic larynx has a richer lymphatic drainage than the glottic larynx. Although surgery and radiotherapy have equal cure rates, the ability to preserve organ function and to treat the adjacent neck nodes means radiotherapy is preferred.

■ Advanced laryngeal cancer (T3–4, N+)

The preferred treatment for many years for advanced laryngeal cancer has been surgery (total laryngectomy and neck dissection) with adjuvant radiotherapy in selected cases. In practice, adjuvant radiation is recommended to the primary site in T4 cancer or where resection margins are close or involved and to the neck in N2–3 disease or in N1 disease with extracapsular nodal spread. Adjuvant radiotherapy is therefore recommended for the majority of patients who have a laryngectomy.

An alternative approach is organ preservation – initial radiotherapy, usually combined with chemotherapy with laryngectomy reserved for recurrence. There are phase III data to support this approach, provided there is careful follow-up to detect recurrence and allow salvage surgery. Without this, (chemo)radiation will produce inferior cure rates compared with laryngectomy.

If the primary tumour invades through the laryngeal cartilage, laryngectomy is preferred. In other cases we recommend initial radiochemotherapy with close follow-up and salvage laryngectomy in case of residual or recurrent disease.

■ Palliative EBRT

If distant metastases are present initially or if the patient is not suitable for curative treatment, palliative EBRT may improve pain and reduce the chance of laryngeal obstruction or tumour ulceration in the neck.

Sequencing of multimodality therapy

Locally advanced laryngeal disease is often treated with surgery, radiotherapy and chemotherapy. Initial laryngectomy may be followed by adjuvant radiotherapy with concomitant chemotherapy for selected patients (see Chapter 8). Concomitant radiochemotherapy can be used as initial treatment with surgery (laryngectomy and/or neck dissection) for residual or recurrent disease.

Induction (neoadjuvant) chemotherapy has been used to predict response to radiation and to select patients for organ preservation. Two to three cycles of cisplatin and 5-fluorouracil are given with assessment of disease response at each cycle. Most patients respond and then have organ preservation with radiotherapy, but if response is poor, a laryngectomy is recommended. The role of concomitant radiochemotherapy after induction chemotherapy is not established.

Exophytic glottic and subglottic tumours may present with stridor. Even if organ preservation is the preferred treatment, surgical debulking may be required initially to preserve a clear airway.

Clinical and radiological anatomy

The larynx is divided into three subsites: the supraglottic larynx (epiglottis, false cords, ventricles, aryepiglottic folds and arytenoids), glottic larynx (true cords) and subglottic larynx (from the under surface of the cords to the inferior border of the cricoid cartilage) (Table 14.1 and Fig. 14.1). Primary tumours can spread mucosally or submucosally between these subsites or to the adjacent oropharynx or hypopharynx. They can invade deep structures including the laryngeal cartilages,

Table 14.1 UICC TNM (6th edn, 2002*) tumour staging for supraglottic and glottic cancer

Supraglottis (subsites – suprahyoid epiglottis, aryepiglottic fold, arytenoids, infrahyoid epiglottis, false cords)

T1	Tumour limited to one subsite with normal vocal cord mobility
T2	Tumour invades mucosa of more than one adjacent subsite of supraglottis or glottis or region outside the supraglottis (e.g. mucosa of base of tongue) without fixation of the larynx
T3	Tumour limited to the larynx with vocal cord fixation and/or invades postcricoid areas, pre-epiglottic tissues, paraglottic space, and/or with minor thyroid cartilage erosion (e.g. inner cortex)
T4a	Tumour invades through the thyroid cartilage and/or invades tissues beyond the larynx e.g. trachea, soft tissues of the neck including deep/extrinsic muscle of tongue, strap muscles, thyroid, oesophagus
T4b	Tumour invades prevertebral space, mediastinal structures or encases carotid artery (i.e. unresectable)

(Continued)

Table 14.1 Continued

Glottis (subsites – vocal cords, anterior commissure, posterior commissure)

T1	Tumour limited to vocal cords with normal mobility
	T1a – limited to one vocal cord
	T1b – involves both vocal cords
T2	Tumour extends to supraglottis and/or subglottis and/or with impaired vocal cord mobility
T3	Tumour limited to the larynx with vocal cord fixation and/or invades paraglottic space, and/or with minor thyroid cartilage erosion (e.g. inner cortex)
T4a	Tumour invades through the thyroid cartilage and/or invades tissues beyond the larynx, e.g. trachea, soft tissues of the neck including deep/extrinsic muscle of tongue, strap muscles, thyroid, oesophagus
T4b	Tumour invades prevertebral space, mediastinal structures or encases carotid artery (i.e. unresectable)

*With permission.

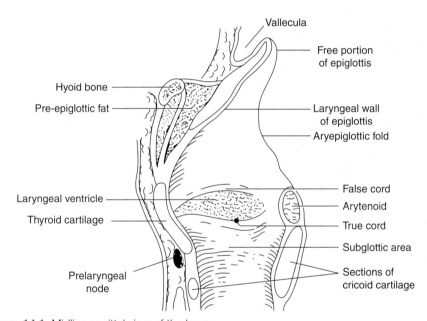

Figure 14.1 Midline sagittal view of the larynx.

pre-epiglottic and paraglottic fat, or into nearby structures such as the carotid sheath or prevertebral muscles.

The glottic larynx has very few lymphatics so early tumours confined to this site are usually N0 and adjacent nodes do not require treatment. The prelaryngeal (Delphian) node lies on the cricothyroid membrane and is usually included in radiotherapy treated volumes incidentally. Tumours originating in the supraglottic larynx can spread to adjacent level II or III nodes unilaterally or bilaterally if the primary tumour crosses the midline. Locally advanced cancers spread to adjacent level II–IV nodes. If there is subglottic involvement, tumours can spread to level IV or midline level VI nodes.

Assessment of primary disease

For early disease, clinical assessment of local invasion and vocal cord mobility is more important than cross-sectional imaging. Most patients have an EUA to obtain biopsies and to evaluate supraglottic and subglottic spread, although a transnasal oesophagoscopy can be used instead. Both oncologist and surgeon should examine the larynx with a nasendoscope or indirect laryngoscopy to visualise the primary tumour and to assess vocal cord mobility (Fig. 14.2).

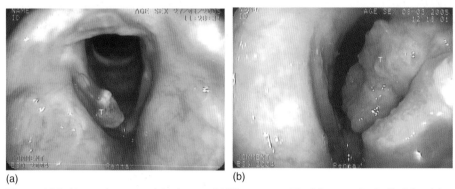

(a)　　　　　　　　　　　　　　　　　(b)

Figure 14.2 Nasendoscopy of the larynx. (a) T1a tumour (T) of the anterior half of the right vocal cord. (b) T3 tumour (T) of the left vocal cord extending into the supraglottic larynx.

T1N0 squamous cell cancer confined to one vocal cord does not require cross-sectional imaging as the risk of deep invasion or nodal spread is very small. All other laryngeal cancer requires cross-sectional imaging with CT or MRI. Invasion of paraglottic fat and laryngeal cartilages may be assessed by CT or MRI (Fig. 14.3). Ultrasound can be useful particularly to help assess cartilage sclerosis where cartilage invasion is suspected but not proven with MRI or CT.

Data acquisition

■ Immobilisation

All patients having radiotherapy should be immobilised in a Perspex or thermoplastic shell fixed to the couch in at least five places. The spine should be straight. The shoulders are immobilised in the shell as inferiorly as possible so that the shoulder tips are inferior to the lower border of the cricoid cartilage thus permitting lateral radiation beams to treat the larynx without the need to angle them inferiorly. Grip bars on the side of the couch may help to achieve this.

■ Simulator

Radiotherapy for early (T1) glottic carcinomas with no extra-laryngeal disease can be planned on a simulator because the position of the primary tumour can be determined – the vocal cords extend horizontally from 10 mm below the thyroid promontory – and lymph nodes do not require treatment. The whole larynx can therefore be treated with opposing lateral beams with the following

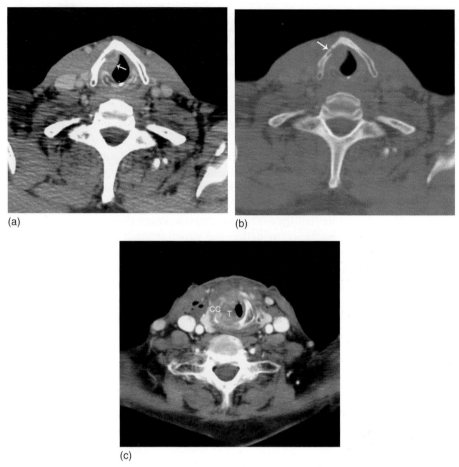

Figure 14.3 Cartilage invasion in laryngeal tumours. (a) Diagnostic CT scan showing tumour (arrowed) with possible invasion of the thyroid cartilage. (b) Same slice with window and level optimised for bone/cartilage to show cartilage invasion. (c) T4a tumour (T) invading through the cricoid cartilage (CC) into the soft tissues of the neck.

borders: superior – mid-body of the hyoid, inferior – inferior margin of cricoid cartilage, anterior – to cover skin, posterior – anterior vertebral column. A 1 cm thick tissue equivalent bolus should be applied anteriorly if tumour extends to the anterior commissure. As the larynx moves superiorly on swallowing, fluoroscopy is used in the simulator to ensure that the glottis remains within the treated volume when the patient swallows.

■ CT scanning

CT slices 3–5 mm thick are obtained from the base of skull to the top of the aortic arch with the patient immobilised in the treatment position. As treatment of locally advanced glottic cancer or adjuvant radiation after a laryngectomy may require lateral beams angled inferiorly, the CT scan in these patients should be extended inferiorly to the carina.

Target volume definition

■ T1 N0 glottic larynx

As conventional treatment with small lateral beams is usually successful and well tolerated, target volumes should be defined with these borders in mind. Records and pictures from nasendoscopy and EUA should be available as small primary vocal cord tumours are difficult to see on CT scan. GTV is defined as the site of primary tumour. CTV is the glottic larynx with a border at least 10 mm superiorly and inferiorly from the GTV. Axially the bilateral mucosal laryngeal surface is included as field change is common. PTV is CTV with a 3–5 mm isotropic margin depending on local assessment of random and systematic errors assuming tumour movement is minimal. Motion can be assessed by watching laryngeal movement with fluoroscopy in the simulator to ensure that the vocal cords remain within the PTV on swallowing.

In practice, it can be easier to define the superior (mid-body of hyoid) and inferior (inferior margin of cricoid) beam borders on the lateral DRR from the planning CT scan and then check on the axial slices that the whole glottic larynx is included within the CTV, assuming a 5 mm penumbra from PTV to beam edge. Using smaller beams defined solely on the basis of GTV-CTV-PTV definition has little therapeutic advantage and increases the possibility of a geographical tumour miss due to intra-fractional motion from swallowing.

■ Other curative radiotherapy

The GTV is defined on the planning CT scan as the primary tumour and any involved lymph nodes. There are no clinicopathological studies to help determine the GTV-CTV70 margin, but in practice the GTV is grown isotropically by 10 mm and then edited to take into account likely patterns of spread and barriers to tumour growth. The high dose CTV70 also includes lymph nodes of normal size that are at high risk of having microscopic tumour involvement – in practice this includes the level III nodes immediately adjacent to the primary tumour.

Table 14.2 Suggested nodal CTVs for laryngeal cancer

Site and stage	CTV70 nodal levels	CTV44 nodal levels
T1 N0 glottis	None	None
T2 N0 glottis	Level III nodes immediately adjacent to tumour	None
T1/2 N0 supraglottis	Level II, III nodes immediately adjacent to tumour	Bilateral level II, III
T3/4 N0/1 glottis	Involved nodal levels + level III nodes immediately adjacent to tumour	Bilateral low level II, levels III–IV. Level VI for subglottic tumours
T3/4 N2/3 glottis	Involved nodal levels + level III nodes immediately adjacent to tumour	Bilateral level II–IV. Level V if >1 node involved in that side of the neck. Level VI for subglottic tumours
N+ supraglottis	Involved nodal levels + level III nodes immediately adjacent to tumour	Bilateral levels II–IV Consider Ib, V depending on site of primary and of involved nodes

The CTV44 in the patient with clinically negative nodes includes all nodes at risk for microscopic metastases as shown in Table 14.2. If adjacent structures are involved, the CTV44 must reflect their lymphatic drainage, e.g. level II nodes if there is tongue base invasion.

■ Adjuvant radiotherapy

The CTV after a laryngectomy is determined by the initial site of the tumour and which local structures were invaded, and by the pattern of lymph node spread found on initial imaging and at neck dissection. A CTV66 can be defined as sites where surgical margins were involved or where there was extracapsular nodal spread but in practice it is often difficult to delineate this volume separately from the CTV60.

Preoperative imaging, clinicopathological correlation, a clear operation note and discussion with the surgeon all help to determine the CTV60, which includes sites at risk of microscopic residual disease. Particular thought should be given to establishing whether there was subglottic invasion as this predicts for recurrence in the tracheostomy site and mandates inclusion of the stoma in the CTV60.

For a pT4N0 tumour that has been completely excised with a bilateral negative selective neck dissection, the CTV60 is the tumour bed alone. For node positive disease, the CTV60 should include all nodal levels which contained disease in the dissected neck. A separate CTV44 can be defined to treat contralateral nodes that are at lower risk of metastases if there has not been a selective neck dissection on that side.

Dose solutions

■ T1 N0 glottic larynx

Conventional

The field borders defined above will provide adequate coverage for early glottic cancers. Opposing lateral beams of approximately 5 cm × 5 cm require 15–45° wedges to compensate for missing tissue anteriorly. A 1 cm tissue equivalent bolus is needed over the apex of the larynx if the anterior commissure is involved.

Conformal

A more conformal dose distribution can be obtained by either using anterior oblique rather than lateral beams or by the addition of an anterior beam which can obviate the need for bolus anteriorly. MLCs are used to conform each beam to the shape of the PTV. In this way dose to the lateral neck is reduced which may reduce the risk of damage to the carotid vessels. However, the adjacent lymph nodes will not receive a therapeutic dose as they would with an opposing beam arrangement (Fig. 14.4). If there is any question of supraglottic involvement the adjacent nodes must be included in the CTV and the volume treated accordingly.

■ Other tumours

Conformal

For a PTV that extends bilaterally and involves midline structures, opposing or slightly angled lateral photon beams may be the only way to provide adequate coverage. The beams are shaped to the PTV contour with MLC leaves to improve

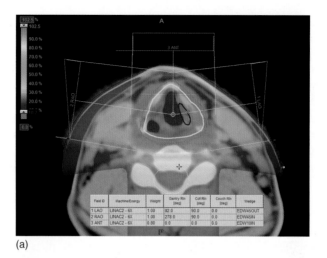

Field ID	Machine/Energy	Weight	Gantry Rtn [deg]	Coll Rtn [deg]	Couch Rtn [deg]	Wedge
1 LAO	LINAC2 - 6X	1.00	82.0	90.0	0.0	EDW45OUT
2 RAO	LINAC2 - 6X	1.00	278.0	90.0	0.0	EDW45IN
3 ANT	LINAC2 - 6X	0.80	0.0	0.0	0.0	EDW10IN

(a)

(b)

Figure 14.4 Conformal radiotherapy for T1a cancer of the left glottis with three beams. (a) Axial slice showing beams and dose distribution. (b) Sagittal slice. The superior beam border is the mid-body of the hyoid bone and the inferior border is the inferior margin of the cricoid cartilage.

the therapeutic ratio. When the PTV extends inferiorly below the shoulders, the opposing lateral beams are angled inferiorly by 10–30° to provide dose to the low neck. Because the contour of the neck changes both from anterior to posterior and also from superior to inferior, the beams are wedged in two planes to provide a conformal distribution. This is impossible with MLCs, so it is necessary to use two identical sized fields for each lateral beam – each with a wedge in a different plane. An anterior beam can also improve the dose distribution in some plans. Even with these modifications it can be difficult to get a uniform dose distribution and particularly to get adequate dose to the inferior part of the PTV.

Where a single PTV anterior to the cord is defined one beam arrangement is used throughout (Fig. 14.5). If a PTV70 and PTV44 are defined two phases are used, usually with similar beam angles but different MLC positions (Fig. 14.6). If the high dose PTV extends posterior to the spinal cord on one side, the lateral beams can sometimes be angled by 20–30° which may also allow some sparing of the contralateral parotid gland if the PTV extends superiorly. For some volumes, matched electron beams may be required to treat the posterior extent of high dose PTVs in phase 2. The posterior border of the opposing photon beams is set just anterior to the spinal cord and the electron energy is chosen to provide as good coverage of the PTV as possible without exceeding spinal cord tolerance.

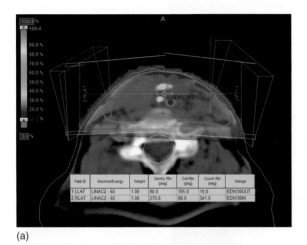

(a)

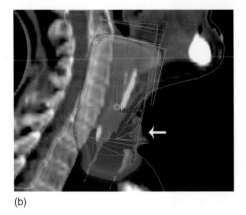

(b)

Figure 14.5 Adjuvant radiotherapy for a pT4N0 laryngeal tumour. (a) Axial view. Tissue planes are difficult to define in the postoperative setting. (b) Sagittal view showing the stoma (arrowed) included within the treated volume.

Complex

IMRT has the potential to produce a more conformal dose distribution to the PTVs particularly if the PTV extends inferiorly below the shoulders or posteriorly behind the spinal cord. It also means matching within the PTV to an anterior neck or posterior electron beam is unnecessary. Dose escalation may then be possible. Parotid sparing can be accomplished if the PTV extends superiorly into level II. A seven beam coplanar arrangement is likely to produce the best plan though five beams may be adequate.

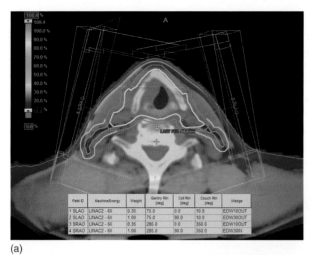

(a)

(b)

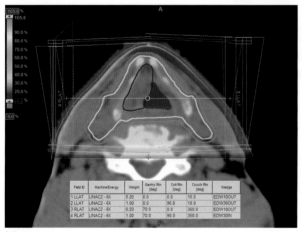

(c)

Figure 14.6 Radiotherapy for T3 N0 carcinoma of the right glottis. Phase 1 lateral beams angled (a) posteriorly and (b) inferiorly. (c) Phase 2 lateral beams to treat the larynx and adjacent level III nodes.

Conventional

Where resources are not available for conformal planning, conventional techniques may be unavoidable with beam arrangements as described above.

Dose-fractionation

■ T1–2 N0 glottic larynx

55 Gy in 20 daily fractions of 2.75 Gy given in 4 weeks.
50 Gy in 16 daily fractions of 3.125 Gy given in 22 days.

■ Other curative treatments

70 Gy in 35 daily fractions given in 7 weeks ± concomitant cisplatin or alternative fractionation, e.g. with concomitant boost.
44 Gy in 22 daily fractions to PTV44 given in 4½ weeks.

■ Adjuvant treatment

60 Gy in 30 daily fractions given in 6 weeks ± concomitant cisplatin.

Treatment delivery and patient care

See Chapter 8. Particular care of the tracheostomy site is needed if the stoma is included in the treated volume. Tracheitis will occur and may make it painful to replace a stoma button. Desquamation anteriorly can make fixing stoma devices difficult. These patients should be assessed weekly throughout treatment by a speech and language therapist. Patients having an intact larynx irradiated will develop varying degrees of laryngitis and need advice to rest their voice until acute effects subside.

Verification

See Chapter 8.

Key trials

EaStER – *Ea*rly *St*age glottic cancer: *E*ndoscopic excision or *R*adiotherapy. Feasibility Study. A randomised, controlled, feasibility study developed by the EaStER trial management group on behalf of the NCRI Head and Neck Cancer Clinical Studies Group (in progress).

Forastiere AA, Goepfert H, Maor M *et al.* (2003) Concurrent chemotherapy and radiotherapy for organ preservation in advanced laryngeal cancer. *N Engl J Med* **349**: 2091–8.

The Department of Veteran Affairs Laryngeal Cancer Study Group (1991) Induction chemotherapy plus radiation compared with surgery plus radiation in patients with advanced laryngeal cancer. *N Engl J Med* **324**: 1685–90.

Information sources

Cellai E, Frata P, Magrini SM *et al.* (2005) Radical radiotherapy for early glottic cancer: Results in a series of 1087 patients from two Italian radiation oncology centers. I. The case of T1N0 disease. *Int J Radiat Oncol Biol Phys* **63**: 1378–86.

Clark CH, Bidmead AM, Mubata CD *et al.* (2004) Intensity-modulated radiotherapy improves target coverage, spinal cord sparing and allows dose escalation in patients with locally advanced cancer of the larynx. *Radiother Oncol* **70**: 189–98.

Pfister DG, Laurie SA, Weinstein GS *et al.* (2006) American Society of Clinical Oncology clinical practice guideline for the use of larynx-preservation strategies in the treatment of laryngeal cancer. *J Clin Oncol* **24**: 3693–704.

Salivary glands

15

Indications for radiotherapy

Most salivary gland tumours arise in the parotid glands, but tumours of the submandibular or other minor salivary glands can also occur. Most tumours are treated with surgery, followed by postoperative radiotherapy when risk of local recurrence is high. Retrospective series suggest the addition of radiotherapy can reduce local recurrence rates from 30 per cent to 10 per cent but there is no effect on overall survival.

Patterns of local and metastatic spread vary with histological subtype. Careful pathological assessment is important to help predict risk of local recurrence and the need for adjuvant radiotherapy. Pre- and postoperative discussions with the surgeon are useful to define extent of surgery and likely sites of macroscopic or microscopic residual disease though some tumours will only be found to be malignant at operation. Tumours close to the facial nerve within the parotid gland may often be excised with positive or very close margins in order to preserve the nerve, with the expectation that adjuvant radiotherapy will be used. Primary skin cancers of the head and neck can metastasise to intraparotid lymph nodes, but radiotherapy for these cancers is considered separately in Chapter 9.

■ High grade tumours (high grade mucoepidermoid, high grade adenocarcinoma, carcinoma arising from pleomorphic adenoma)

Adjuvant radiotherapy to the tumour bed is recommended for all high grade salivary tumours except for T1 tumours completely excised with clear margins. Ipsilateral neck levels Ib, II and III should be treated prophylactically in view of the high risk of occult neck node metastases, unless a negative selective neck dissection has been performed. In node-positive patients, adjuvant radiotherapy is recommended for N2/3 disease or in the presence of extracapsular spread. Tumours of intermediate grade should be managed as high grade cancers.

■ Low grade tumours (low grade mucoepidermoid, low grade adenocarcinoma, acinic cell carcinoma)

Adjuvant radiotherapy is recommended where excision margins are positive or close (<5 mm) after discussion with the surgeon and pathologist. The deep excision margin close to the facial nerve is usually most critical. The risk of occult neck metastases is smaller than for high grade tumours, so prophylactic treatment of the N0 neck is not recommended.

■ Adenoid cystic carcinoma

These tumours have a relatively high local recurrence rate and a propensity for perineural spread, therefore adjuvant radiotherapy is recommended for all adenoid cystic cancers except in rare T1 tumours without pathological evidence of perineural invasion.

■ Pleomorphic adenoma

Pleomorphic adenomas, though histologically benign, can be difficult to control locally with surgery alone. Radiotherapy is indicated if excision margins are positive and no further surgery is possible (e.g. tumour close to the facial nerve). Radiotherapy should also be considered to prevent further recurrences in patients who have had a pleomorphic adenoma excised on more than one occasion previously, particularly if there is a short interval between recurrences relative to the life expectancy of the patient, or if further surgery would compromise cosmesis or function.

Sequencing of multimodality therapy

Adjuvant radiotherapy should ideally commence 4–6 weeks after surgery as long as adequate wound healing has occurred. There is no proven role for concomitant chemotherapy.

Clinical and radiological anatomy

Parotid tumours usually arise in the portion of the gland lateral to the plane of the facial nerve – the superficial lobe – though there is no anatomical distinction between the superficial and deep lobes. They can invade locally throughout the gland, compromising facial nerve function if trunks of the nerve are invaded. Extraparotid extension can occur laterally into skin or medially into the pterygopalatine fossa and lateral parapharyngeal space, resulting in trismus or invasion of the carotid sheath. Bone invasion is uncommon. Adenoid cystic carcinomas in particular can invade nerve fibres spreading up the facial nerve towards the stylomastoid foramen.

The parotid gland contains several intraparotid lymph nodes. The superficial intraparotid nodes are on the external surface of the gland, and the deep nodes are found within the gland, mainly adjacent to the external carotid artery and external jugular vein. Parotid tumours can spread via the intraparotid nodes to the subparotid nodes in the retrostyloid space and thence to the retropharyngeal nodes, or directly to level II nodes (Fig. 15.1).

Tumours of the submandibular salivary gland can invade locally or perineurally in the marginal branch of the facial nerve, the lingual nerve, nerve to mylohyoid and hypoglossal nerve. Lymphatic drainage is to level Ib nodes lying adjacent to (but rarely within) the salivary gland and then to ipsilateral level II nodes.

There are minor salivary glands submucosally throughout the upper aerodigestive tract and malignant salivary tumours can occur in any site. The hard palate is the most common location for such tumours which spread to the same lymph nodes as squamous cell carcinomas at those sites.

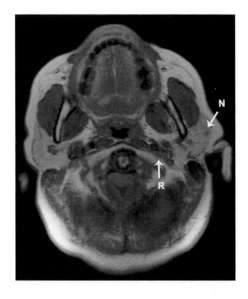

Figure 15.1 Axial T1-weighted MRI showing intraparotid lymph node (N), and the location of the subparotid nodes in the retrostyloid space (R).

Assessment of primary disease

Clinical examination can reveal invasion of local structures such as the skin, facial nerve (palsy) or pterygoid muscles (trismus) or spread to draining lymph nodes. Fine needle aspiration either in clinic, or under ultrasound guidance, usually provides confirmation of malignancy.

Cross-sectional imaging is performed to assess extent of the primary tumour particularly at the deep margin adjacent to the parapharyngeal space and to assess local lymph nodes. MRI is preferred to CT as primary tumours are better defined and nerve enhancement can be assessed. Scans should include imaging of the skull base. Cross-sectional preoperative imaging should be obtained on all patients with malignant tumours to enable more accurate postoperative volumes to be defined for radiotherapy.

Data acquisition

■ Immobilisation

Patients should be immobilised lying supine with the neck slightly extended to move the orbits superiorly and reduce the chance of beams exiting through the eye. A Perspex or thermoplastic shell with at least five fixation points should ideally be used even if the neck is not included in the treatment volume, as systematic and random errors will be smaller and CTV-PTV margins can be tighter.

■ CT scanning

CT slices are obtained from the skull base to the hyoid in patients not requiring neck radiotherapy, or from the skull base to the arch of the aorta if the neck is to be irradiated. Slices should be no more than 5 mm thick and ideally 3 mm.

Fusion of planning MRI and CT images can be particularly helpful where there is extensive perineural invasion which necessitates inclusion of the skull base in the target volume.

■ Simulator

CT scanning is preferred to simulator-based planning to allow individualised ipsilateral beam arrangements to conform better to the PTV and avoid critical structures and mucosa.

Target volume definition

■ Parotid

The planning CT (and MRI if performed) should be carefully evaluated to detect macroscopic residual disease or lymphadenopathy. Preoperative imaging and discussions with the surgeon and pathologist are important. As radiotherapy is usually given adjuvantly after surgery, no GTV is defined unless there is macroscopic residual disease. The CTV60 is contoured as the sites of possible microscopic disease. Particular attention is given to the deep excision margin which is likely to be close or involved if the facial nerve has been preserved. As a minimum, the medial extent of the CTV60 should be to the lateral surface of the internal jugular vein, but if the deep lobe of the parotid is thought to contain tumour, the parapharyngeal space should be included (Figs 15.2 and 15.3). The lateral extent of the CTV60 will be close to the surface of the skin. The position of the contralateral parotid on the planning CT can be a useful guide to the superior and inferior limits of the CTV60.

In adenoid cystic carcinomas, the CTV60 should include the course of the facial nerve up to the stylomastoid foramen at the skull base. In recurrent pleomorphic adenomas, the CTV should be individualised depending on the location of recurrent disease as defined by preoperative imaging and surgical discussions.

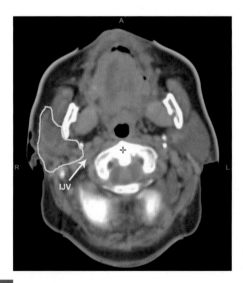

Figure 15.2 CTV for a small high grade tumour completely excised by a superficial parotidectomy with a close deep margin adjacent to the facial nerve. Arrow indicates internal jugular vein.

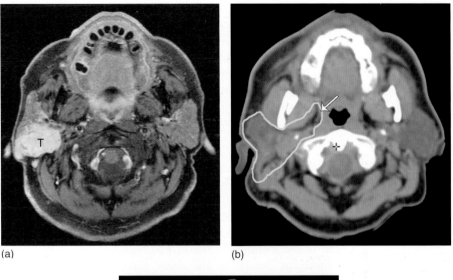

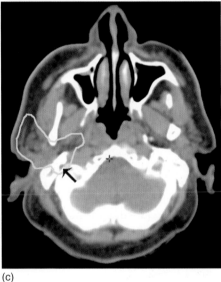

Figure 15.3 Target volume definition for an adenoid cystic tumour of the deep lobe of the parotid gland. (a) Axial T1-weighted contrast-enhanced MRI showing primary tumour (T). (b) Corresponding planning CT scan showing CTV including the parapharyngeal space (arrowed). (c) Axial planning CT slice close to skull base. The course of the facial nerve up to the stylomastoid foramen (arrowed) is included in the CTV.

If there are indications for neck radiotherapy adjuvantly after a neck dissection, the levels to be treated are included in the CTV60. If there are indications (high grade tumour) for prophylactic neck radiotherapy, the ipsilateral level Ib, II and III nodes should be included in the treated volume. While a separate CTV44 can be defined to give these sites a prophylactic dose, the proximity of the nodes to the parotid bed means that including them in the CTV60 and treating the whole volume in one phase is a more pragmatic approach.

Sites where resection margins are involved, or where there was extracapsular nodal extension, should be defined in a CTV66 – though again it may be more appropriate to treat the whole CTV to this dose rather than to define separate dose levels.

The CTV is expanded isotropically to form the PTV by a margin determined for each department by the observed random and systematic errors – usually 3–5 mm.

The contralateral parotid gland does not usually receive sufficient dose to cause xerostomia but it should be contoured as an organ at risk if the mean dose to the gland is expected to be >24 Gy. The inner ear should be defined as an OAR, as reducing dose to the cochlear apparatus may reduce the risk of deafness.

■ Other sites

Similar principles can be applied for volume definition for tumours of the submandibular or minor salivary glands. In adenoid cystic carcinomas the nerve innervating the primary tumour site should be included up to the skull base. In adenoid cystic carcinomas of the submandibular gland this should include the lingual nerve (a branch of the mandibular nerve, V3) back to the foramen ovale and the marginal mandibular branch of the facial nerve to the stylomastoid foramen. For tumours arising in or close to midline (e.g. hard palate), prophylactic lymph node volumes should be outlined bilaterally if lymph nodes are to be included in the CTV.

Dose solutions

■ Conformal

Two or three ipsilateral photon beams will usually provide homogeneous dose distribution to the CTV without exceeding the tolerance of adjacent critical structures. The anterior oblique beam angle is chosen according to the shape of the anteromedial edge of the PTV while trying to minimise dose to the mucosa of the oral cavity and oropharynx. The posterior oblique angle is chosen according to the contour of the posterolateral edge of the PTV and should be lateral to the spinal cord and brainstem (Fig. 15.4). The exit dose from this beam should be inferior to the contralateral eye. This is usually achieved by immobilising the patient with the neck slightly extended but half beam blocking may be needed if the PTV extends more superiorly. An additional lateral photon beam may provide a more homogeneous distribution but will increase dose to the contralateral parotid gland and possibly to the spinal cord. Alternatively, a lateral electron beam can be used but current algorithms make the calculation of mixed photon and electron beams less reliable. All beams should be shaped to the PTV contour with MLCs.

The PTV may come close to the skin surface, in which case it can be difficult to cover the lateral surface of the PTV unless tissue equivalent bolus is used. However, bolus is only recommended if there is a risk of microscopic residual disease in the skin. This is an uncommon situation as involved skin is usually resected and a myocutaneous flap used to fill the defect. This new skin will not contain microscopic disease. However, if a Perspex shell is used it should not be cut out over the treated volume.

Hotspots in the mandible of >107 per cent should be avoided to reduce the risk of osteoradionecrosis. Excessive dose in the temporomandibular joint (TMJ)

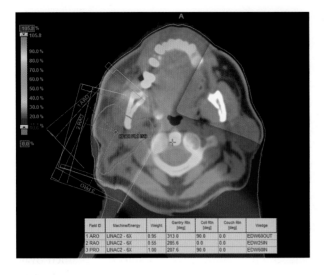

Figure 15.4 Axial planning CT slice showing three-beam plan for adjuvant radiotherapy of a parotid tumour.

Field ID	Machine/Energy	Weight	Gantry Rtn [deg]	Coll Rtn [deg]	Couch Rtn [deg]	Wedge
1 ARO	LINAC2 - 6X	0.95	313.0	90.0	0.0	EDW60OUT
2 RAO	LINAC2 - 6X	0.55	285.6	0.0	0.0	EDW25IN
3 PRO	LINAC2 - 6X	1.00	207.6	90.0	0.0	EDW60IN

should also be avoided to reduce the risk of long-term TMJ dysfunction and trismus. The cochlear dose should be kept below 50 Gy if possible to reduce the risk of long-term sensorineural hearing damage.

If level III and IV nodes are to be treated as an adjuvant to neck dissection, a matched anterior neck beam can be used. The match plane should be inferior to any preoperative lymphadenopathy to avoid a junction through microscopic residual disease.

■ Complex

IMRT planning studies have reported reduced dose to the cochlea. An equispaced nine-beam coplanar technique has been described, but this risks increasing dose to the contralateral parotid. An ipsilateral four-beam IMRT planning solution has also been used but may not be better than a 3D-conformal beam arrangement.

Neutron therapy

The one small RCT of fast neutron therapy versus conventional radiotherapy for unresectable salivary gland cancers reports a better local control rate with neutrons at the risk of increased late toxicity.

■ Conventional

The irregularly shaped PTV will be treated best with conformal radiotherapy to reduce dose to organs at risk, but an ipsilateral anterior and posterior oblique wedged beam arrangement can be planned conventionally. Care should be taken to avoid organs at risk, especially exit dose to the contralateral eye.

Dose-fractionation

■ Adjuvant

60 Gy in 30 daily fractions given in 6 weeks.
66 Gy in 33 fractions for positive margins or extracapsular nodal spread.

■ Recurrent pleomorphic adenoma

50 Gy in 25 daily fractions given in 5 weeks.

There are no data to support the use of altered fractionation regimens for salivary gland tumours.

Treatment delivery and patient care

The amount of oral cavity and oropharynx included in the treatment volume may predict the degree of swallowing problems seen during treatment. Treatment of mucositis should be given within a multidisciplinary team, which reviews the patient weekly. Advice on jaw exercises can reduce the risk of trismus and TMJ dysfunction.

Conductive hearing loss due to middle ear effusions can occur during radiotherapy and take several months to improve after treatment has finished. If subjective hearing loss persists 2 months after treatment, an audiogram should be performed. If there is evidence of conductive hearing loss, a grommet may be indicated.

Verification

In addition to the procedures outlined in Chapter 8, if the posterior oblique beam is shown on BEV to exit close to the contralateral eye, lens doses should be measured by TLD on the first day of treatment to ensure tolerance is not exceeded.

> **key trials**
>
> COchlear Sparing Therapy And conventional Radiation COSTAR – A multicentre randomised study of cochlear sparing intensity modulated radiotherapy versus conventional radiotherapy in patients with parotid tumours. Available at www.ncrn.org.uk (accessed 4 December 2008).
>
> Laramore GE, Krall JM, Griffin TW et al. (1993) Neutron versus photon irradiation for unresectable salivary gland tumors: final report of an RTOG-MRC randomized trial. Int J Radiat Oncol Biol Phys **27**: 235–240.

Information sources

Chen AM, Garcia J, Lee NY et al. (2007) Patterns of nodal relapse after surgery and postoperative radiation therapy for carcinomas of the major and minor salivary glands: what is the role of elective neck irradiation? Int J Radiat Oncol Biol Phys **67**: 988–94.

Terhaard CHJ, Lubsen H, Rasch CRN et al. (2005) The role of radiotherapy in the treatment of malignant salivary gland tumours. Int J Radiat Oncol Biol Phys **61**: 103–11.

Sinuses: maxilla, ethmoid and nasal cavity tumours

16

Indications for radiotherapy

Tumours arising in the sinonasal area usually present with symptoms of local invasion and the importance of local extent is reflected in the T stage (see Table 16.1).

Lymphatic spread and distant metastases are unusual so surgery and radiotherapy to the primary site are the main treatments. Fifty per cent of tumours appear to arise in the maxilla with 25 per cent each in the nasal cavity and ethmoids. Primary tumours of the frontal or sphenoid sinus are very rare.

Table 16.1 UICC TNM (6th edn, 2002*) tumour staging for nasal cavity and paranasal sinuses

	Maxillary sinus	Nasal cavity or ethmoid sinus
T1	Tumour limited to the mucosa with no erosion or destruction of bone	Tumour restricted to one subsite of nasal cavity or ethmoid sinus,[†] with or without bony invasion
T2	Tumour causing bone erosion or destruction, including extension into hard palate and/or middle nasal meatus, except extension to posterior wall of maxillary sinus and pterygoid plates	Tumour involves two subsites in a single site or extends to involve an adjacent site within the nasoethmoidal complex, with or without bony invasion
T3	Tumour invades any of the following: bone of posterior wall of maxillary sinus, subcutaneous tissues, floor or medial wall of orbit, pterygoid fossa, ethmoid sinuses	Tumour extends to invade the medial wall or floor of the orbit, maxillary sinus, palate, or cribriform plate
T4a	Tumour invades any of the following: anterior orbital contents, skin of cheek, pterygoid plates, masticator space, cribriform plate, sphenoid or frontal sinuses	Tumour invades any of the following: anterior orbital contents, skin of nose or cheek, minimal extension to anterior cranial fossa, pterygoid plates, sphenoid or frontal sinuses
T4b	Tumour invades any of the following: orbital apex, dura, brain, middle cranial fossa, cranial nerves other than maxillary division of trigeminal nerve V2, nasopharynx, clivus	Tumour invades any of the following: orbital apex, dura, brain, middle cranial fossa, cranial nerves other than V2, nasopharynx, clivus

*With permission.
[†]Subsites are: septum, floor, lateral wall and vestibule of nasal cavity and left and right ethmoid sinuses.

Squamous cell cancers are the commonest histological subtype (50 per cent) and radiotherapy is often combined with chemotherapy in advanced disease on the basis that there is additional benefit from combined treatment in other head and neck squamous cell cancers.

There are many other tumour types that all have slightly different clinico-pathological characteristics. Adenoid cystic cancers have a propensity for perineural spread so radiotherapy volumes need to include the course of the relevant nerve to the skull base. Olfactory neuroblastomas (aesthesioneuroblastoma) arise in the olfactory epithelium of the superior nasal cavity and can invade the cribriform plate and anterior cranial fossa. This is important when planning both surgery (craniofacial resection) and radiotherapy.

Malignant melanomas can arise from the nasal cavity mucosa, especially the lateral wall. Depth of invasion does not correlate well with prognosis. Sinonasal melanomas behave unpredictably but almost inevitably recur at some point, often locally. This means a more palliative approach should be considered in the elderly or those with poor performance status. Adenocarcinomas usually start in the middle meatus or ethmoid sinus, and are related to exposure to hardwood dust. Other rarer tumours include chondrosarcomas and sinonasal undifferentiated carcinomas (SNUC).

■ Adjuvant radiotherapy

Whilst surgery is the treatment of choice for almost all sinonasal malignancies, adjuvant radiotherapy is recommended in most cases as it is difficult to resect these tumours *en bloc* with clear margins. There is non-randomised trial evidence that radiotherapy improves local recurrence rates for all tumour types. The exception is completely resected T1 disease where recurrence rates are likely to be low. It may also be appropriate not to irradiate after surgery for sinonasal melanoma, reserving radiotherapy for the almost inevitable recurrence.

Combined surgery and postoperative radiotherapy lead to optimal 5-year survival rates of 50 per cent in maxillary sinus squamous cell cancers, 60 per cent in ethmoid adenocarcinoma, 75 per cent in olfactory neuroblastoma and 30 per cent in sinonasal melanoma.

■ Primary radiotherapy

If complete resection is considered impossible because of invasion of local structures (e.g. cranial fossae, masticator space) or if the patient declines surgery, primary radiotherapy is used to obtain local control and, occasionally, cure.

■ Palliative radiotherapy

Mucosal melanomas and other locally advanced sinonasal tumours in patients with poor performance status are treated with palliative radiotherapy as cure is unlikely. This approach should be discussed with individual patients.

Sequencing of multimodality therapy

Adjuvant radiotherapy should begin after adequate surgical healing – usually within six weeks of operation. Concomitant chemotherapy with cisplatin may be given in stage III and IV squamous cell carcinomas, particularly if disease is unresectable or if excision margins are positive.

If primary radiotherapy is given, disease should be reassessed 4–6 weeks later by a surgeon to see if resection is then possible.

Clinical and radiological anatomy

The nasal cavity, ethmoid sinuses and maxillary sinuses are interconnected mucosa-lined spaces in close proximity to the orbit and anterior cranial fossa (Fig. 16.1). Most tumours present with symptoms from spread outside the sinuses. An understanding of the 3D anatomy is important to assess disease and to determine target volumes for radiotherapy.

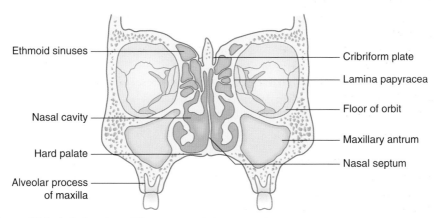

Ethmoid sinuses
Nasal cavity
Hard palate
Alveolar process of maxilla

Cribriform plate
Lamina papyracea
Floor of orbit
Maxillary antrum
Nasal septum

Figure 16.1 Anterior view of the paranasal sinuses.

Maxillary tumours can extend through the anterior wall to invade the cheek or posteriorly into the pterygopalatine fossa and masticator space (infratemporal fossa) causing trismus, and from there to the middle cranial fossa. Inferior extension into and through the floor of the maxilla may result in loose teeth or an oroantral fistula.

It is relatively easy for tumour to grow into the orbit superiorly through the inferior orbital fissure or for ethmoid tumour to grow into the orbit through the thin lamina papyracea. Ethmoid tumours can also grow superiorly through the cribriform plate and into the anterior cranial fossa and anteriorly into the nasal cavity.

MRI with gadolinium enhancement is the imaging modality of choice as it can assess local extent and differentiate tumour from retained secretions. CT may provide additional information if cribriform plate erosion or early orbital involvement is suspected.

Lymph node involvement is seen in less than 20 per cent of tumours but the neck should be examined clinically and radiologically. Tumours invading the anterior nose and cheek have a higher risk of lymphatic spread than those contained within the sinuses, with level Ib and II nodes most likely to be involved. Lymphatic spread is more common in tumours invading adjacent mucosal surfaces such as the nasopharynx.

Metastases at presentation are uncommon but all patients should have a chest radiograph and appropriate investigation of symptoms suggestive of metastases.

Assessment of primary disease

Owing to the late presentation, it can be difficult to determine the exact primary site so possible spread to all the above sites should be assessed clinically and radiologically. Clinical assessment includes nasendoscopy to assess the nasal cavity and examination of the oral cavity to check for inferior extension. Pterygopalatine fossa extension may lead to trismus, infraorbital canal involvement to facial pain and paraesthesia and orbital cavity spread to proptosis and diplopia, all of which should be sought.

Several surgical approaches are possible and need to be understood to define target volumes in the adjuvant setting.

A lateral rhinotomy allows access to the medial maxilla, the nasal cavity and the ethmoid, sphenoid and frontal sinuses. It has been superseded for many tumours by a midfacial degloving approach. In this operation, a sublabial incision allows the soft tissues of the face to be elevated to provide greater bilateral access though access to the frontal sinus is more limited.

A craniofacial approach enables assessment and resection of the anterior skull base at the cribriform plate with *en-bloc* resection of tumour involving the ethmoids. If there is tumour invading the medial wall of the orbit but not the periosteum (i.e. no tumour within the orbital cavity), part of the orbital periosteum can be resected. This enables the eye to be spared but presents a challenge in planning radiotherapy. Frozen sections are used to define margins of excision. Surgery for selected patients is performed endoscopically. Tumours are removed piecemeal but with frozen sections to assess margins. The technique is not suitable when the orbit and skull base are thought to be at risk.

Data acquisition

■ Immobilisation

Patients should be immobilised supine in a Perspex or thermoplastic shell. If the neck is not irradiated, the shoulders do not need to be immobilised. If the low neck nodes are to be treated (level III–V) the neck should be extended to allow treatment of most of the neck nodes with an anterior beam, avoiding the oral cavity and pharynx where possible.

A mouth bite is used to depress the tongue and oral cavity away from the treated volume and reduce acute morbidity. Patients should be asked to look straight ahead to avoid rotating the lens or retina, particularly if the orbital cavity is included in the treated volume. Wax plugs in the nostrils are used if the tumour extended inferiorly in the nasal cavity to enable a more uniform dose distribution.

■ CT scanning

A CT scan is performed with 3 mm slices from 2 cm superior to the superior orbital ridge to the hyoid bone (but extended to include the low neck if neck nodes are to be treated). The whole head should be imaged if non-coplanar beams are to be used in the treatment plan (see below).

Fused CT-MRI images can be useful in the definition of the optic pathways and skull base. MRI also allows retained secretions to be differentiated from tumour where resection has been incomplete.

■ Simulator

3D CT-planned conformal radiotherapy is recommended for all patients, given the complex anatomy of this region. If this is not available, orthogonal simulator films are taken and volumes defined on these films using knowledge of tumour extent and patterns of spread.

Target volume definition

Where resection is not possible or has been incomplete, the GTV is outlined but defining the CTV is the most important step for most patients.

The proximity of these tumours to critical structures such as the optic nerves and chiasm, brainstem, and lacrimal glands mandates meticulous CTV definition so that radiotherapy can be targeted to sites at highest risk of relapse in individual tumours and reduce the risk of long-term radiation damage. The importance of discussion between the surgeon, pathologist and radiation oncologist in defining sites at greatest risk of recurrence after surgery cannot be overemphasised. Preoperative imaging should be viewed beside the CT planning dataset to ensure that initial sites of disease are covered.

The CTV should encompass all initial sites of disease (presurgery GTV), the mucosa of adjacent compartments of the sinonasal complex and a 10 mm margin at least from initial sites of GTV where no good bony barrier to invasion exists (e.g. masticator space, cribriform plate and infraorbital fissure) (Fig. 16.2).

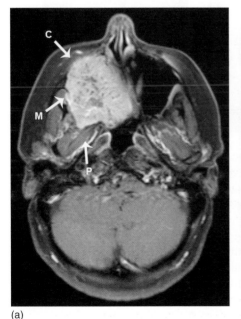
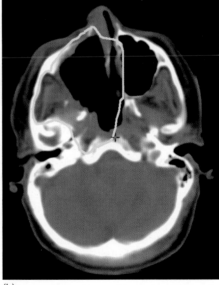

(a)   (b)

Figure 16.2 Definition of CTV for a pT4a carcinoma of the maxilla resected with clear margins. (a) Preoperative T1-weighted contrast-enhanced MRI showing primary tumour invading the cheek (C), masticator space (M) and lateral pterygoid muscle (P). (b) Corresponding planning CT slice showing CTV.

For most tumours, the CTV will include the ipsilateral maxillary sinus and nasal cavity and the ethmoid sinuses bilaterally. The superior extent can be modified for a very inferior tumour. Where the primary involved the maxilla, consideration should be given to including the pterygopalatine and masticator space. When a maxillary tumour has invaded inferiorly, the hard palate should be included in the CTV so as to allow a 10 mm margin around original disease.

The CTV for tumours involving the ethmoid sinuses should include the sphenoid sinus. Where initial disease came close to the orbit or invaded the lamina papyracea, the CTV should include that portion of the medial and inferior orbital wall (Fig. 16.3). The orbital cavity should be included in the CTV if the orbital wall has been breached by tumour or if tumour has grown superiorly through the inferior orbital fissure. Where a craniofacial excision has been carried out, the CTV should extend 10 mm superior to the cribriform plate or 10 mm superior to initial sites of disease, whichever is greater. Olfactory neuroblastomas arise from the cribriform plate and particular attention should be paid to the CTV at this site.

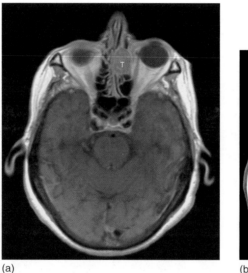 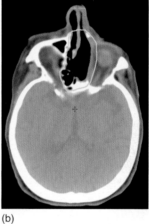

(a)   (b)

Figure 16.3 CTV for an olfactory neuroblastoma invading the lamina papyracea but not into the orbit. (a) Preoperative T1-weighted contrast-enhanced MRI showing primary tumour (T) close to the left orbit. (b) Corresponding planning CT slice showing CTV including the medial portion of the orbital wall.

If the primary was close to or invading the nasopharynx, the adjacent ipsilateral retropharyngeal nodes should be included in the CTV. When cervical node radiotherapy is indicated, the intraparotid nodes, level Ib and superior level II nodes can be included in the CTV but including these nodes will make a complex volume harder to treat adequately. As local relapse in the primary site is usually the greatest risk, the nodes are often not treated in sinonasal tumours.

The CTV is expanded isotropically (usually by 3–5 mm but determined by local audit) to form the PTV.

Organs at risk to be outlined include the lenses, lacrimal glands (in the superolateral orbit and upper eyelid), optic nerves and chiasm, spinal cord, brainstem and pituitary gland. Some centres also expand these structures (in particular the optic nerves) by 2–3 mm to create a PRV to account for systematic and random errors. The direction of such errors is likely to be in the same direction as changes in the PTV so adding a 3 mm margin to both the CTV and the OAR may be unnecessary.

Dose solutions

■ Conformal

The commonest beam arrangement for sinonasal tumours uses an anterior beam to provide most of the dose with an ipsilateral or bilateral wedged lateral beams added to provide extra dose to the posterior part of the PTV (Fig. 16.4). This arrangement cannot provide a uniform dose distribution. Hot-spots of >110 per cent are usually found anteriorly and inadequate posterior coverage occurs in spite of the lateral beams. MLCs are used to shape each beam to the PTV. The lateral fields have their anterior border behind the lens and can be angled 5° posteriorly to avoid exiting through the contralateral lens. As a result, not all the PTV will be within the lateral beams.

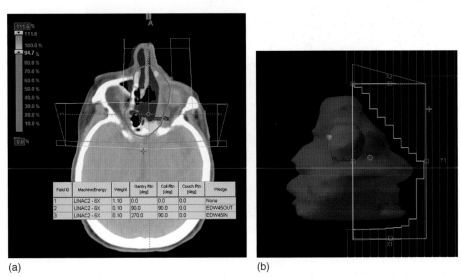

Field ID	Machine/Energy	Weight	Gantry Rtn [deg]	Coll Rtn [deg]	Couch Rtn [deg]	Wedge
1	LINAC2 - 6X	1.10	0.0	0.0	0.0	None
2	LINAC2 - 6X	0.10	90.0	90.0	0.0	EDW45OUT
3	LINAC2 - 6X	0.10	270.0	90.0	0.0	EDW45IN

(a)   (b)

Figure 16.4 Conformal radiotherapy for sinonasal tumours. (a) Beam arrangement. Colour wash scale is set from 95 per cent to demonstrate the hot spot anteriorly and the underdosing posteriorly. (b) BEV of left lateral beam. This beam is to add dose to the posterior part of the PTV only. Left eyeball green; lens yellow.

The course of the optic nerves becomes more medial at the posterior part of the orbital cavity as they exit through the optic canal. At this point, the nerves commonly overlap the PTV. The authors recommend a dose limit of 50 Gy (in 2 Gy fractions) for the optic nerve and chiasm, but where there is particularly high risk of local recurrence (which could itself cause blindness) 55 Gy can be accepted to one optic nerve. In practice, this necessitates a two-phase technique. The whole PTV is treated to 50 Gy. Then the MLCs are moved to ensure the optic nerve doses remain acceptable, although inevitably the posterolateral part of the PTV will not be in the treated volume.

Where the orbital contents are included in the CTV (or after an orbital exenteration) equally weighted anterior and lateral wedged beams are used.

■ Complex

IMRT provides a more conformal dose distribution to the unusual PTVs in sinonasal cancer. Five- or seven-field coplanar beams have been used but these arrangements will increase dose to the orbital contents. A non-coplanar arrangement of three to five sagittal midline beams with right and left lateral beams avoids entry or exit of beams through the eyes and provides a uniform dose distribution (Figs 16.5–16.7). Where the PTV overlaps the optic nerve, there must still be either an acceptance of increased risk of blindness or a reduction in PTV coverage.

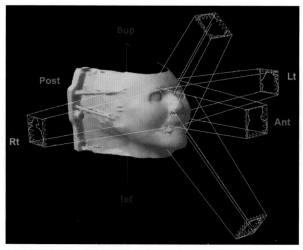

Figure 16.5 Beam arrangement for IMRT of sinonasal tumours.

■ Conventional

The shape of the PTV means that simple conventional planning will not be able to produce adequate dose to the PTV and spare critical normal structures.

Dose-fractionation

■ Adjuvant

60 Gy in 30 daily fractions given in 6 weeks.
66 Gy in 33 daily fractions if possible where there is residual disease.

■ Palliative

36 Gy in 6 fractions of 6 Gy treating once weekly.

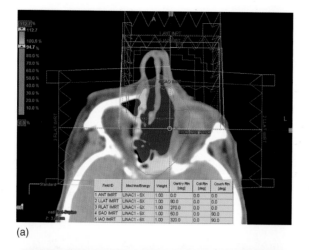

Field ID	Machine/Energy	Weight	Gantry Rtn [deg]	Col Rtn [deg]	Couch Rtn [deg]
1 ANT IMRT	LINAC1 - 6X	1.00	0.0	0.0	0.0
2 LLAT IMRT	LINAC1 - 6X	1.00	90.0	0.0	0.0
3 RLAT IMRT	LINAC1 - 6X	1.00	270.0	0.0	0.0
4 SAO IMRT	LINAC1 - 6X	1.00	50.0	0.0	90.0
5 IAO IMRT	LINAC1 - 6X	1.00	320.0	0.0	90.0

(a)

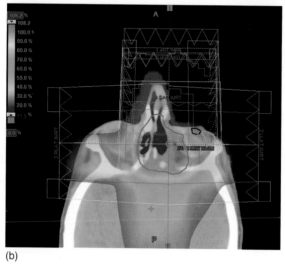

(b)

Figure 16.6 IMRT dose solution for a sinonasal tumour. (a) Note the more homogeneous coverage of the PTV than the conformal solution (Fig. 16.4) provides. Colourwash scale is set from 95 per cent. (b) Dose colourwash to illustrate relative sparing of the left lacrimal gland (pink) and lens (blue).

Treatment delivery and patient care

Patients are seen weekly during treatment in a multidisciplinary clinic. Exercises to reduce trismus (e.g. Therabite™) are recommended if there is pre-existing trismus or where the masticator muscles are in the treated volume. Prophylactic feeding tubes should be considered when the patient has trismus and the treated volume includes a significant portion of the oral cavity (e.g. in maxillary sinus tumours). Careful oral hygiene is essential with prompt treatment of oral *Candida* infections.

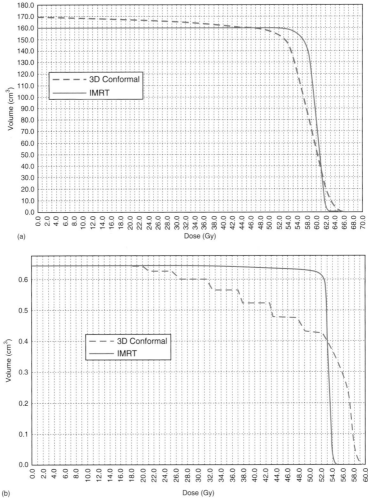

Figure 16.7 DVHs comparing plans shown in Figure 16.4 (three-dimensional conformal) and 16.6 (IMRT). Prescribed dose 60 Gy in 30 fractions. (a) PTV. (b) Ipsilateral (left) optic nerve. Note that in the conformal plan, dose to the nerve exceeds tolerance (55 Gy) and the prescribed dose would have to be reduced.

Where the cornea is within the treated volume, ophthalmic review should be carried out both during and after radiotherapy. Lubricating eye ointments can be applied during the day and at night. If there is a pre-existing facial nerve palsy, the eyelid should be taped shut at night to avoid a dry eye.

Pituitary function tests should be carried out annually during follow-up to evaluate late radiotherapy effects to the pituitary gland.

Verification

Portal images are compared with DRRs as for other head and neck tumours with *in vivo* dosimetry on the first day of treatment.

■ None in this rare cancer.

Information sources

Claus F, De Gersem W, De Wagter C *et al.* (2001) An implementation strategy for IMRT of ethmoid sinus cancer with bilateral sparing of the optic pathways. *Int J Radiat Oncol Biol Phys* **51**: 318–31.

Dirix P, Nuyts S, Vanstraelen B *et al.* (2007) Malignancies of the nasal cavity and paranasal sinuses: long-term outcome with conventional or three-dimensional conformal radiotherapy. *Int J Radiat Oncol Biol Phys* **69**: 1042–50.

Lund VJ (2003) Tumours of the upper jaw and anterior skull base. In: Rhys Evans PH, Montgomery PQ, Gullane PJ (eds) *Principles and Practice of Head and Neck Oncology*. Martin Dunitz: London, 337–54.

Mendenhall WM, Amdur RJ, Hinerman RW *et al.* (2005) Head and neck mucosal melanoma. *Am J Clin Oncol* **28**: 626–30.

Mendenhall WM, Mendenhall CM, Riggs CE Jr *et al.* (2006) Sinonasal undifferentiated carcinoma. *Am J Clin Oncol* **29**: 27–31.

17 Orbit

Indications for radiotherapy

■ Intraocular tumours

Metastases to the vascular choroidal layer (or uvea) – particularly from breast, lung or gastrointestinal tumours – are the commonest intraocular tumours. They usually present with reduced visual acuity and are treated with palliative radiotherapy.

The most frequent primary intraocular tumour is choroidal melanoma. Tumours arising in the choroid have a 30 per cent chance of metastasis at 5 years while rarer iris or conjunctival melanomas have a much lower risk. Tumour size is the most important prognostic factor. Small melanomas are usually asymptomatic and can be difficult to differentiate from various benign conditions. Small tumours ($\leq$5 mm diameter and $\leq$3 mm thick) can therefore be observed or treated with iodine-125 or ruthenium-106 plaque brachytherapy, protons or other local treatments such as laser photocoagulation or surgical excision. Large tumours (>16 mm diameter or >10 mm thick) are treated with enucleation. Preoperative radiation does not improve cure rates. Where there is extrascleral extension, prognosis is poor but enucleation and postoperative radiotherapy can be considered to optimise local control.

A large RCT has shown equivalent cure rates for enucleation and iodine-125 plaque brachytherapy for tumours up to medium size. The plaque is temporarily sutured to the sclera underlying the melanoma and left in place for 3–7 days. Doses of 400 Gy to the base of the tumour and 80–100 Gy to the apex can be achieved. Fractionated proton therapy, available only in specialised centres, gives similar local control rates.

Radiotherapy can be used for cure of retinoblastoma but because there is a high incidence of second malignancies, chemotherapy is often used to allow radiation dose to be reduced. IMRT and proton therapy can produce more conformal dose distributions than standard EBRT.

Conjunctival lymphomas present as salmon-coloured patches on the sclera. They are confined to the orbit in 70 per cent of patients and are treated with radiotherapy. If there is systemic disease chemotherapy is also used. Mucosal associated lymphoid tissue (MALT) lymphomas of the conjunctiva can also be treated with topical chemotherapy or intralesional interferon or can be observed.

■ Extraocular tumours

Orbital lymphomas respond well to radiotherapy either given as sole treatment in stage I disease or following chemotherapy. Primary lacrimal gland carcinomas and orbital sarcomas are treated with excision and postoperative radiotherapy.

Radiotherapy is useful for basal and squamous cell carcinomas arising from the skin and lower eyelid. Superficial photons or electrons are used for early disease whereas EBRT can be used as an alternative to exenteration in more advanced disease or can be considered following exenteration if excision margins are close or involved.

■ Benign disease

Graves' disease is an autoimmune lymphocyte activation causing infiltration and oedema of the extraocular muscles. Radiation is an effective way to reduce local inflammation and compressive symptoms, especially when combined with systemic steroids. It can similarly be used for orbital pseudotumour – an idiopathic orbital inflammation.

Clinical and radiological anatomy

The eye is composed of three layers. An outer fibrous layer is formed by the sclera posteriorly and the cornea anteriorly. The inner layer is the sensory retina with vision concentrated at the fovea which is lateral to the optic nerve and directly posterior to the lens. In between these is the vascular layer – the uvea or choroid – which supplies the retina. The iris is the outer continuation of the vascular layer and the lens sits just behind it, suspended from the ciliary body. The eye has no lymphatic drainage (Fig. 17.1).

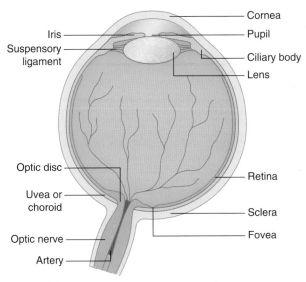

Figure 17.1 Anatomy of the eye.

The extraocular structures often need to be considered and contoured as critical structures in radiotherapy. The optic nerve can clearly be seen on cross-sectional imaging and leaves the orbit via the optic canal to form the optic chiasm. The lacrimal gland sits mainly in the lacrimal fossa – the under-surface of the orbital plate of the frontal bone – but also has a palpebral portion within the upper eyelid. It can be difficult to see on imaging (see Fig. 16.6b, p. 193). Tears from the eye drain through the nasolacrimal duct within the nasolacrimal canal which runs from the lacrimal sac to the inferior nasal meatus between the inferior concha and nasal cavity floor. Tumour invasion, surgery or radiation to the duct can cause epiphora.

The conjunctiva is a clear membrane of lymphoid tissue that covers the sclera and the inner surface of the eyelids producing protective mucus and tears.

The orbit is conical and formed by the fusion of several bones, the thinnest of which is the lamina papyracea of the ethmoid bone which forms part of the medial wall. Tumour can grow into the middle cranial fossa through the superior orbital fissure and optic canal or into the pterygopalatine fossa and masticator space via the inferior orbital fissure.

Only the eyelids, conjunctiva and lacrimal glands have lymphatic drainage and they drain to the preauricular node.

Assessment of primary disease

The oncologist and ophthalmologist should jointly assess any intraocular tumour after the pupil has been dilated. Extraocular tumour is best assessed by cross-sectional imaging with CT or MR scans with coronal and sagittal reconstructions. Clinical examination can also help define extraocular spread into the superior orbital fissure (which causes cranial nerve palsies of VI and then of III, IV and V_1) or into the pterygopalatine fossa and masticator space via the inferior orbital fissure (causing trismus). Careful examination of eye movements can help distinguish invasion of the external ocular muscles from cranial neuropathies. Invasion of the ethmoid sinuses or the nasopharynx can be assessed at nasendoscopy.

Data acquisition

■ Immobilisation

The proximity of target volumes to several critical normal structures means excellent immobilisation is vital. A custom-made thermoplastic or Perspex shell is created with the patient supine and the chin in a neutral position.

■ Simulator

The dimensions of the eye vary by only 1–2 mm between subjects, with a vertical diameter of 23 mm and a slightly larger anteroposterior diameter. Palliative EBRT beams for choroidal metastases can therefore be defined in the simulator. A 4×4 cm beam is marked onto the shell with the anterior margin at the outer canthus and the centre of the field in line with the pupil. The beam is angled posteriorly by 5° to avoid exit through the contralateral lens. Dose is either prescribed to D_{max} or to the depth of the metastasis if known from imaging (Fig. 17.2). An alternative is to use a direct anterior 4×4 cm beam centred on the pupil and to treat with the eye open to minimise lens dose. For treatment of bilateral choroidal metastases, opposing beams are used, again angled 5° posteriorly.

The direct anterior beam used to treat conjunctival lymphomas can also be defined in the simulator. If the lymphoma is confined to the conjunctiva, electrons or orthovoltage photons can be used. If diagnostic imaging reveals tumour tracking posterior to the globe, MV photons are preferred (Fig. 17.3).

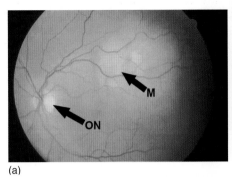
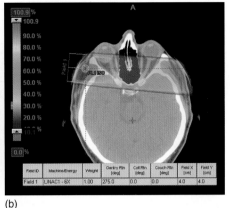

(a)   (b)

Figure 17.2 Palliative radiotherapy for choroidal metastasis. (a) Photograph of a choroidal metastasis (arrowed); optic nerve (ON). (b) Dose colourwash illustrating the dose distribution created by a 4 × 4 cm lateral beam angled 5° posteriorly.

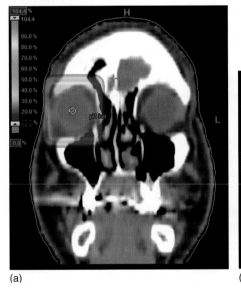
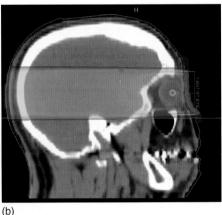

(a)   (b)

Figure 17.3 A 6 MV photon beam to treat conjunctival lymphoma. (a) Anterior view. (b) Sagittal view. Note tissue equivalent bolus used to increase the surface dose.

In Graves' disease small opposed lateral beams can be defined in the simulator to treat the retro-orbital tissues. No target volumes are defined in benign disease. Beam borders are specified by the 50 per cent isodose at the front of the pituitary fossa and the 10 per cent isodose at the posterior lens edge. Beams are angled 5° posteriorly to avoid the contralateral lens (Fig. 17.4).

■ CT scanning

As non-coplanar beams are sometimes required, the volume imaged should extend from the vertex of the skull to the hyoid bone. Slices should be no more than

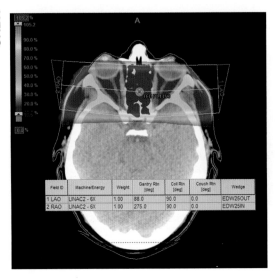

Figure 17.4 Beam arrangement and dose distribution for treatment of the retro-orbital tissues in Graves' disease.

3 mm thick. Intravenous contrast is not necessary. Fused CT and MR images can be particularly helpful to define the optic chiasm and any skull base involvement.

Target volume definition

■ Intraocular tumours

For choroidal metastases, conjunctival lymphoma, melanoma or retinoblastoma, disease can be adequately defined in the simulator as described above.

■ Extraocular tumours

The variety of rare extraocular tumours makes it difficult to give general recommendations for target volume definition following surgery or chemotherapy. Preoperative or pre-chemotherapy imaging should be available at the time of volume definition so that all original sites of disease are included in the CTV. Discussion with the surgeon and pathologist may help to define locations at greatest risk of recurrence. The CTV should take account of likely patterns of spread: for example for tumours invading behind the eye in the orbital cavity, the whole orbit should be included in the CTV. A 3 mm isotropic margin is added to produce a PTV.

It is tempting to edit the target volumes away from critical structures with the assumption that tolerance of these structures will be exceeded unless the PTV size is reduced. The complexity of possible planning solutions – conformal or with IMRT – means that the compensation needed is hard to predict. We strongly recommend that tumour target volumes are not influenced by critical structures and vice versa. Any compromise needed can thus be assessed using dose distributions and DVHs to choose the plan providing the best solution. The optic nerves, chiasm, lenses, retinas, lacrimal glands and pituitary should all be contoured as OAR.

Dose solutions

■ Intraocular tumours

For treatment to the choroid or retina, planning scan data can be used to create virtual simulation images to define the beam size and angle to minimise lens dose.

■ Extraocular tumours

A 3D planning scan with 3D conformal planning is the technique of choice for all curative extraocular tumour treatments because of the inevitable proximity of critical optic structures to the PTV and the need to identify dose to organs at risk. Postoperative radiotherapy for carcinomas and sarcomas ideally requires doses of at least 60 Gy (66 Gy to sites of residual macroscopic disease) so the location and tolerance of critical structures needs to be considered from the start of the planning process.

Fractionated doses of more than 10 Gy have a high risk of inducing a cataract but this late effect is treatable surgically. Lacrimal gland damage can occur with doses over 32 Gy and as a dry eye causes serious morbidity, great care should be taken to avoid this. Corneal ulceration is uncommon at doses below 48 Gy and can be minimised by patients being treated with the eye open to avoid any build-up effect of the overlying eyelid and by good eye care. Retinopathy can occur with doses over 50 Gy and is more common in diabetic patients. Particular care should be taken to avoid excess dose to the fovea. Optic nerve and chiasm doses should be kept below 55 Gy.

A variety of beam arrangements can be considered depending on the PTV. Anterior and lateral wedged beams will usually produce adequate PTV coverage but the lacrimal gland, retina and optic nerve will usually lie within the treated volume and the lens dose will exceed tolerance in spite of the lateral beam position being chosen to be posterior to the lens. It is the preferred beam arrangement after an enucleation (Fig. 17.5).

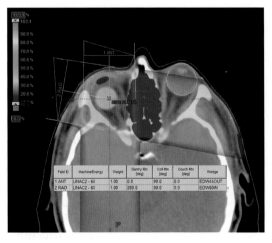

Field ID	Machine/Energy	Weight	Gantry Rtn [deg]	Coll Rtn [deg]	Couch Rtn [deg]	Wedge
1 ANT	LINAC2 - 6X	1.00	0.0	90.0	0.0	EDW45OUT
2 RAO	LINAC2 - 6X	1.00	280.0	90.0	0.0	EDW60IN

Figure 17.5 Adjuvant radiotherapy to the orbit after an enucleation. The lateral beam is angled to avoid the contralateral lens.

Another solution is to use superior and inferior wedged beams in the sagittal plane (Fig. 17.6). The borders can be chosen to spare the cornea anteriorly but the lacrimal gland is again difficult to avoid. If the PTV is entirely behind the

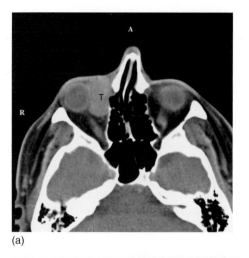

(a)

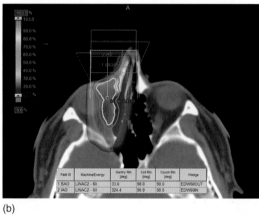

Field ID	Machine/Energy	Gantry Rtn [deg]	Coll Rtn [deg]	Couch Rtn [deg]	Wedge
1 SAO	LINAC2 - 6X	33.0	90.0	90.0	EDW60OUT
2 IAO	LINAC2 - 6X	324.4	90.0	90.0	EDW60IN

(b)

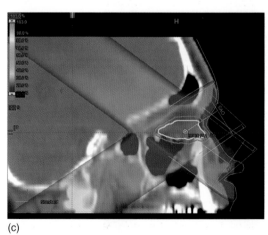

(c)

Figure 17.6 Treatment of residual orbital lymphoma after chemotherapy. (a) Diagnostic pre-chemotherapy CT scan showing tumour (T). (b) Corresponding slice on planning CT scan after chemotherapy showing the CTV, PTV and dose distribution. (c) Sagittal view to show beam angles and dose distribution.

globe, as in some extraorbital lymphomas, either a single lateral beam is used or superior and inferior wedged beams in the coronal plane are angled behind the globe.

It is usual for the oncologist to have to accept some compromise in PTV dose to keep all critical structures within tolerance or to accept an increased risk of late effects from delivering an adequate dose. This decision will be influenced by the risk and likely site of recurrence and should be discussed with the radiotherapy team and the patient. It may be necessary to use two phases of treatment with the whole PTV treated in phase 1 and some compromise in phase 2 to keep within tolerance. Both phases should be planned at the same time.

IMRT may offer some advantage to conformal planning in these complex volumes with a combination of coronal and lateral beams as for ethmoid tumours. Particular care must be taken not to exceed tolerance of the contralateral orbital structures when the number of beams is increased.

■ Benign disease

As both eyes are usually treated and a relatively low dose required, lateral beams angled posteriorly to avoid the lenses can be defined using the CT dataset to help to choose beam angles as for choroidal metastases.

Dose-fractionation

■ Choroidal metastases

20 Gy in 5 daily fractions of 4 Gy given in 1 week.

■ Conjunctival lymphoma

30 Gy in 15 daily fractions given over 3 weeks.

■ Orbital lymphoma

40 Gy in 20 daily fractions (no chemotherapy).
30–36 Gy in 15–18 daily fractions after chemotherapy depending on the bulk of any residual disease.

■ Postoperative radiotherapy (sarcoma, carcinoma, melanoma)

60 Gy in 30 daily fractions given in 6 weeks.

Consider
66 Gy in 33 daily fractions given in 6½ weeks to sites of residual disease.

■ Thyroid eye disease

20 Gy in 12 daily fractions given in 2½ weeks (1 Gy for first fraction, 1.73 Gy thereafter).

Treatment delivery and patient care

Patients should be advised on meticulous eye care and use of lubricating drops throughout treatment. There should be prompt assessment and treatment of any conjunctivitis or corneal damage. Close liaison with the ophthalmic team during treatment is therefore essential. A full ophthalmic assessment including plotting of visual fields should be carried out before radiotherapy so that any late effects can be detected.

Patients should be instructed to keep their eyes open and look directly at the beam to spare the front of the eye as much as possible.

Verification

TLD is used to confirm dose to the contralateral anterior eye.

Other points

Proton and plaque therapy are available in national specialised centres and referral protocols should be readily available for consultation by any oncologist responsible for an ophthalmological practice.

key trials

Collaborative Ocular Melanoma Study Group (2006) The COMS randomized trial of iodine 125 brachytherapy for choroidal melanoma: V. Twelve-year mortality rates and prognostic factors: COMS report No. 28. *Arch Ophthalmol* **124**: 1684–93.

Hawkins BS, Collaborative Ocular Melanoma Study Group (2004) The Collaborative Ocular Melanoma Study (COMS) randomized trial of pre-enucleation radiation of large choroidal melanoma: IV. Ten-year mortality findings and prognostic factors. COMS report number 24. *Am J Ophthalmol* **138**: 936–51.

Information sources

Wei RL, Cheng JW, Cai JP (2008) The use of orbital radiotherapy for Graves' ophthalmopathy: quantitative review of the evidence. *Ophthalmologica* **222**: 27–31.

Central nervous system

18

Indications for radiotherapy

This chapter will discuss the following tumours from the WHO classification (Box 18.1).

> ### Box 18.1   WHO classification of brain tumours*
>
> - Tumours of neuroepithelial tissue (of which astrocytomas, ependymomas and oligodendrogliomas are commonest). These are graded I–IV
> - Tumours of cranial or paraspinal nerves
> - Tumours of the meninges
> - Lymphomas and haemopoietic malignancies
> - Tumours of the sellar region
> - Germ cell tumours
> - Metastatic tumours
>
> *With permission.

Primary brain tumours are uncommon and comprise only 1.6 per cent of cancers. Metastatic spread to the brain from primary cancers elsewhere in the body is much more common. The variable behaviour of intracranial tumours depends on site and histology. Some cause problems by their intracranial extension alone (gliomas, meningiomas, pituitary tumours, metastases) while others (such as lymphomas, germ cell tumours and primitive neuroendocrine tumours [PNET]) have a predilection for leptomeningeal spread.

Gliomas

Gliomas constitute 40 per cent of all primary CNS tumours. They arise from glial cells and are classified by cell type into astrocytomas, ependymoma and oligodendroglioma. Tumours of mixed cell type can also occur. Grading (I–IV) is determined by pathological examination with grade I–II classified as low grade astrocytomas, grade III as anaplastic gliomas and grade IV as glioblastoma multiforme.

Low grade gliomas

Low grade gliomas (LGG) comprise a heterogeneous group of tumours which often occur at a younger age and present with more insidious symptoms than high grade tumours (HGG). Prognosis is variable and is adversely affected by age >40, size >6 cm, corpus callosum involvement and histology of astrocytoma rather than oligodendroglioma or mixed tumour.

Survival may be prolonged for many years so that treatment related sequelae are of more significance than for HGG. Low grade gliomas should be excised completely wherever possible. Surgery alone gives 5-year progression free survival rates of 65–80 per cent. If resection is incomplete, studies have shown that EBRT given immediately after surgery improves progression-free survival and control of seizures when compared with no EBRT, but there is no difference in overall survival. Trials of early versus delayed radiotherapy have shown similar outcomes, and the neuro-oncology team and the patient must weigh up the risks and benefits of further treatment in each individual situation. However, taking into account age, performance status, site of tumour, and patient choice, immediate treatment may be indicated because of the risk of transformation to higher grade. Larger volume of residual tumour is associated with a shorter time to tumour progression. In young patients (<2–3 years) radiotherapy may be deferred until recurrence because of the increased risk of toxicity.

Comparison of radiotherapy doses of 50.4 Gy with dose escalation to 64.8 Gy has shown increased toxicity with no improvement in disease control. There is no proven benefit for chemotherapy, but studies are underway comparing EBRT as sole treatment, or temozolomide alone or in combination with EBRT.

High grade gliomas

These tumours behave very aggressively with a median survival without treatment of only 3–6 months. Because of their infiltrative nature and proximity to critical structures, complete surgical resection is very rarely possible, but prognosis is improved in proportion to the degree of completeness of excision. Surgery can be followed by radiotherapy within 4–6 weeks of uncomplicated recovery. Radiotherapy following surgery extends median survival to 9–12 months. Dose escalation above 60 Gy does not improve outcomes. Chemotherapy with low dose temozolomide (75 mg/m^2 daily) during radiotherapy and for six courses afterwards (200 mg/m^2 given for 5 days every 28 days) gives an increase in median and progression-free survival of 2.5 months and survival at 2 years of 26.5 per cent compared with 10.5 per cent with EBRT alone.

Glioblastoma multiforme can be divided into two prognostic groups on the basis of performance status, age of the patient and treatment. Elderly patients with good performance status may be treated as above but patients over the age of 70 with poor performance status should be considered for biopsy and short course EBRT for palliation of symptoms only, because of poor results of aggressive treatment.

Studies have shown no benefit from dose escalation, hyperfractionation, addition of radiosensitiser, or wide compared with local irradiation; 90 per cent of recurrences occur within 1–3 cm of the original site. For high grade tumours, survival after treatment is of the order of 3 years for grade III, and 12 months for grade IV.

■ Clinical and radiological anatomy

Gliomas can arise throughout the central nervous system including the spine and optic nerve. In adults, most are supratentorial in the cerebral cortex but in children, an infratentorial site is more common. Tumours expand and infiltrate within the brain and may cross the corpus callosum, but extracranial spread does not occur. They are best evaluated with MRI but the infiltrative nature of HGG makes it difficult to determine tumour margins accurately.

■ Assessment of primary disease

Gliomas may present with symptoms of raised intracranial pressure, including headache, nausea and vomiting, cognitive or behavioural problems, focal neurological deficits or epilepsy. Spinal cord gliomas can cause pain, weakness, or numbness in the extremities, and glioma of the optic nerve may present with visual loss. A full general and neurological examination is needed to detect extent of impairment. PS should be recorded. Early discussion is needed between neurologist, radiologist, neurosurgeon and oncologist to agree an appropriate plan for each individual. Since neurosurgical services are often located in specialised centres, videoconferencing can be very helpful.

Whole brain or spinal CT will reveal the site of the tumour and show areas of low density (necrosis) or calcification. However, MRI with gadolinium enhancement is the investigation of choice.

T1-weighted sequences show low signal density and T2-weighted a high signal density in comparison with the rest of the brain. For grade III tumours, a contrast-enhanced CT will show a low density tumour with ring enhancement. There is heterogeneity within the tumour and associated oedema. For grade IV tumours, oedema will be seen outside the ring enhancement.

Grade cannot be predicted accurately by imaging and 40 per cent of tumours diagnosed as LGG will be HGG after biopsy. PET and various functional MRI approaches may give additional information.

Postoperative MRI is used to assess completeness of resection. If EBRT is given in a different hospital, good liaison between surgeon and oncologist following resection is important to maintain continuity of care for the patient.

■ Data acquisition

Immobilisation

The patient lies supine with the head immobilised in an individual Perspex or thermoplastic shell. More rigorous immobilisation with a stereotactic frame and mouth bite is possible.

CT scanning

MRI is more sensitive than CT scanning for demonstrating tumour extent. Tumours are non-enhancing with low signal intensity on T1-weighted and high signal on T2. Active tumour lies mainly within areas of T2 hyperintensity but can extend up to 2 cm from it. Since MRI cannot be used for planning treatment alone, CT planning scans using intravenous contrast are taken with 1–3 mm slices from the vault to the base of the skull. Pre-and postoperative MR images are then co-registered with the CT planning scans and the target volumes delineated.

■ Target volume definition

GTV

Grade I–II

The initial preoperative GTV seen on T2-weighted MRI is outlined on fused MR/CT planning images and includes areas of peritumoural oedema shown as low density on CT scan (Fig. 18.1).

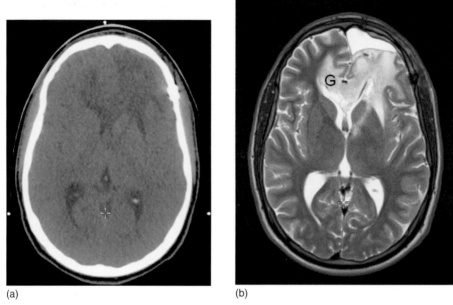

(a)   (b)

Figure 18.1 Comparison of (a) CT and (b) fused T2-weighted MR/CT images for low grade glioma (G) to illustrate value of fusion. Note fluid in postoperative cavity anteriorly.

Grade III–IV

The GTV is delineated at the contrast-enhancing edge of the tumour (not oedema) on postsurgical gadolinium enhanced T1-weighted MRI scans fused with planning CT (Fig. 18.2).

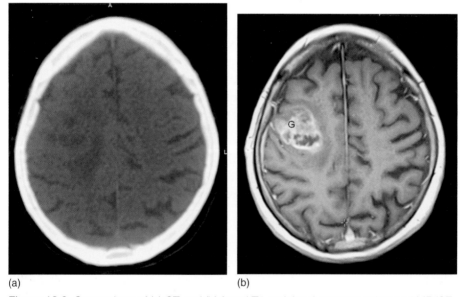

(a)   (b)

Figure 18.2 Comparison of (a) CT and (b) fused T1-weighted contrast-enhanced MR/CT images for high grade glioma (G) to illustrate value of fusion.

For palliative treatment, the GTV includes gross visible tumour as seen on a CT planning scan.

CTV

Two CTVs are defined according to dose to be delivered and reflect degree of infiltration dependent on tumour grade:

Grade II
CTV54 = GTV + 15 mm

Grade III
CTV45 = GTV + 25 mm
CTV54 = GTV + 15 mm

Grade IV
CTV50 = GTV + 25 mm
CTV 60 = GTV + 15 mm

For palliative treatments a single phase CTV margin of 15 mm is added.

PTV

A 5 mm margin is added to the CTV taking into account departmental measurements of set-up accuracy.

Volumes must be tailored to minimise dose to OAR, such as optic chiasm, and take account of natural barriers to spread such as bone and falx.

OAR

These will vary according to the site of the primary tumour. They should be outlined and a PRV added. A clinical decision about relative risks and benefits is needed if PTVs and PRVs volumes overlap.

■ Dose solutions

Conventional

Simple coplanar beam arrangements or opposing beams defined on the simulator using 6 MV photons may be appropriate for palliative treatments, but CT scanning is needed to define the GTV.

Conformal

Using CT scanning and MLCs, volumes are tailored to avoid as much normal tissue as possible. Three beam arrangements are often used which may be non-coplanar and should be wedged as appropriate to obtain a satisfactory dose distribution (Figs 18.3 and 18.4).

Complex

Better dose homogeneity across the tumour may be achieved using forward planning IMRT with segmentation or 'field in field' arrangements. Full IMRT may produce optimal plans to meet normal tissue dose constraints if these would limit effective doses to tumour when long-term survival is expected (such as treatment of optic glioma in children).

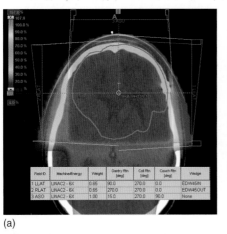
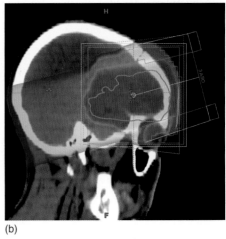

(a)   (b)

Figure 18.3 Treatment plan for low grade gliomas as in Figure 18.1 showing (a) axial and (b) off axis sagittal non-coplanar beams to avoid the eyes.

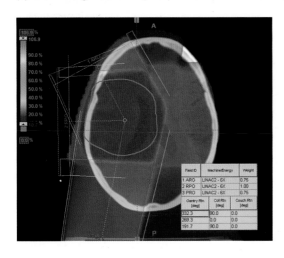

Figure 18.4 Treatment plan for high grade glioma as in Figure 18.2 showing axial dose distribution.

■ Dose-fractionation

Grade II/III

CTV 45
45 Gy in 25 daily fractions of 1.8 Gy given in 5 weeks.

CTV 54
9 Gy in 5 daily fractions of 1.8 Gy given in 1 week.

Grade IV

CTV 50
50 Gy in 25 daily fractions given in 5 weeks.

CTV 60
10 Gy in 5 daily fractions given in 1 week.

Adjustments to this treatment approach may be made in the light of known prognostic factors:

Grade IV, PS 0–1 age <70

As above (60 Gy) with temozolomide 75 mg/m^2 daily throughout treatment.

Grade IV, PS 0–1 Age >65

40 Gy in 15 daily fractions gives equivalent control rates to higher dose radiotherapy without temozolomide and may be preferred.

Grade IV, PS 2 or age >70 or any palliative treatment

30 Gy in 6 fractions over 2 weeks.

■ Treatment delivery and patient care

During the first days of treatment, there may be an increase in peritumoral oedema, which may require adjustment or introduction of steroid dosage to prevent headache and vomiting. Antiemetics may also be required. Consideration to cutting out parts of shells to reduce skin dose, for example over the ears, may help to prevent skin erythema and irritation, but adequate immobilisation must be maintained. Shells may need to be adjusted with changes in steroid dose which affect the amount of swelling of the patient's face. Hair loss from the irradiated area including sites of exit of the beam will start after about 2 weeks of treatment and will be permanent in high dose volumes.

Regular weekly review is essential to monitor response and check medication. This should include assessment of seizure control. Rapid deterioration during treatment may lead to discontinuation of radiotherapy. Patients and relatives often require considerable psychological support from the treatment team during this period. If temozolomide is used, blood counts should be checked weekly.

■ Verification

EPIs are taken on the first 3 days of treatment and then once weekly to ensure accuracy of set-up. Diodes or TLDs are used to check delivered dose.

Other glial tumours

Oligodendrogliomas are treated as described above, according to prognostic factors. Choroid plexus carcinomas may be treated palliatively with short-term improved control. With a dose of 54 Gy, symptoms of gliomatosis cerebri may be improved for about 6 months.

Medulloblastoma and infratentorial primitive neuroepithelial tumour

These tumours are discussed together because the radiotherapy technique of treatment is similar. Craniospinal radiotherapy (CSRT) is also used in the treatment of some non-germinomatous germ cell tumours and lymphomas. These tumours are rare, optimal treatment is still under investigation and patients should be cared for by multidisciplinary teams in specialist centres and entered into clinical trials whenever possible.

■ Indications for radiotherapy

Medulloblastoma and infratentorial PNET are treated with a multimodality approach. Surgery should be as complete as possible without causing disability. Because of the risk of subarachnoid seeding of tumour, surgery is followed by CSRT with a boost to the posterior fossa or primary tumour site, and by combination chemotherapy. Although radiotherapy can be deferred in very young children, most cures are only achieved with the addition of radiotherapy, and reduced doses, hyperfractionated regimens and reduced volumes have been associated with poorer control rates. Control rates with concurrent radiotherapy and chemotherapy followed by multiagent chemotherapy for 1 year are higher than with surgery and radiotherapy alone.

For medulloblastoma or PNET in adults, the role of chemotherapy is less well established.

■ Sequencing of multimodality therapy

Surgery is considered as essential first treatment and is followed as soon as recovery permits (usually 2–3 weeks) by radiotherapy and, for medulloblastoma, with modified concurrent and consequent chemotherapy. Local failure remains the commonest problem.

■ Clinical and radiological anatomy

Medulloblastoma arises from the roof of the fourth ventricle in the posterior fossa in the midline. CT scanning commonly shows a well-circumscribed hyperdense tumour projecting into the fourth ventricle. There may be enlargement of the other ventricles because of compression. Cysts and necrosis may show as areas of low density. MRI shows more clearly the point of origin of medulloblastoma from the roof of the fourth ventricle. On T1-weighted images the tumour is iso- or hypodense. Leptomeningeal disease is seen as an irregular thin layer of enhancement.

■ Assessment of disease

Full neurological, endocrinological and general examination should be performed as a baseline to facilitate documentation of response and late effects. Various tests such as audiometry and echocardiography are indicated depending on which chemotherapy regimen is used. Initial lumbar puncture may reveal positive cytology. Bone scan is indicated to rule out metastases if there are suggestive symptoms or neuraxis involvement.

Within 12–48 hours postoperatively, the patient may develop the posterior fossa syndrome, characterised by mutism, cerebellar dysfunction, supranuclear cranial nerve palsy and hemiparesis. Resolution may take several weeks and if the patient's condition is poor, EBRT may have to be deferred.

Preoperative MRI of brain and whole neuraxis is performed to assess tumour extent and operability, and to detect any metastatic disease within the spine. Postoperative MRI should be performed within 48–72 hours after surgery to determine extent of residual disease, as after this time disease is difficult to distinguish from postsurgical artefacts.

■ Data acquisition

Immobilisation

Conventional
Formerly the patient was treated prone with an individual facial support and a shell down over the shoulders to immobilise the head, neck and shoulders.

Conformal
Improved technology has now made it possible to treat the patient in the supine position and this is preferred as it is more comfortable and reproducible and is safer if general anaesthesia is required. The patient lies on a carbon-fibre couch top with neck extended with a vacuum moulded bag to support the head and shoulders. An individually made Perspex or thermoplastic shell covers the face and shoulders and is attached onto the couch top. Indexed knee rests are used to ensure that the spine is straightened and hips are also fixed in a foam form. The sides of these hip rests act as arm rests to lift the arm above the spine. Anterior and lateral tattoos are placed at the point of hip fixation.

CT scanning
With the patient in the supine treatment position, whole body images are obtained with 5 mm slices from the vault of the skull to the bottom of the sacrum, with 3 mm slices through the primary tumour.

Simulator
The initial volume includes the whole brain and extends to the inferior border of the third or fourth cervical vertebra to allow an adequate margin below the primary tumour in the posterior fossa, to facilitate the matching of the spinal beam and to avoid the spinal beam exiting through the mouth.

Spine
The spine is treated from the fourth or fifth cervical vertebra to the fourth sacral foramina to include the theca and sacral nerve roots.

Primary tumour
The volume is reduced to cover the primary tumour.

■ Target volume definition

CT scanning
Using CT scanning with co-registration of MR images, the GTV-T (preoperative extent of primary tumour and any residual disease after surgery) is outlined.

Two CTVs are defined:

CTV35 whole brain and spine.
CTV54 posterior fossa, or GTV-T + 1 cm margin.

PTV is determined according to departmental protocols, usually:

PTV = CTV + 3–5 mm.

All OAR for both CTV35 and 54 such as the ear, optic chiasm, pituitary, thyroid, lungs, kidneys, ovaries or testes are outlined for DVH evaluation.

Conventional

For conventional treatment, opposing lateral beams with the lower border at C3–4 are applied to cover the whole brain, with a collimator rotation of 7–10° to match the divergence of the posterior spinal beam. A template is made to facilitate lead shielding of extracranial structures (such as eyes, teeth, etc.) or MLC shielding is designed. It is important to check that cribriform plate, anterior and temporal lobes are adequately treated. The lower border of the cranial field is tattooed. Lateral and posteroanterior simulator films of the vertebral column are then taken. The position of the spinal cord is marked on the lateral film and the dose at its central axis calculated over its entire length, which extends from the junction with the cranial field to the fourth sacral foramina. A wax compensator may be required to improve homogeneity over this length. The width of the spinal beam ranges from 4 cm in small children to 6 cm in adults (to cover the lateral spinal roots).

For the second phase of treatment, the anterior border passes behind the posterior clinoid process avoiding the pituitary gland. The inferior border lies at the bottom of the first cervical vertebra, and the superior and posterior borders are set to cover the contents of the posterior fossa (Fig. 18.5).

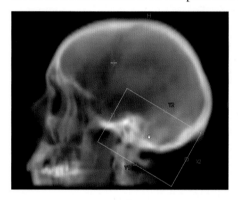

Figure 18.5 Lateral BEV for posterior fossa treatment for medulloblastoma.

■ Dose solutions

Complex

Beams are designed to cover first the whole brain and spine (CTV 35) (Fig. 18.6) and then the posterior fossa (CTV54) defined on axial CT scans and are angled posteriorly to avoid the external auditory meatus and cochlea. MLC is used to shield the face. Multiple segmented beams are used to ensure a homogeneous dose throughout the length of the spine and to prevent overdose at sites of beam junction between skull and spine. Using beam segments, forward planned IMRT, asymmetrical jaws and dynamic wedges, several boost fields can be added to the posterior spine to top up areas of underdose. Tomotherapy™ may improve sparing of critical structures but there is concern about whole body dose, especially in children.

Conformal

Whole brain irradiation is delivered using opposing lateral beams. By using MLC with 5 mm leaves if available, the face is shielded from the lateral beams and the

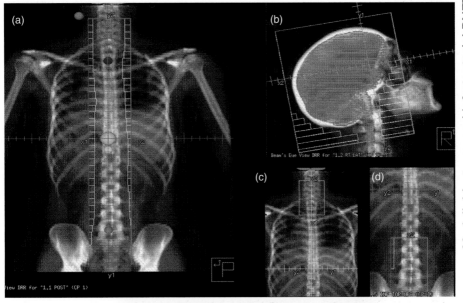

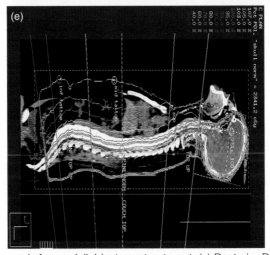

Figure 18.6 Whole neuraxis for medulloblastoma treatment. (a) Posterior DRRs showing spinal beam, (b) whole brain, (c) and (d) segment beams to create homogeneous dose along whole spine. (e) Isodose distribution. Courtesy of Helen Taylor and Dr F Saran, Royal Marsden Hospital.

kidneys from the posterior spinal beam. Use of posterior oblique beams, rather than opposing laterals, for treatment to the posterior fossa, makes it possible to avoid the ears to reduce the likelihood of deafness. Compensation may be applied at the skull vault and neck. If the uncompensated distribution of dose over the length of the spine exceeds the ICRU recommended limits of +7 per cent/−5 per cent, a physical compensator of aluminium, wax or Perspex may be used to even out the overdose superiorly and the underdose inferiorly.

Conventional

Whole brain and posterior fossa

Treatment is given isocentrically using a linear accelerator and opposing lateral beams as defined in the simulator. The position of the lower cranial border is shifted by 1 cm every seven treatments to change the level of the junction with the spinal field.

Spinal field

Despite the use of an FSD extended up to 140 cm, two adjacent fields are commonly required to cover the spinal cord in adults and older children. The technique for calculating the gap at beam junctions is described in Chapter 2. Both this and the craniospinal beam junction are moved caudally every seven treatments. Using a 6 MV linear accelerator it is not possible to spare anterior abdominal structures but shielding can be used to cover the kidneys.

■ Dose-fractionation

The doses in both phases of the cranial treatment are prescribed to the midplane of the posterior fossa volume. Doses received at the midplane of the whole brain volume are also documented. If there is a variation of more than ±5 per cent between the two central doses, compensators must be used with the conventional technique. The spinal dose is prescribed to the central spinal axis (the middle of the spinal cord).

35 Gy to whole brain and spine in 21 daily fractions of 1.66 Gy given in 4½ weeks.
19 Gy boost to posterior fossa in 12 daily fractions of 1.6 Gy given in 2½ weeks.

■ Treatment delivery and patient care

The patient is aligned using lasers and shell markings with palpation of the spine and visualisation of the gaps between head and spine (in the prone set-up). With a supine treatment position, gaps are more difficult to visualise and checking spine alignment requires a suitable insert in the couch so that spines can be palpated. A radio-opaque marker can be placed at the inferior margin of the lateral beams in the anterior midline for visualisation with on board imaging or EPIs.

Hair loss begins with doses of 10–20 Gy and 80 per cent of those receiving 50 Gy will have permanent hair loss over the occiput. Raised intracranial pressure should be relieved before radiotherapy starts, but steroids may nevertheless be required to control vomiting during treatment. The mutism syndrome may make it difficult for the patient to cooperate. Antiemetics may be required. A general anaesthetic may be needed to treat very young patients but use of the supine position and appropriate preparation with play therapy reduces the number for whom it is necessary. If anaesthesia is used, care must be taken to maintain adequate nutrition. Skin reactions, especially over the ears, can be reduced by cutting out the shell. Deafness is a late effect of radiotherapy especially given in conjunction with platinum-based chemotherapy, but may be reduced by the use of conformal techniques which exclude the ear from the full posterior fossa dose. Blood counts should be monitored at least weekly. Other side effects may include a period of somnolence after radiotherapy, which is self-limiting.

Long-term follow-up should be ensured to diagnose and remediate any late effects such as hypothyroidism or pituitary insufficiency.

■ Verification

Beams and shielding are verified with portal films. TLDs or diodes are used on the first day of treatment to measure doses including to the lens of the eye. MV or kV imaging online is used where available before treatment to check set-up.

Ependymoma

■ Indications for radiotherapy

Ependymomas may arise at any site in the neuraxis. In children, 90 per cent are intracranial and are commonest in the posterior fossa. Spinal lesions are more common in adults. Extent of resection is the most important prognostic factor. Supratentorial lesions with complete gross resection in patients older than 3 years and with benign histology have the best prognosis and require only surgery. Local failure is the commonest problem and CSRT is not necessary for non-metastatic disease. Radiotherapy is considered if resection has been incomplete and the patient is over 3 years old, if the tumour has been grossly resected but there are adverse histological features, or if the lesion is infratentorial. Children who have not received radiotherapy at the time of surgery may be treated for tumour relapse.

■ Clinical and radiological anatomy

Ependymomas arise from the floor of the fourth ventricle and extend laterally. They spread by seeding in the leptomeninges. Tumours may contain calcification and are best defined as hypodense lesions on T1-weighted MR images.

■ Assessment of disease, data acquisition

See section on gliomas.

■ Target volume definition

The GTV is defined as the tumour and any residual tumour shown on pre- and postoperative MRI fused with CT planning scans.

CTV = GTV + 10–15 mm.
PTV = CTV + 5 mm.

The optic chiasm is the main OAR.

■ Dose solutions

Treatment may be delivered conformally with three to four beams or a full IMRT solution.

■ Dose-fractionation

Primary brain

54 Gy in 30 daily fractions of 1.8 Gy given in 6 weeks.

Primary spinal tumours

50.4 Gy in 28 daily fractions of 1.8 Gy given in 5½ weeks.
For metastatic disease, CSRT is given.

Craniospinal

35 Gy in 21 daily fractions of 1.66 Gy given in >4 weeks, with a boost to individual sites of spinal disease up to 50.4 Gy.

Primary tumour

As above.

Meningioma

■ Indications for radiotherapy

These tumours arise from the meninges, most commonly adjacent to the falx, along the sphenoid ridge, in the olfactory grooves, the sylvian region, cerebellopontine angle, and the spinal cord. Most are benign (grade I) but atypical (grade II) and malignant (grade III) types also occur. Surgery is the treatment of choice. Radiotherapy is indicated when surgery is impossible, if there is infiltration of adjacent tissue, biopsy shows grade II or III histology or the patient is suffering a second or subsequent relapse after surgery. When radiotherapy is indicated, there is evidence that it is best given early rather than deferred.

■ Clinical and radiological anatomy

Tumours are usually well defined and localised although they may spread along the dura. They may lie flat (en plaque) along the meninges or be lobulated and indent the adjacent brain. Resectability is in part determined by the relationship to adjacent structures, particularly major blood vessels, such as the superior sagittal sinus, anterior and middle cerebral arteries and cavernous sinus, and must be evaluated for each site. Spread through bone and foramina into the orbit, temporal fossa and other sites may make radical excision very difficult.

CT scans usually show a well-defined hyperdense mass which enhances with intravenous contrast. Calcification and lower density is seen in about 25 per cent of tumours. Evidence of bone involvement may be seen. Oedema may be a prominent feature. MRI is useful to demonstrate the attachment of the tumour to the dura and relationship to vascular structures.

■ Assessment of primary disease

Full clinical and radiological examination as described above is carried out to assess operability or need for radiotherapy. Tumours may be asymptomatic or may present with focal seizures, neurological impairment or more rarely with signs of raised intracranial pressure.

■ Data acquisition

Immobilisation

See glioma. Stereotactic frames may be used when treatment with protons or stereotactic techniques is used.

CT scanning

With the patient immobilised, CT scans are obtained from the skull vault to the base of brain or the first cervical vertebra depending on site of origin of the tumour, with 1–3 mm slice thickness for fusion with MR images.

■ Target volume definition

If surgery is not performed, the whole tumour with any spread along the meninges or through bone must be encompassed within the GTV. Gadolinium-enhanced T2-weighted MR images are co-registered with CT planning scans and GTV delineated by contouring areas of enhancement. CTV is created by adding a 5 mm margin. Normal barriers to spread (such as bone) may in fact be invaded and this must be taken into account if any editing of volumes is done.

After macroscopic surgical removal, information from surgeon and pathologist must be taken into account in designing volumes. CTV is defined using presurgical MR images fused with CT scans to identify areas at greatest risk of recurrence, which are the point of attachment to the dura and any meningeal extensions, and intravascular or bony involvement. Invasion into the brain is rare and therefore volume of brain tissue included in the CTV should be minimal. A variable margin (from 1 mm to 5 mm) which will increase with grade of tumour should be added around these areas to allow for microscopic spread. A PTV margin is added according to departmental protocols and measurements and is usually 5 mm.

OAR are defined according to the primary site and a PRV created and edited as appropriate.

■ Dose solutions

Conventional

Conventional planning and treatment with opposing beams only has a place in the palliative treatment of recurrent tumours where long-term control is not expected.

Conformal

Conformal planning and treatment delivery are essential because of the proximity of critical normal organs. An arrangement of three 6 MV beams is commonly used, chosen to avoid normal structures as much as possible with MLC shielding and wedges to improve dose distribution.

Complex

Small meningiomas may be most appropriately treated by proton therapy or stereotactic techniques for which referral to a specialised treatment centre may be necessary. For other tumours, a non-coplanar beam arrangement with appropriate MLC shielding and wedges should be used.

■ Dose-fractionation

60 Gy in 33 daily fractions of 1.8 Gy given in 6½ weeks.
Reduced doses of 51 Gy in 30 daily fractions of 1.7 Gy over 6 weeks may be used for tumours adjacent to optic nerves, chiasm or spinal cord.

■ Treatment delivery and patient care

See general recommendations above. Most patients are in good general condition and few complications arise during treatment other than skin reactions.

■ Verification

See above.

Primary CNS lymphoma

■ Indications for radiotherapy

Ninety per cent of intracranial lymphomas are diffuse large B cell tumours. They are associated with immune-suppression or compromise, or Epstein–Barr virus infection. They invade the perivascular space and in 30 per cent there is spread into the cerebrospinal fluid (CSF) and meninges.

High dose methotrexate, which crosses the blood–brain barrier, in conjunction with systemic chemotherapy is the most effective treatment. The role of radiotherapy is still unclear although it is known to be effective treatment. CHOP (cyclophosphamide, vincristine, doxorubicin and prednisolone) chemotherapy given after cerebral radiotherapy added no further benefit. A study by the EORTC used high dose methotrexate, teniposide, carmustine, and intrathecal therapy before 40 Gy of whole brain radiotherapy. The overall response rate at the end of treatment was 81 per cent, but these results were associated with significant acute chemotherapy-related toxicity (10 per cent death rate). It is difficult to use these results to guide treatment since the commonest age group with this condition (patients >65) were excluded from the study. Most trials reported to date have noted the deleterious effect of increasing age on outcome.

In patients in whom complete remission is obtained with chemotherapy, there appears to be no significant difference in overall or progression-free survival when radiotherapy is added. Chemotherapy, with radiotherapy deferred until further relapse, is now recommended, except where there is residual disease after chemotherapy when whole brain radiotherapy is given.

■ Clinical and radiological anatomy

Lymphoma infiltrates widely throughout the brain and shows on contrast-enhanced MRI or CT scanning as a homogeneous poorly defined low density mass.

■ Assessment of disease

Patients present with symptoms from tumour mass effect, or from discrete deposits on cranial or spinal nerves or with ocular involvement in the vitreous. Complete examination should exclude lymphoma outside the brain and full neurological testing and slit lamp eye examination should be performed.

Data acquisition, target volume definition, dose solutions and verification are described in the section on whole brain irradiation for intracranial metastases below.

■ Dose-fractionation

Whole brain

40 Gy in 20 daily fractions of 2 Gy given in 4 weeks
  or
45 Gy in 25 daily fractions of 1.8 Gy given in 5 weeks.

CNS irradiation for acute leukaemia

■ Indications for radiotherapy

Patients with high risk disease and those with CNS disease at presentation, who are assigned by a current protocol to receive cranial irradiation, have treatment to the cranial meninges with extensions retro-orbitally and into the foramen magnum, after complete remission has been achieved by systemic and intrathecal chemotherapy.

Palliative treatment is rarely given but may be beneficial for facial nerve involvement or spinal cord compression when the volume is determined by the extent of disease.

■ Radiotherapy

A thermoplastic or other type of shell is used to immobilise the patient in the supine position and the outer bony canthi of both orbits are marked with wire or lead pellets before simulation or virtual simulation. Two opposing lateral beams are used to cover the whole cranium extending to the lower border of the second cervical vertebra (Fig. 18.7). The posterior part of the orbit is included because of the reflection of the meninges along the optic nerve. The anterior orbit and nasopharynx are shielded with MLCs or a custom-made block. The exit dose to the contralateral eye may be reduced by angling beams posteriorly by 5° or, preferably, by placing the central axis of the beam at the anterior orbital margin with appropriate shielding. Lasers are used to check alignment and portal images are taken on the first day of treatment to ensure correct positioning of the beams and shielding. Lithium fluoride TLDs or diodes are used to measure the dose to the eyes, which should not exceed 10 per cent of the MPD.

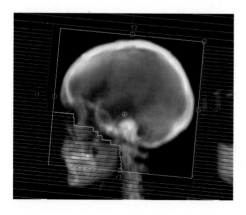

Figure 18.7 Opposing lateral beams on virtual simulation for cranial treatment for lymphoma/leukaemia, with whole brain covered including cribriform plate and cervical vertebrae.

■ Dose-fractionation

24 Gy in 15 daily fractions of 1.6 Gy given in 3 weeks (designed to attain the highest antileukaemic dose and minimise effect on developing brain).

■ Treatment delivery and patient care

Most patients will already have alopecia from chemotherapy. Acute skin reactions are mild. Patients may have headaches or nausea during treatment because of concomitant chemotherapy. Most experience somnolence at 6 weeks after treatment and should be warned that lethargy, nausea and anorexia are self-limiting and do not require special treatment. Blood counts should be checked regularly according to protocol.

Tumours of the sellar region

■ Indications for radiotherapy

Pituitary adenoma (in adults) and craniopharyngioma (commonly in children or young adults) are benign tumours for which surgery is the primary treatment of choice. For pituitary tumours, radiotherapy may be indicated for residual or progressive tumour after surgery or for recurrence, but individual assessment should be made by the multidisciplinary team. For good risk craniopharyngiomas, surgery is followed by careful surveillance. If resection is incomplete, radiotherapy is indicated for poor risk tumours larger than 2–4 cm, where there has been a breach of the floor of the third ventricle, or where the patient has hydrocephalus or the hypothalamic syndrome. Radiotherapy is also indicated after cyst aspiration, partial trans-sphenoidal resection, shunting or debulking.

■ Clinical and radiological anatomy

Pituitary adenomas arise in the anterior pituitary gland within the sella, whereas craniopharyngiomas are primarily suprasellar although 50 per cent have an intrasellar component. Clinical presentation is related either to endocrine or hypothalamic dysfunction or to the effects of extension outside the site of origin with compression of surrounding brain tissue.

Contrast-enhanced MRI is the investigation of choice to demonstrate relationship to the optic chiasm superiorly (Fig. 18.8a) and the sphenoid sinus inferiorly. Pituitary macroadenomas will show low signal on T1-weighted images but there may be high signal in areas of haemorrhage. In craniopharyngiomas, CT will show calcification in a majority of tumours and 70–75 per cent have a cystic component, which will show high signal intensity on T2-weighted MR images. There will be contrast enhancement of solid areas.

■ Assessment of primary disease

Patients are seen initially by endocrinologist and neurosurgeon and discussed when appropriate in a multidisciplinary meeting with the oncologist. Before radiotherapy, there must be a full ophthalmological and endocrinological assessment and neurological examination.

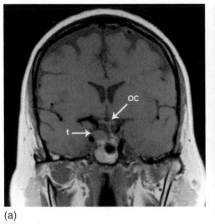
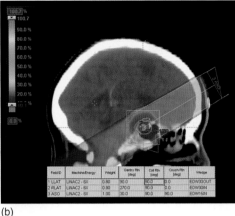

(a)   (b)

Figure 18.8   (a) MRI showing pituitary tumour (t) and relation to optic chiasm (oc).
(b) Sagittal dose distribution showing optic chiasm (yellow).

■ Data acquisition

Immobilisation

The patient is immobilised in a Perspex shell or relocatable frame with the head in a neutral position.

CT planning

CT scans are obtained with 3 mm slice thickness from the skull vault to the first cervical vertebra with intravenous contrast, and co-registered with postoperative gadolinium-enhanced T1-weighted MR images or planning MR scan.

Target volume definition

Any abnormality showing enhancement on T1-weighted MR images postoperatively is outlined as GTV for pituitary tumours. For craniopharyngioma GTV is defined as the cystic and solid elements of the tumour defined by pre- and postoperative MRI. Decompression of large tumour masses may lead to alterations in normal anatomy and post-decompression changes must be taken into account. For pituitary adenomas, no GTV to CTV margin is needed as there is no microscopic spread, but for craniopharyngioma a GTV-CTV margin of 3–5 mm is allowed because of the tendency of the tumour to adhere to surrounding structures.

A CTV to PTV margin is added according to departmental protocols, but is usually 5 mm.

■ Dose solutions

Conformal

Using CT planning, MLCs are used to shape a superior oblique and opposing lateral beams (Fig. 18.8b), or other beam arrangement to the target volume.

Complex

Three to six non-coplanar conformal beams are used to try to reduce dose to optic structures and temporal lobes. Higher energies than 6 MV may be appropriate to reduce dose to temporal lobes. Stereotactic techniques may be used for small intrasellar lesions.

Conventional

An anterior and two opposing lateral beams are chosen to cover the target volume, angled to avoid optic structures.

■ Dose-fractionation

Craniopharyngioma or large pituitary adenomas

50–54 Gy in 30 daily fractions of 1.67–1.8 Gy given in 4–5 weeks.

Small pituitary adenomas

48 Gy in 25 daily fractions of 1.8 Gy given in 5 weeks.

MRI at weeks 3 and 5 may make it possible to reduce the volumes if tumour shrinkage is confirmed.

Cystic recurrences of craniopharyngioma may be treated with aspiration and intracystic instillation of radioactive colloids such as Y-90 (half-life 2.67 days, range 11 mm) to give a planned dose of 200–300 Gy.

■ Treatment delivery and patient care

Steroid and other endocrine replacement therapy is given as necessary. Visual function should be carefully monitored each week as reaccumulation of fluid in a cystic component of a craniopharyngioma may require urgent neurosurgical decompression.

■ Verification

See above.

Intracranial germ cell tumours

■ Indications for radiotherapy

These tumours, which arise from primitive germ cell precursors, comprise 2–5 per cent of primary CNS tumours; 75 per cent occur between the ages of 10 and 20 years. All histological types of germ cell tumours may be seen, but 57 per cent are germinomas (analogous to seminomas).

Introduction of effective chemotherapy regimens has led to reduction in radiotherapy volumes and dose. A series of international trials has indicated that cure rates of nearly 100 per cent can be achieved in germinomas with chemotherapy and radiotherapy. Outcomes in non-germinomatous germ cell tumours are poorer (65–70 per cent 5-year survival) and are improved when chemotherapy and surgical excision are followed by radiotherapy if complete remission is not obtained. CSRT is reserved for patients with disseminated disease. Children are treated within agreed international protocols which must be consulted.

■ Sequencing of multimodality therapy

Primary treatment is with cisplatin-based chemotherapy. If complete remission is achieved, focal radiotherapy to the primary tumour site and ventricles is given starting within 3–6 weeks of the end of chemotherapy. If there is residual disease, surgical excision is performed before radiotherapy. For disseminated disease, chemotherapy is given before CSRT.

■ Clinical and radiological anatomy

Germ cell tumours may be unifocal in the pineal or suprasellar region or bifocal in both areas (Fig. 18.9). There may be CSF involvement (M1) or macroscopic metastases (M2/3). Tumours may be secreting or non-secreting.

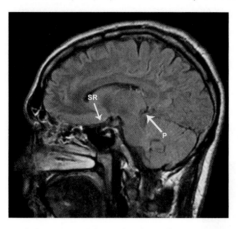

Figure 18.9 MRI to show sites of origin of germ cell tumours in the suprasellar region (SR) and pineal gland (P).

MRI will demonstrate primary tumour extent, and special techniques including magnetic resonance spectroscopy, diffusion-weighted or diffusion tensor imaging may make it possible to distinguish germ cell from non-germ cell tumours.

Spread from the primary site is first to the ventricular system and thence to the leptomeninges. Metastases to other sites occur late with uncontrolled CNS disease.

■ Assessment of disease

Symptoms and signs at presentation depend on site and size of tumour. There may be raised intracranial pressure, lethargy, visual loss, hormone abnormalities or hypothalamic disturbance.

Factors predicting unfavourable outcome include older age, metastases at presentation, elevated markers (β-hCG or α-fetoprotein [AFP]), histological subtype and residual disease after initial chemotherapy.

Diagnosis may be possible without surgery if the characteristic position of the tumour is associated with elevations in β-hCG or AFP in blood or CSF. If biopsy is needed to confirm the diagnosis, it may be achieved endoscopically with or without a procedure designed to restore CSF flow. MRI of the spine and CSF cytology are required to exclude disseminated disease.

Full endocrine and visual assessment should be carried out as well as baseline measurement of blood counts and renal and liver function before chemotherapy.

■ Data acquisition

Immobilisation

The patient lies supine and is immobilised in a Perspex or thermoplastic shell, with the shoulders as low as possible and the neck in a neutral position. Foot restraints and a vacuum moulded bag to immobilise the body may also be helpful.

CT scanning

CT scans are taken of the whole brain from the vault of the skull to the first cervical vertebra and are fused with MR images taken pre- and postoperatively.

■ Target volume definition

The pre-chemotherapy/surgery GTV is defined by contrast-enhanced T1- and T2-weighted MR scans. CT may demonstrate fatty or calcified areas better and fused images may be used. The patient should be in remission at the time of radiotherapy so that there is no residual GTV. Two CTVs are designed, the first corresponding to the pre-chemotherapy tumour extent and the second to the potential sites of spread within the ventricular system (whole ventricular radiotherapy; WVRT). The WVRT CTV should be grown by 5–10 mm to create the PTV (Fig. 18.10). OAR should be outlined (eyes, parotid, pituitary gland, supra- and infratentorial brain) and PRVs designed with 3 mm margins to reduce the incidence of late effects.

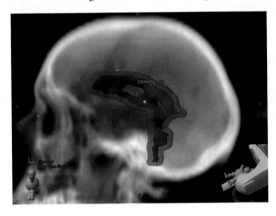

Figure 18.10 Lateral DRR showing outlining of CTV and PTV for whole ventricular radiotherapy.

CSRT

See medulloblastoma.

■ DOSE SOLUTIONS

Conventional

Opposing lateral beams may be used to cover the PTV with shielding to other areas of the brain.

Conformal

Conformal solutions are preferred, using either two opposing, or three or four beam non-coplanar arrangements. DVHs are created and OAR doses are minimised with MLC shielding.

Complex

IMRT solutions may permit sparing of supratentorial brain and pituitary gland and make it possible to give a simultaneous integrated boost to the primary tumour site during WVRT. Care must be taken that the use of five to seven non-coplanar beams does not result in unwanted radiation to normal areas of brain.

■ Dose-fractionation

Germinomas

If CR after chemotherapy – WVRT (CTV 24)
24 Gy in 15 daily fractions of 1.6 Gy given in 3 weeks.

If PR after chemotherapy, an additional boost – primary tumour bed (CTV40)
16 Gy in 10 daily fractions of 1.6 Gy given in 2 weeks to give a total dose of 40 Gy in 25 fractions of 1.6 Gy given in 5 weeks.

Non-germinomatous GCT

WVRT
24 Gy in 15 daily fractions of 1.6 Gy given in 3 weeks.

Primary tumour bed
An additional dose of 25.2 Gy in 14 daily fractions of 1.8 Gy given in 2.5–3 weeks.

Metastatic
CSRT
30 Gy in 15 daily fractions given in 3 weeks.

Boost to primary tumour
25.2 Gy in 14 daily fractions of 1.8 Gy.

These doses are still being investigated and current protocols should be checked.

■ Treatment delivery and patient care, verification

See medulloblastoma.

Cerebral metastases

■ Indications for radiotherapy

Forty per cent of intracranial neoplasms are metastatic, arising in order of frequency from lung, breast, melanoma, renal, and colon cancers. They are increasing in frequency with improved treatment of the primary tumour leading to longer survival.

If CT scan or MRI confirms a single metastasis, surgery is the treatment of choice. Postoperative whole brain radiotherapy with or without a local boost improves progression-free survival. More commonly, MRI will reveal multiple metastases and radiotherapy is then indicated. Median survival after whole brain irradiation for multiple metastases is 3–6 months depending on the number of lesions and the tumour type as well as performance status. The side effects of radiotherapy, which include hair loss, and possibly headache, nausea, or other symptoms, are unfortunate with such a short survival period but quality of life is nevertheless often much improved.

Stereotactic radiosurgery may be appropriate to treat small solitary or few metastases and gives a median survival of 11 months. Highly collimated beams are focused on the tumour to give a high dose treatment (17–18 Gy) in a single session. It may be used after surgical excision for focal treatment to the area of metastasis. Details of this technique are beyond the scope of this book.

■ Sequencing of multimodality treatment

If chemotherapy is required for systemic disease in a sensitive tumour, radiotherapy can be deferred unless symptoms of intracranial disease worsen. Following surgical treatment of a single metastasis, radiotherapy, either focally or to the whole brain, may be added to improve cure rates, especially if there is any concern about whether clear margins have been achieved.

■ Assessment of disease

The need for treatment of secondary tumours in the brain must be assessed in the light of the extent of the primary tumour and other metastatic disease, and the general condition of the patient. MRI is more sensitive in detecting intracranial metastases and should be used if surgery is envisaged for single metastases. Routinely, contrast-enhanced CT scanning may be more readily available and is adequate.

■ Data acquisition

Immobilisation

The patient lies supine in a thermoplastic shell with the neck in a comfortable neutral position.

Simulator

Unless focal EBRT is being given after surgical resection of a single metastasis, planning can be adequately done with the simulator or, if available, virtual simulation to define borders of treatment volumes (Fig. 18.11). Focal higher dose treatment can be planned using the general principles outlined above.

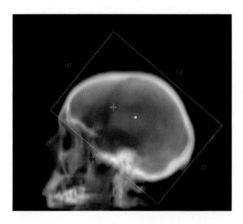

Figure 18.11 Lateral DRR with BEV for whole brain irradiation.

■ Target volume definition

Diagnostic images can be fused with CT planning scans to define GTV accurately if focal EBRT is planned. If whole brain irradiation is given, beams are defined in the simulator to cover the whole skull from vertex to a line joining the external auditory meatus with the outer canthus of the orbit (Reid's base line). If there is any evidence of involvement of the skull base this line will need to be 1–2 cm lower to ensure tumour is included in the treatment volume.

■ Dose solutions

Simple opposing lateral beam arrangements are used for whole brain irradiation with wedging if necessary to improve dose distribution. For focal treatment, plans are drawn up after CT scanning for optimal dose to tumour and minimal dose to normal tissues, often using non-coplanar arrangements.

■ Dose-fractionation

Whole brain irradiation

12 Gy in 2 daily fractions given on consecutive days.
20 Gy in 5 fractions of 4 Gy given in 1 week.
30 Gy in 10 fractions of 3 Gy given in 2 weeks.

Focal irradiation alone

40 Gy in 20 daily fractions given in 4 weeks
   or
17 Gy by stereotactic radiotherapy.

---

key trials

Borgelt B, Gelber R, Kramer S *et al.* (1980) RTOG 7361 1973–1976; The palliation of brain metastases: final results of the first two studies by the Radiation Therapy Oncology Group. *Int J Radiat Oncol Biol Phys* **6**:1–9.

Cairncross G–RTOG 9402, Phase III intergroup randomised comparison of radiation alone vs pre-radiation chemotherapy for pure and mixed anaplastic oligodendrogliomas.

EORTC Brain Tumor Group Phase III trial on concurrent and adjuvant temozolomide chemotherapy in non-1p/19q deleted anaplastic glioma. The CATNON intergroup trial. www.eortc.be

Mead GM, Bleehen NM, Gregor A *et al.* (2008) Medical Research Council randomised trial in patients with primary cerebral non-Hodgkin lymphoma: cerebral radiotherapy with and without cyclophosphamide, doxorubicin, vincristine, and prednisone chemotherapy. *Neurology* **29**: 401–2A.

Mirimanoff RO, Mason W, van den Bent M *et al.* (2007) Is long term survival in glioblastoma possible? Updated results of the EORTC/NCIC phase III randomised trial on radiotherapy (RT) and concomitant and adjuvant temozolomide versus RT alone. *Int J Radiat Oncol Biol Phys* **69**(3S): 2.

Information sources

Brandes AA, Franceschi E, Tosoni A *et al.* (2000) Long-term results of a prospective study on the treatment of medulloblastoma in adults. *Cancer* **15**: 1359–70.

Chang CH, Housepian EM, Herbert C Jr (1969) An operative staging system and a megavoltage radiotherapeutic technic for cerebellar medulloblastomas. *Radiology* **93**: 1351–9.

Cochrane Database of Systematic Reviews (2002) Chemotherapy in adult high-grade glioma: a systematic review and meta-analysis of individual patient data from 12 randomised trials. Issue 4. Art. No.: CD003913. Available at: www.cochrane.org/reviews/en/ab003913.html (accessed 1 December 2008).

Gerstner ER, Carson KA, Grossman SA, Batchelor TT (2003) Long-term outcome in PCNSL patients treated with high-dose methotrexate and deferred radiation. *J Clin Oncol* **21**: 4483–8.

Kleihues P, Burger PC, Scheithauer BW (1993) The new WHO classification of brain tumours, *Brain Pathol* **3**: 255–68.

Laperriere N, Zuraw L, Cairncross G (2002) The Cancer Care Ontario Practice Guidelines Initiative Neuro-Oncology Disease Site Group. Radiotherapy for newly diagnosed malignant glioma in adults: a systematic review. *Radiother Oncol* **64**: 259–73.

Louis DN, Ohgaki H, Wiestler OD *et al.* (2007) The 2007 WHO Classification of Tumours of the Central Nervous System. *Acta Neuropathol* **114**: 97–109. (See also BrainLife.org: WHO Classification ⩾ 2007 WHO Classification.)

Nieder C, Astner ST, Grosu A-L (2007) The role of postoperative radiotherapy after resection of a single brain metastasis. *Strahlenther Onkol* **183**: 576–80.

Ogawa K, Shikama N, Toita T *et al.* (2004) Longterm results of radiotherapy for intracranial germinoma: A multi-institutional retrospective review of 126 patients. *Int J Radiat Oncol Biol Phys* **58**: 705–13.

Poortmans PMP, Kluin-Nelemans H C, Haaxma-Reiche H *et al.* (2003) High-dose methotrexate-based chemotherapy followed by consolidating radiotherapy in non–AIDS-related primary central nervous system lymphoma: European Organization for Research and Treatment of Cancer Lymphoma Group Phase II Trial 20962. *J Clin Oncol* **44**: 1210–16.

Shawl EG, Seiferheld W, Scott C *et al.* (2003) Re-examining the radiation therapy oncology group (RTOG) recursive partitioning analysis (RPA) for glioblastoma multiforme (GBM) patients. *Int J Radiat Oncol Biol Phys* **57**: S135–6.

Stupp R, Hegi ME, Gilbert MR, Chakravarti A (2007) Chemotherapy in malignant glioma: standard of care and future directions. *J Clin Oncol* **25**: 4127–36.

Wolden SL, Wara WM, Larson DA *et al.* (1995) Radiation therapy for primary intracranial germ cell tumors. *Int J Radiat Oncol Biol Phys* **32**: 943–9.

Thyroid and thymoma

19

Thyroid

■ Indications for radiotherapy

Well-differentiated thyroid cancer (WDTC – papillary, follicular)

Total thyroidectomy and thyroid remnant ablation with iodine-131 is the recommended initial treatment for most follicular and papillary tumours. As patients are usually young and have an excellent prognosis, the possible late effects of radiotherapy should be carefully considered before advocating treatment.

Adjuvant EBRT is indicated for incompletely excised or inoperable WDTC (usually T4a or T4b) that does not concentrate iodine-131 sufficiently. The area of incomplete excision is usually in the thyroid bed but occasionally in the neck where there is extracapsular lymph node spread or invasion of local structures. Less well-differentiated follicular or papillary cancers (in particular Hürthle cell neoplasms) take up iodine poorly.

Occasionally recurrences in the neck or thyroid bed will be inoperable due to invasion of local structures and will not concentrate iodine. EBRT is then indicated to improve local control unless the patient has uncontrollable distant metastases. Radiotherapy can effectively palliate metastases, for example in the bones or mediastinum.

Medullary thyroid cancer

Surgery is the principal treatment for medullary cancer. There is no role for iodine-131. Radiotherapy is indicated if there is inoperable or macroscopic residual local disease unless there are uncontrollable distant metastases. It should also be considered in patients with microscopic residual disease though careful follow-up with calcitonin and carcinoembryonic antigen measurements, and neck imaging, may be appropriate.

Anaplastic thyroid cancer

Many patients with anaplastic cancer are elderly, have poor performance status and significant local symptoms. Good supportive and palliative care is paramount but radiotherapy can be used for local control and to relieve or prevent compression of critical structures such as the trachea and oesophagus.

Occasionally anaplastic carcinoma is operable. Adjuvant radiotherapy should then be considered to improve local control as there are rare long-term survivors with this disease.

■ Sequencing of multimodality therapy

In follicular and papillary cancer, total thyroidectomy is followed by radio-ablation of the thyroid remnant by iodine-131 where possible or by EBRT for residual disease if there is no iodine-131 uptake.

In anaplastic cancer where surgery is possible, postoperative radiotherapy may be followed by adjuvant doxorubicin-based chemotherapy to reduce the risk of distant metastases. In the palliative setting, concurrent radiochemotherapy has been advocated in patients with good performance status and no distant metastases but this approach increases acute toxicity without a proven survival advantage. If palliation of local symptoms is paramount, radiotherapy is indicated and palliative chemotherapy can be considered subsequently for distant metastases.

■ Clinical and radiological anatomy

Most WDTC is confined to the thyroid gland and is therefore completely excised with a total thyroidectomy. Tumours can invade beyond the capsule into the soft tissues of the neck, trachea, oesophagus, larynx, neck vessels or recurrent laryngeal nerve and in these tumours a microscopically complete excision is unusual. With anaplastic tumours, local structures have usually been invaded at presentation.

Lymphatic drainage is initially to the midline level VI nodes in the anterior neck which extend from the hyoid to the suprasternal notch. Subsequent drainage is to levels III–V and then to the supraclavicular nodes, or inferiorly to nodes in the tracheo-oesophageal groove or superior mediastinum. This region is sometimes termed level VII and extends from the suprasternal notch to the brachiocephalic veins. The term superior mediastinal nodes is used to avoid confusion due to the different numbering of mediastinal node levels and those in the neck (Fig. 19.1). Papillary cancer has a relatively high risk of lymph node metastasis though the prognostic significance of this is debated. Extracapsular lymph node spread is a risk factor for local recurrence.

■ Assessment of primary disease

Routine imaging is not required before surgery for WDTC unless there is clinical suspicion of local invasion or lymphadenopathy. A CT scan without contrast (iodinated contrast may inhibit uptake of therapeutic iodine-131) or MRI may then be of value to document local extent and help plan surgery and possible radiotherapy. If the patient is hoarse, nasendoscopy is used to assess vocal cord movement and hence involvement of the recurrent laryngeal nerve.

Medullary cancer should be treated in a centre with specialist expertise. Preoperative assessment should include genetic and biochemical tests to look for multiple endocrine neoplasia.

If treatment is contemplated for anaplastic cancer, a contrast-enhanced CT or MR scan of the neck should be performed as well as a CT scan of the chest and mediastinum because of the high incidence of distant metastases.

All patients in whom radiotherapy is being considered should be discussed within a specialist thyroid multidisciplinary team. A full discussion with the surgeon is vital to be able to define sites at highest risk of local recurrence.

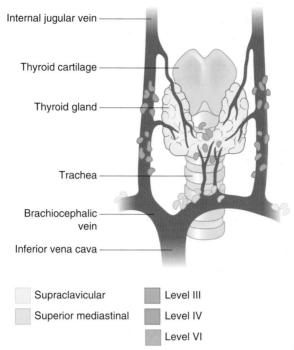

Figure 19.1 Lymphatic drainage of the thyroid gland.

Supraclavicular
Superior mediastinal
Level III
Level IV
Level VI

■ Data acquisition

Immobilisation

Patients should be immobilised in a custom-made Perspex or thermoplastic shell fixed to the couch top in at least five places. The neck is extended to move the oral cavity superiorly and to reduce dose to the mandible and salivary glands. The shoulders should be as low as possible.

CT scanning

Slices 3–5 mm thick are obtained from the base of skull to the carina to allow assessment of lymphadenopathy. If the target volume is smaller (for example the thyroid bed only) the extent of the scan can be reduced. Intravenous contrast should be avoided if iodine-131 is being considered but otherwise can be helpful to delineate vascular structures.

Simulator

Rapidly growing anaplastic carcinomas may require urgent radiotherapy if there is tracheal compression and this is often achieved most quickly using a simulator for planning. Palpable disease is marked with lead wire and parallel opposed anterior–posterior fields defined to cover the tumour and adjacent lymph nodes if required (see target volumes). If a dose which exceeds spinal cord tolerance is prescribed, a CT-planned phase 2 treatment is needed.

■ Target volume definition

Papillary, follicular and medullary cancer

A careful discussion with the surgeon and pathologist is essential to define the sites at highest risk of local recurrence. Any macroscopic residual disease is contoured as GTV. Any sites where tumour was excised with a known positive margin (e.g. from the trachea or vessels) should also be contoured as GTV to facilitate CTV definition.

The CTVs will depend on the sites of residual disease, excision margins and the extent and risk of lymph node involvement. If tumour is inoperable or EBRT is given because of local invasion, the GTV is expanded by 10 mm isotropically to form the CTV66 and then edited to account for natural tumour barriers, e.g. bone. The CTV66 is copied to form the CTV60 and edited to include the sites of preoperative tumour. If a level VI node dissection revealed no tumour and there are no lateral cervical nodes, there is no indication for lymph nodes to be included in the CTV60. If there were positive level VI nodes but the lateral cervical nodes were not dissected or nodes were not assessed surgically then level VI, the superior mediastinal nodes, and bilateral level IV and lower level III nodes adjacent to the thyroid bed should be included in the CTV60.

If EBRT is indicated because of extracapsular nodal spread, the CTV60 should be defined individually depending on the extent of disease and surgery. It will usually include the level VI, bilateral level III–V, and supraclavicular and superior mediastinal nodes. If level III nodes were involved, then level II nodes may also be included but this will increase both acute mucosal toxicity and the risk of late effects, particularly xerostomia.

The CTV is expanded by 3–5 mm to form the PTV, depending on local assessment of systematic and random errors and likely organ motion.

Anaplastic thyroid cancer

If radiotherapy is adjuvant to surgery the CTV is defined as for WDTC above. Most radiotherapy is palliative and there needs to be a careful balance between trying to cover all sites of possible disease and maintaining quality of life by minimising acute toxicity. The GTV is defined as the primary tumour and involved lymph nodes (>10 mm short axis diameter). The GTV is expanded by 10 mm isotropically to form the high dose CTV55. This CTV is edited to reflect local patterns of tumour spread (e.g. including adjacent muscles if invaded but edited off bone and air).

A low dose CTV35 may also be defined by expanding the CTV55 to include uninvolved nodes in levels III, IV, V and VI and the inferior part of level II and in the supraclavicular fossae and superior mediastinum.

There may be significant shrinkage of tumour during a long course of radiotherapy so it may be necessary to redefine the CTV on a new planning CT scan during treatment. The CTV is expanded by 3–5 mm to form the PTV depending on local assessment of systematic and random errors and likely organ motion.

When a short palliative course (20 Gy in 5 fractions or 30 Gy in 6 fractions) is used, a 10 mm margin is added to the GTV to produce the PTV (Fig. 19.2).

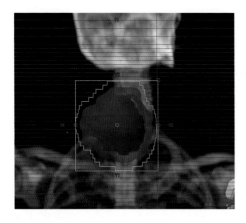

Figure 19.2 Palliative radiotherapy for anaplastic thyroid cancer. Anterior and posterior opposing beams with MLC shielding to reduce acute toxicity.

■ Dose solutions

Conformal

The proximity of the PTV to critical structures such as spinal cord and oesophagus makes a conformal approach desirable in all patients with WDTC or medullary cancer and in anaplastic tumours where a high dose is used.

Adjuvant treatment of WDTC, medullary and anaplastic cancer

The PTV is best covered by an antero-oblique wedged pair arrangement with the beam angles chosen to avoid exit through the spinal cord. An additional anterior beam may improve coverage but at the expense of increasing spinal cord dose. Beams may need to be angled caudally if coverage of the superior mediastinal nodes is needed. A wedge in the superoinferior dimension can reduce inhomogeneities in this plane caused by the PTV being more superficial at the superior end (Fig. 19.3).

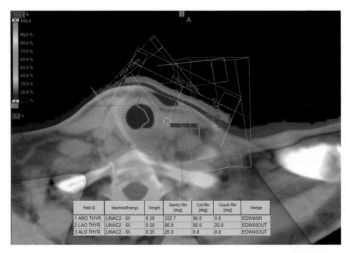

Field ID	Machine/Energy	Weight	Gantry Rtn [deg]	Coll Rtn [deg]	Couch Rtn [deg]	Wedge
1 ARO THYR	LINAC2 - 6X	0.50	322.7	90.0	0.0	EDW45IN
2 LAO THYR	LINAC2 - 6X	0.50	80.9	90.0	20.0	EDW60OUT
3 ALO THYR	LINAC2 - 6X	0.25	25.0	0.0	0.0	EDW45OUT

Figure 19.3 Adjuvant radiotherapy for a small left-sided anaplastic thyroid cancer following a total thyroidectomy without involved lymph nodes. The tumour came close to the skin surface so bolus was used.

Anaplastic cancer

The PTV35 is treated with a pair of anterior and posterior opposed beams with MLC shielding. The PTV55 is treated as for well-differentiated tumours above. Both phases should be planned together so as not to exceed spinal cord tolerance.

If the high dose PTV includes both the thyroid bed and level II or III nodes, it is very difficult to treat the whole PTV in continuity without using IMRT. A pair of lateral opposing beams angled caudally will not be able to treat posterior nodes (cord tolerance would be exceeded) and will risk underdosing the PTV in the low neck. The thyroid bed may be treated with two antero-oblique wedged beams matched to electrons superiorly to treat the nodes.

Complex

IMRT can provide better target volume coverage than conformal radiotherapy for thyroid cancer when the concave PTV surrounds the spinal cord. It is of particular value when lateral cervical nodes are included in the PTV. It can also allow simultaneous treatment of different volumes to different doses depending on the risk to each. A five- or seven-beam inverse-planned technique is used.

Conventional

Where a palliative dose is being given (usually for anaplastic carcinoma), opposing anterior and posterior beams can be defined on the simulator to cover the target volume with an appropriate margin to the beam edge. MLC shielding can reduce dose to adjacent normal structures.

■ Dose-fractionation

WDTC or medullary cancer
60 Gy in 30 daily fractions given in 6 weeks to PTV60.
66 Gy in 33 daily fractions given in 6½ weeks to PTV66 if defined.

Anaplastic cancer
20 Gy in 5 daily fractions of 4 Gy given in 7 days.
30 Gy in 6 fractions of 5 Gy given in 2 weeks.
55 Gy in 20 daily fractions of 2.75 Gy given in 4 weeks if high dose treatment appropriate (35.75 Gy in 13 fractions to PTV35, 19.25 Gy in 7 fractions to PTV55).

■ Treatment delivery and patient care

Patients should be treated daily without hyperfractionation for missed treatments. Weekly review is critical to manage acute effects proactively. As mucositis of the pharynx and oesophagus are inevitable, dietetic advice should be provided to maintain weight and calorie intake throughout treatment. Enteral feeding with a nasogastric or gastrostomy tube may be necessary if weight falls more than 10 per cent from baseline. Pain should be managed with paracetamol, non-steroidal anti-inflammatory drugs and oral or transdermal opiates as needed. Steroids may be necessary at the start of treatment in anaplastic cancer to reduce local oedema if there is airway compromise.

■ Verification

Portal images should be taken on days 1–3 and weekly thereafter to ensure any day-to-day set-up variation is within tolerance. If there is significant shrinkage of tumour, a repeat CT scan may be required to evaluate the 3D dose distribution of the original beam arrangement within the new contour. A new plan should be considered if there is an increased dose to critical structures or the PTV dose is reduced.

Thymus

■ Indications for radiotherapy

Thymic tumours are usually clinically staged according to the Masaoka system (Table 19.1) which reflects local invasion. Pathological classification (WHO) separates thymic carcinomas (WHO C) from thymic epithelial tumours (WHO B – true thymoma), but clinical staging is more useful to predict prognosis and guide treatment decisions. Surgery is the treatment of choice for thymic tumours. There are no phase III studies investigating adjuvant treatment or to guide therapy for unresectable disease.

Table 19.1 The Masaoka clinical staging system* for thymoma

Stage I	Macroscopically and microscopically completely encapsulated (includes tumour invading into but not through the capsule)
Stage II	A: microscopic transcapsular invasion
	B: macroscopic invasion into the surrounding fatty tissue or grossly adherent to but not through mediastinal pleura or pericardium
Stage III	Macroscopic invasion into neighbouring organs (e.g. pericardium, great vessels, lung)
	A: without invasion of great vessels
	B: with invasion of great vessels
Stage IVA	Pleural or pericardial dissemination
Stage IVB	Lymphogenous or haematogenous metastases

*With permission.

Adjuvant radiotherapy is recommended following incomplete excision of stage II and III tumours but an observational approach is appropriate if excision has been complete. In unresectable stage III or IV disease, chemotherapy and radiotherapy are indicated followed by surgery where feasible.

■ Sequencing of multimodality therapy

Combined modality treatment with surgery, radiotherapy and chemotherapy (cisplatin, doxorubicin and cyclophosphamide) is recommended to provide optimal local control and survival in unresectable thymic tumours but the best sequence of treatment is not known. Preoperative chemotherapy may shrink a tumour to allow resection and postoperative radiotherapy. Preoperative radiation with or without chemotherapy has also been advocated to try to allow subsequent resection or as sole treatment. If resection is known to be incomplete, radio-opaque clips placed at sites of residual disease during surgery can be helpful for volume definition.

■ Clinical and radiological anatomy

The thymus sits in the anterior mediastinum behind the sternum. Fifty per cent of thymic tumours invade through the capsule and thence into local structures including the mediastinal pleura, pericardium or great vessels. Lymph node spread is uncommon. Tumours can metastasise to the pleura or to distant sites.

■ Assessment of primary disease

CT or MR imaging of the mediastinum is used to define local invasion. Mediastinoscopy can also be useful to assess resectability.

■ Data acquisition

Immobilisation

Patients lie supine with their arms above the head immobilised with a T bar or similar device. A custom-shaped vacuum bag can be used to aid immobilisation.

CT scanning

Slices 5 mm thick are obtained from the inferior cricoid cartilage to the bottom of the thoracic cavity. Intravenous contrast can be helpful to delineate vascular structures in the mediastinum.

■ Target volume definition

When adjuvant radiotherapy is used, discussion with the surgeon and pathologist is very important to define sites at risk of local recurrence. A GTV is defined if there is residual macroscopic disease. The GTV is expanded isotropically by 10 mm to form the CTV60 encompassing sites of residual disease. The CTV50 is formed by copying the CTV60 and enlarging it to include the sites of preoperative disease, i.e. the operative bed.

If there is no GTV, it can be helpful to contour any clips marking positive microscopic margins. The CTV50 is then contoured as the sites of preoperative disease with a 10 mm isotropic margin with particular attention paid to locations where the surgeon has marked residual disease with clips, or where there is felt to be an incomplete resection. After resection of a large tumour the postoperative anatomy may be very different from that on preoperative imaging (Fig. 19.4).

If primary radiotherapy is the sole treatment for unresectable disease, the initial GTV is defined on the planning CT. If chemotherapy has been given, the CTV should incorporate all initial sites of disease and possible sites of microscopic invasion which may include the mediastinum and adjacent mediastinal pleura and pericardium.

The CTV is expanded by 5 mm to form the PTV though this depends on local assessment of systematic and random errors and likely organ motion.

■ Dose solutions

Three coplanar beams usually provide adequate PTV coverage without exceeding tolerance of the lungs, heart or spinal cord. Examples include two antero-oblique beams with an additional anterior or postero-oblique beam depending on the PTV.

Inverse planned IMRT may provide useful solutions for these rare tumours.

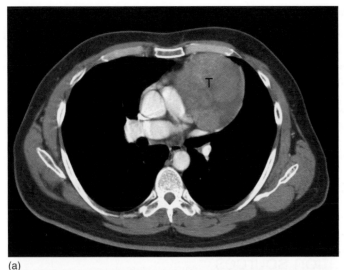

(a)

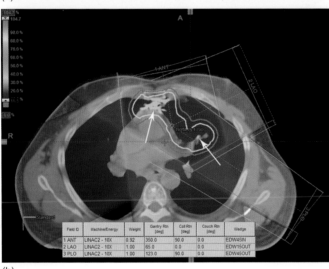

Field ID	Machine/Energy	Weight	Gantry Rtn [deg]	Coll Rtn [deg]	Couch Rtn [deg]	Wedge
1 ANT	LINAC2 - 10X	0.92	350.0	90.0	0.0	EDW45IN
2 LAO	LINAC2 - 10X	1.00	65.0	0.0	0.0	EDW15OUT
3 PLO	LINAC2 - 10X	1.00	123.0	90.0	0.0	EDW45OUT

(b)

Figure 19.4 Adjuvant radiotherapy for a Masaoka IIA (WHO B) thymoma. (a) Preoperative diagnostic CT showing thymoma (T). (b) Corresponding slice on planning CT showing CTV, PTV and beam arrangement. Note the radio-opaque clips used to mark sites at high risk of microscopic residual disease (arrowed).

■ Dose-fractionation

Adjuvant radiotherapy in stage II/III disease
50 Gy in 25 daily fractions given in 5 weeks to PTV50.
60 Gy in 30 daily fractions given in 6 weeks to PTV60 if defined.

Primary radiotherapy for unresectable disease
60 Gy in 30 daily fractions given in 6 weeks.

Pre-operative radiotherapy
45 Gy in 25 daily fractions of 1.8 Gy given in 5 weeks.

■ Treatment delivery and patient care

Treatment is usually well tolerated without severe acute effects but oesophagitis can occur and should be managed with analgesia and dietary advice (see Chapter 24).

■ Verification

Portal images should be taken on days 1–3 and weekly thereafter to ensure any day-to-day set-up variation is within tolerance.

key trials

■ There are no phase III trials of radiotherapy in these tumours.

Information sources

■ Thyroid

British Thyroid Association, Royal College of Physicians (2007) In: Perros P (ed.) *Guidelines for the Management of Thyroid Cancer*, 2nd edn. Report of the Thyroid Cancer Guidelines Update Group, Royal College of Physicians, London. Available at: www.british-thyroid-association.org/news/Docs/Thyroid_cancer_guidelines_2007.pdf (accessed 8 December 2008).

Cooper DS, Doherty GM, Haugen BR *et al.* (2006) The American Thyroid Association Guidelines Taskforce. American Thyroid Association management guidelines for patients with thyroid nodules and differentiated thyroid cancer. *Thyroid* **16**: 109–42.

Meadows KM, Amdur RJ, Morris CG *et al.* (2006) External beam radiotherapy for differentiated thyroid cancer. *Am J Otolaryngol* **27**: 24–8.

Pacini F, Schlumberger M, Dralle D *et al.* (2006) European consensus for the management of patients with differentiated carcinoma of the follicular epithelium. *Eur J Endocrinol* **154**: 787–803.

Pasieka J (2003) Anaplastic thyroid cancer. *Curr Opin Oncol* **15**: 78–83.

Schwartz DL, Rana V, Shaw S *et al.* (2008) Postoperative radiotherapy for advanced medullary thyroid cancer – local disease control in the modern era. *Head Neck* **30**: 883–8.

■ Thymoma

Giaccone G (2005) Treatment of malignant thymoma. *Curr Opin Oncol* **17**: 140–6.

Masaoka A, Monden Y, Nakahara K *et al.* (1981) Follow-up study of thymomas with special reference to their clinical stages. *Cancer* **48**: 2485–92.

Zhu G, He S, Fu X *et al.* (2004) Radiotherapy and prognostic factors for thymoma: a retrospective study of 175 patients. *Int J Radiat Oncol Biol Phys* **60**: 1113–19.

Lung

20

Indications for radiotherapy

■ Non-small cell lung cancer

Curative treatment – stage I/II

Although surgery offers the best cure rates for early stage non-small cell lung cancer (NSCLC), some patients may be medically unfit for surgery due to comorbidity (e.g. insufficient functional lung reserve for a lung resection) or may elect to have radiotherapy rather than surgery after an informed discussion. In these patients curative radiotherapy alone gives a 5-year survival of 20 per cent although studies from single institutions report cure rates of up to 50 per cent. Cure is more likely for early stage or smaller tumours. WHO PS >1 and significant weight loss (>10 per cent) predict for poorer outcome, presumably because they indicate occult distant metastases. There are no phase III trials comparing surgery with radiotherapy for these patients and indirect comparisons are difficult because patients having radiotherapy are likely to have significant comorbidity and poorer PS. There are also no phase III trials of curative radiotherapy compared with lower palliative dose radiation or observation. In patients with a short life expectancy for other reasons, both these alternatives should be considered.

In patients with poor lung function (forced expiratory volume in one second [FEV1] <1.0 L) a balance between attempting cure and maintaining lung function must be sought. Although there is no agreed lower cut-off below which radiation is contraindicated, a curative dose of radiotherapy is likely to significantly impair lung function in patients with an FEV1 of <0.6 L or grade 4 dyspnoea on the Medical Research Council (MRC) scale.

With the increased use of CT and PET imaging and screening programmes in lung cancer, the incidence of small primary lung cancers is likely to rise. Dose escalation approaches such as stereotactic radiotherapy should be considered for these patients.

Curative treatment – stage IIIA/IIIB

Surgery is only possible for a minority of stage III patients. Curative radiotherapy is indicated in patients with PS 0–1 and <10 per cent weight loss in the preceding 3 months where disease can be safely encompassed in a radical radiotherapy volume. It produces 2-year survival rates of 10–25 per cent. Contralateral mediastinal (IIIB) disease increases both the risk of occult distant metastases and the morbidity of radiotherapy. Curative radiotherapy should only be offered to patients in this category if they have good performance status, little comorbidity and relatively small volume disease. There are no firm pretreatment volume or functional indicators to predict which tumours can be encompassed but radiotherapy should be attempted with caution in patients with stage III disease and FEV1<1.0 L or MRC dyspnoea score 3 or 4.

The addition of either sequential or concomitant chemotherapy to radiation improves cure rates and should be considered in patients able to tolerate combined treatment. Hyperfractionated regimens such as the CHART protocol of 54 Gy in 36 fractions delivered with three fractions a day on 12 consecutive days offer a small advantage over conventional fractionation but have been difficult to implement.

The brain is a common site of relapse in patients treated for IIIA/B disease, but prophylactic cranial radiotherapy is not widely used. There is evidence that it reduces the incidence of brain metastases but no evidence that survival is improved. Results of a further randomised trial (RTOG 0214) are awaited.

Palliative radiotherapy

The majority of patients treated with palliative radiotherapy for lung cancer obtain symptomatic benefit particularly for cough, chest pain or haemoptysis. The optimal fractionation schedule is unclear but longer regimens produce a more durable response and a small survival advantage compared to shorter regimens. They should be considered for patients with PS 0–1 who are not suitable for curative radiotherapy. Other patients should be treated with one or two fractions. There is no evidence to support the use of palliative radiotherapy in asymptomatic patients.

Intravascular stents relieve the symptoms of SVCO faster than radiation or chemotherapy and should be considered first. Nonetheless SVCO is effectively palliated by EBRT in 60 per cent of patients with NSCLC and 80 per cent with SCLC. Palliative radiotherapy should also be considered for symptomatic distant metastases in sites such as bone, lung or skin.

Adjuvant radiotherapy

Although for many cancers radiotherapy is used as an adjunct to surgery in patients at high risk of local recurrence, it is not recommended routinely in NSCLC. Meta-analyses have shown an improvement in local control but an adverse effect on overall survival, particularly in stage I/II disease. Most studies used non-conformal techniques and lower doses of radiotherapy than would be considered today, so the benefits of modern conformal radiotherapy as an adjunct to surgery are unclear.

Adjuvant radiotherapy should be considered after surgery where there is microscopic residual disease (positive resection margins) or unexpected mediastinal lymphadenopathy at operation.

Neoadjuvant radiotherapy

Some centres recommend radiotherapy in combination with chemotherapy for tumours that are borderline operable. However, there are only two phase III trials (both from the 1970s) comparing the addition of preoperative radiation to surgery and neither showed a benefit. There is no role for neoadjuvant radiotherapy outside a clinical trial.

■ Small cell lung cancer

Curative thoracic radiotherapy

Radiotherapy should be considered for patients with SCLC who have tumour that can be encompassed within a curative radiotherapy volume. Four to six cycles of chemotherapy combined with radiotherapy are recommended because of the high incidence of systemic metastases and the relative chemo-sensitivity of SCLC. If patients are unable to tolerate chemotherapy, radiation alone is given if all sites of disease can be encompassed.

Thoracic radiotherapy has proven benefit (2-year survival improved from 13 per cent to 19 per cent) if given after chemotherapy to patients with a partial or complete response with the aim of treating all sites of initial disease. In practice, this is mainly patients with limited stage disease, excluding those with a malignant pleural effusion. There is also an RCT supporting the use of thoracic radiotherapy in extensive disease if there is a complete response outside the chest and a complete or partial response in the chest. Radiotherapy should therefore be considered in this situation.

There is also evidence to support starting thoracic radiotherapy early in the course of chemotherapy (concurrently with cycle 1 or 2) in patients with limited stage disease.

Smoking during thoracic radiotherapy for SCLC has been shown to affect outcomes adversely so cessation advice and support should be provided.

Palliative thoracic radiotherapy

There are no trials of palliative radiotherapy in SCLC, but the relative radiosensitivity suggests benefits should be at least equivalent to those in NSCLC. As most patients with good PS will receive chemotherapy, short fractionation schedules (one or two fractions) are recommended for patients with thoracic symptoms. There are no data comparing palliative chemotherapy with palliative radiotherapy – treatment should be chosen on the basis of which is likely to provide better palliation for the individual patient.

Prophylactic cranial radiotherapy in patients with SCLC

In patients with limited stage disease, prophylactic cranial radiotherapy (PCI) reduces the incidence of brain metastases and has a small benefit in overall survival. The additional acute toxicity of PCI and possible effects on long-term cognitive function need to be balanced against this small benefit for individual patients. It is given after curative chemotherapy and radiotherapy as long as there has been a complete or near-complete response. If thoracic radiation follows chemotherapy, the brain and chest can be irradiated at the same time.

PCI has also been shown to improve 1-year survival from 13 per cent to 27 per cent in patients with extensive disease who respond to chemotherapy and should be considered in this group.

Sequencing of multimodality therapy

■ NSCLC stage I/II treated with radiotherapy

Patients in this group undergoing radiotherapy will usually have single modality treatment. Adjuvant chemotherapy after surgery confers a survival benefit in resected stage IB–IIIA disease. A similar benefit could be expected for the few patients with stage IB–II disease having potentially curative radiotherapy who are fit enough to undergo chemotherapy, but there is no clinical trial evidence to support this.

■ NSCLC stage IIIA/B treated with radiotherapy and chemotherapy

Chemotherapy and radiation can be combined sequentially or concomitantly. Sequential regimens use three to four cycles of platinum based chemotherapy followed 3–4 weeks later by radiotherapy. Concomitant regimens use cisplatin-based chemotherapy in various schedules concurrent with radiotherapy and usually have further courses of chemotherapy either before or after concurrent treatment.

No one regimen has been shown to be conclusively superior although there are trials showing improved survival with concomitant compared with sequential regimens at the expense of increased acute toxicity (mainly oesophagitis and myelosuppression).

■ NSCLC adjuvant radiotherapy and chemotherapy after surgery

Where radiotherapy is indicated as an adjunct to surgery it should ideally begin 4–6 weeks postoperatively or when wound healing is adequate. There are phase III trial data to support the use of adjuvant chemotherapy in resected stage IB–IIIA NSCLC and radiotherapy was given to some patients in these trials on a non-randomised basis. For some patients adjuvant chemotherapy and adjuvant radiotherapy may both be indicated but there are no data on which to base sequencing of these treatments. The risks of local recurrence and systemic metastases should be assessed on an individual basis and radiotherapy or chemotherapy started first as appropriate. As the majority of patients having adjuvant radiotherapy will have positive excision margins we recommend adjuvant radiotherapy should be given first, followed 3–6 weeks later by consideration of adjuvant chemotherapy if indicated.

■ NSCLC palliative therapy

Patients may have indications for both palliative chemotherapy and radiotherapy. Sequencing depends on the balance of local and systemic symptoms and the likely benefits of each treatment. If significant local symptoms exist there is no good reason to delay radiotherapy as the response is likely to be good.

■ Superior sulcus (Pancoast) tumours

Tumours in the superior sulcus are often considered separately from other lung cancers and there is support for initial radiotherapy or chemoradiotherapy followed by surgery from several phase II studies and retrospective series, with 5-year survival rates of 15–40 per cent. The optimal management of these tumours is unclear but there is no evidence that surgery improves cure rates when added to (chemo) radiotherapy in NSCLC overall. We therefore recommend managing patients with superior sulcus tumours in the same way as other NSCLC patients.

■ Small cell lung cancer

The optimal timing of chemotherapy and radiotherapy for SCLC is still debated. Starting radiotherapy after chemotherapy will result in smaller treatment volumes and therefore reduced toxicity. It will also mean that patients who respond unusually poorly to chemotherapy will be spared the toxicity of radiation. There is, however, increasing evidence that starting radiotherapy early (concurrent with cycle 1 or 2) improves survival, suggesting that the overall treatment time may be important. We recommend radiation concurrent with cycle 2 in patients of excellent performance status with relatively small volume disease. The advantage of a shorter overall treatment time is only seen if optimal chemotherapy can still be given after the increased toxicity of early radiation.

Clinical and radiological anatomy

All pathological subtypes of lung cancer have a high rate of regional lymph node and distant metastases, so histology alone is not a good predictor of spread. SCLC often presents with large volume mediastinal lymphadenopathy and distant metastases are common. Squamous cell carcinomas are more frequently confined to the thorax than other subtypes and may cavitate.

Primary lung tumours spread within lung parenchyma where they are relatively asymptomatic. Satellite tumour nodules may be visible on imaging. Spread within major airways can cause obstruction, and distal collapse or atelectasis which can be difficult to differentiate from tumour (Fig. 20.1). Tumour may invade the chest wall, mediastinal structures, major vessels or the heart. Although invasion does not preclude curative radiotherapy if the treated volume is small enough, it is a predictor for distant metastasis.

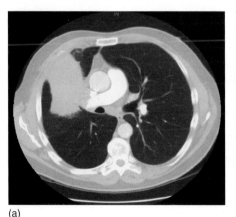
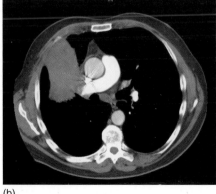

(a)   (b)

Figure 20.1 Tumour can be difficult to differentiate from distal collapse and consolidation on a contrast-enhanced CT scan with either (a) lung windowing or (b) soft tissue windowing.

Lung tumours first spread to lymph nodes within the lung – the subsegmental, segmental, lobar and interlobar nodes, which lie close to the division of bronchi, arteries or veins. These are rarely visible on imaging but are often removed at surgery when involvement may help define adjuvant radiotherapy volumes. Hilar nodes are situated at each hilum outside the reflection of the pleura. Adjacent tracheobronchial nodes are inside the reflection but cannot be differentiated from hilar nodes on CT.

The lymph node stations of the mediastinum are best divided into tracheobronchial, paratracheal, aorto-pulmonary, anterior mediastinal, subcarinal and para-oesophageal nodes (Fig. 20.2). There are numerical classification systems for mediastinal nodes based on surgical series.

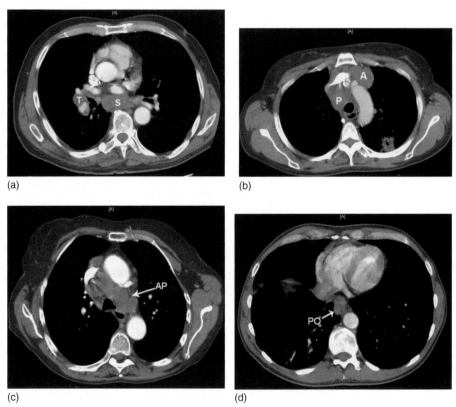

(a) (b)

(c) (d)

Figure 20.2 Enlarged mediastinal lymph nodes on diagnostic CT scans:
(a) tracheobronchial (T) and subcarinal (S), (b) paratracheal (P) and anterior mediastinal (A),
(c) aorto-pulmonary window (AP), and (d) para-oesophageal (PO).

N staging in the TNM system reflects involvement of ipsilateral hilar (N1), ipsilateral mediastinal (N2) or contralateral mediastinal or supraclavicular (N3) nodes (Tables 20.1 and 20.2).

The right lung drains systematically to hilar and adjacent mediastinal nodes (e.g. right upper paratracheal for upper lobe tumours, right lower paratracheal and subcarinal for middle and lower lobes). Left lower lobe tumours drain to the para-oesophageal, subcarinal, left paratracheal and aorto-pulmonary nodes. In contrast the left upper lobe can also drain to the right paratracheal nodes. Skip metastases to the mediastinal nodes when hilar nodes are negative occur in up to 15 per cent of tumours.

The criterion for nodal involvement on CT is a short axis diameter of ≥10 mm, but 15 per cent of nodes smaller than 10 mm contain tumour if removed and over 30 per cent of 2 cm nodes are pathologically negative. The likely pattern of nodal spread, number of enlarged nodes, node shape and presence of obstructive pneumonitis or other lung pathology (e.g. sarcoidosis) all need to be considered when assessing nodes on cross-sectional imaging as well as size. Primary tumour size is also correlated with N stage.

Table 20.1 UICC TNM (6th edn, 2002) staging of lung cancer*

T1	Tumour 3 cm or less in greatest dimension, surrounded by lung or visceral pleura, without bronchoscopic evidence of invasion more proximal than the lobar bronchus (i.e. not in the main bronchus)
T2	Tumour with any of the following features of size or extent: ■ More than 3 cm in greatest dimension ■ Involves main bronchus, 2 cm or more distal to the carina ■ Invades the visceral pleura ■ Associated with atelectasis or obstructive pneumonitis that extends to the hilar region but does not involve the entire lung
T3	Tumour of any size that directly invades any of the following: chest wall (including superior sulcus tumours), diaphragm, mediastinal pleura, parietal pericardium; or tumour in the main bronchus less than 2 cm distal to the carina, but without involvement of the carina; or associated atelectasis or obstructive pneumonitis of the entire lung
T4	Tumour of any size that invades any of the following: mediastinum, heart, great vessels, trachea, oesophagus, vertebral body, carina; or separate tumour nodules in the same lobe; or tumour with malignant pleural effusion
N1	Metastasis to ipsilateral peribronchial and/or ipsilateral hilar lymph nodes, and intrapulmonary nodes including involvement by direct extension of the primary tumour
N2	Metastasis to ipsilateral mediastinal and/or subcarinal lymph nodes
N3	Metastasis to contralateral mediastinal, contralateral hilar, ipsilateral or contralateral scalene, or supraclavicular lymph node(s)

* With permission.

Table 20.2 UICC TNM (6th edn, 2002) stage groupings for lung cancer*

IA	T1	N0	M0
IB	T2	N0	M0
IIA	T1	N1	M0
IIB	T2	N1	M0
	T3	N0	M0
IIIA	T1–3	N2	M0
	T3	N1	M0
IIIB	T1–4	N3	M0
	T4	N0–3	M0
IV	Any T	Any N	M1

* With permission.

Assessment of primary disease

Initial assessment and imaging aims to identify disease that is either operable or treatable within a curative radiotherapy volume. The primary tumour is imaged with chest radiograph and contrast-enhanced CT with particular attention to differentiating tumour from distal collapsed lung and to assessing mediastinal invasion. CT imaging for staging should include the low neck nodes, liver and adrenal glands. MRI may be useful to look for local invasion of the brachial plexus in superior sulcus tumours. A flexible or rigid bronchoscopy is used to determine endobronchial tumour extent as well as to obtain histology. Cytological confirmation of a possibly malignant effusion may be necessary if it would alter management.

CT will allow assessment of mediastinal lymph nodes on size criteria but this has a relatively high false negative (40 per cent) and false positive (20 per cent) rate. The number of visible nodes, their shape and location can provide further information. If available, a PET-CT can be used to assess enlarged mediastinal nodes as well as distant metastases, and should be considered in all patients eligible for curative treatment for NSCLC (Fig. 20.3). Enlarged mediastinal nodes that are visible on PET-CT should ideally be confirmed on biopsy at mediastinoscopy as there is still a significant false positive rate though the false negative rate is small. If a NSCLC is N0 on CT, a staging PET will still detect occult mediastinal nodes in some patients. Overall PET-CT will change the treatment in patients eligible for curative radiotherapy in up to 40 per cent of cases.

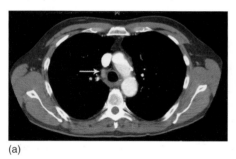 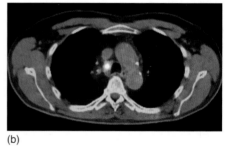

(a)   (b)

Figure 20.3 Diagnostic PET-CT can change treatment volumes by identifying involved mediastinal lymph nodes. (a) Contrast-enhanced CT showing a right paratracheal node 9 mm in short axis diameter (arrowed). (b) Corresponding slice on PET-CT showing increased uptake. This node should be contoured as GTV.

Distant metastases in the liver, adrenals or bones are assessed using the staging CT scan and PET-CT if performed. Bone scans and brain imaging are useful in the presence of unexplained bone pain or neurological symptoms but are not performed routinely.

Data acquisition

■ Immobilisation

Patients should be positioned supine with arms immobilised above the head in a comfortable, reproducible position to allow a greater choice of beam angle. The patient holds on to a T-bar device with their elbows supported laterally (Fig. 20.4). A knee support provides a more comfortable and therefore reproducible set-up.

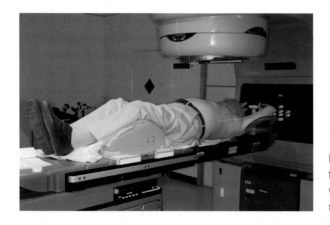

Figure 20.4 Immobilisation for thoracic radiotherapy with a T-bar, lateral elbow supports and a knee rest.

If treatment delivery is prolonged (e.g. with respiratory gating or stereotactic radiotherapy) a vacuum bag should be used to reduce movement.

■ Simulator

If AP beams are to be used for palliation, the borders can be defined in the simulator. The beam centre is marked with a reference tattoo and a photograph of the borders, drawn on the skin, is taken to aid set-up for treatment. Fluoroscopy can be used to view tumour movement but the accuracy of assessment in two dimensions is not enough to predict margins required.

■ CT scanning

CT scans are obtained from the cricoid cartilage to the superior aspect of the L2 vertebra to allow the lung DVH to be calculated. Ideally 3–5 mm slices are used both to aid volume definition and to create high quality DRRs to aid verification. A separate simulator verification visit can then be omitted. An isocentre is tattooed in the CT scanner, as are lateral reference points. Intravenous contrast may help define mediastinal extent of disease but is not essential if a contrast-enhanced diagnostic CT scan is available.

A co-registered PET scan can be used to aid volume definition. Defining volumes on a PET-CT image may help distinguish tumour from collapsed lung. Relatively poor spatial resolution, movement artefact and difficulty in defining the edge of a PET positive mass make this an experimental technique at present.

■ Tumour motion

A free breathing 'slow' CT scan with a single slice scanner is the simplest method of acquiring 3D data for planning. Depending on the speed of image acquisition, some motion will be accounted for with a single CT dataset. Target volumes are then defined taking into account possible organ motion based on population studies.

Whilst some tumours move several centimetres in one or more planes in a respiratory cycle, others are relatively stationary. Moreover, it is difficult to predict from the location of a tumour how much movement there will be. There are several ways to account for individual tumour motion: imaging the tumour at extremes of motion thus incorporating motion into the CT data, limiting mobility by breath-holding or diaphragmatic compression, tracking respiration with respiratory gating and tracking the tumour itself with IGRT.

A very slow CT dataset (4 s per slice) taken during normal breathing will effectively provide a composite image of the tumour as it moves so that volumes defined on the CT scan already take motion into account. Image quality may be reduced making accurate GTV definition more difficult. Fast images taken at maximum inspiration and expiration can be co-registered with a free breathing scan, enabling margins of tumour movement in each plane to be determined so that extremes of motion are encompassed. These techniques allow individualisation of margins while the patient is treated breathing normally.

Several techniques to limit respiratory movement have been researched including breath-holding and abdominal compression but they are difficult to reproduce reliably for each fraction of treatment as they are poorly tolerated by patients. In addition, this approach is time consuming and requires patient education with audio and/or visual cues.

Respiratory gating uses a fiducial marker on the chest wall to switch the CT scanner (and linear accelerator) on in a certain phase of respiration. This approach assumes that an external marker of respiration correlates with internal tumour movement which is not always the case. The baseline thoracic volume can also vary from day to day so a relative measure of tidal volume may not correlate with an absolute position of a tumour.

A 4D CT scan uses a fast multi-slice scanner correlated to the respiratory cycle. Several CT datasets are therefore obtained, each at a different point in the respiratory cycle. A composite GTV including all positions of the tumour in the respiratory cycle can thus be created allowing individual tumour motion to be accounted for in volume definition.

Target volume definition

■ Curative

To define the GTV accurately it is important to have all diagnostic imaging available – ideally on a separate workstation adjacent to the planning computer. Clinical information and bronchoscopy or mediastinoscopy reports should be available. In the case of adjuvant radiotherapy, a discussion with the surgeon and pathologist is essential to define sites at highest risk of relapse. Clips placed at surgery at sites of incomplete excision are valuable, but must not be confused with clips used to ligate vessels. Uncertainty in GTV definition can be reduced by a radiologist and oncologist collaborating to define the GTV.

The parenchymal extent of the GTV should be defined with CT images viewed on a standardised lung window setting (Fig. 20.5). The spiculated edge of the tumour is included within the GTV. Anatomical knowledge, contrast CT scans and radiologist input can help differentiate tumour from normal structures such as pulmonary vasculature and the azygous vein. Tumour can be very difficult to differentiate from adjacent lung collapse or atelectasis.

CT images should be viewed on a mediastinal window setting to define mediastinal extent of disease and any involved lymph nodes. Contrast-enhanced images (planning or diagnostic scan) and PET-CT if available may help define local mediastinal extent.

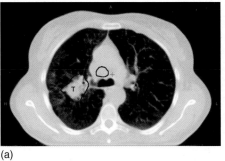
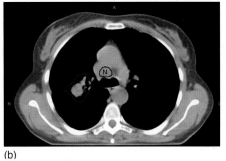

(a)   (b)

Figure 20.5 GTV definition with the appropriate window setting on a planning CT scan. (a) Lung window setting to define the primary tumour (T) within the lung. (b) Same slice on mediastinal window setting to define any invasion into the mediastinum and involved nodes (N). Note primary tumour appears smaller.

If chemotherapy is used before radiation the GTV should include all sites of disease at presentation, e.g. any enlarged nodes that have shrunk to less than 10 mm with treatment.

The GTV is grown isotropically to produce a CTV. There is evidence to suggest that an 8 mm margin from GTV to CTV is adequate to cover microscopic disease in lung tissue. The CTV is edited to take account of natural barriers to tumour spread (e.g. uninvolved bone or great vessels). It is extended to encompass likely patterns of spread and to encompass the original GTV if neoadjuvant chemotherapy has been used. In practice this usually produces a variable GTV-CTV margin throughout the volume but adding an isotropic margin which is then edited will be less prone to systematic errors than manually defining the CTV (Fig. 20.6). Elective nodal irradiation is not recommended as most recurrences after radiotherapy are within the primary tumour or as distant metastases rather than as isolated nodal recurrences.

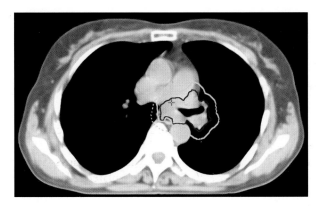

Figure 20.6 Defining the CTV in lung cancer. The GTV is grown isotropically by 8 mm (dashed line) and then edited to take account of natural tumour barriers and likely patterns of spread to create the final CTV.

CTV to PTV margins depend on tumour motion and day-to-day set-up errors. The latter should be measured in each department and should be approximately 5 mm in each direction. The margin added for tumour motion will vary from zero in the case of perfect IGRT using implanted fiducial markers, to a standard solution if individual motion is not accounted for. In practice, margins of 7 mm axially and 12 mm longitudinally are added to account for tumour motion and set-up errors. While this may not reflect extremes of movement for all tumours, larger margins may make it difficult to keep within dose constraints for critical normal structures. Some centres advocate margins as small as 5 mm for GTV-CTV and CTV-PTV, on the basis that local control in lung cancer is primarily determined by the dose that can be delivered to the GTV rather than to the edge of the PTV.

The spinal cord is contoured on axial slices throughout the PTV and an isotropic 5 mm margin applied to produce a PRV. The oesophagus is contoured throughout the PTV if the tumour is close to or involves the mediastinum. Automatic contouring tools can be used to contour the lungs. A lung minus PTV structure is then constructed by subtraction.

■ Palliative

If CT planning is used, the GTV is defined as above and a 10 mm margin applied to produce a PTV on the basis that larger margins would reduce the therapeutic ratio in the palliative setting. If beams are defined on the simulator, the diagnostic CT images can still be used to define a virtual GTV which can be superimposed onto the simulator radiograph. A 15 mm margin from this virtual GTV to the beam edge will give the same effect.

Dose solutions

■ Conventional

Palliative therapy given in one or two fractions can be defined in the simulator as above. Anterior and posterior photon beams are used with dose prescribed to the midplane. MLC shielding may reduce the dose to normal lung tissue; 6 MV photons are adequate unless the separation at the centre is more than 28 cm, in which case a higher energy (e.g. 10 MV) is needed.

■ Conformal

There are several challenges to covering the PTV within ICRU targets while maintaining toxicity at acceptable levels. The location and size of the PTV and its proximity to critical structures, particularly the oesophagus and spinal cord, often necessitate a compromise in choosing the most acceptable plan for an individual patient.

When curative radiotherapy is used for stage I or II disease a three-field conformal plan is commonly used. Many tumours are closer to the chest wall than to the mediastinum and ipsilateral beams will minimise the dose to contralateral normal lung tissue and normally provide a homogeneous dose distribution (Fig. 20.7). Beam angles are chosen to reduce lung dose with anterior oblique, posterior oblique and lateral beams often used. Wedges compensate for the obliquity of the beams in relation to the chest wall, and MLC shielding is used to conform each beam shape to the PTV.

In stage IIIA disease a similar three-field conformal plan is often used. The beam angles are chosen using the BEV tool while viewing the PTV, spinal cord PRV and oesophagus contour so as to reduce dose to the spinal cord and oesophagus as much as possible and with the aim of minimising lung dose.

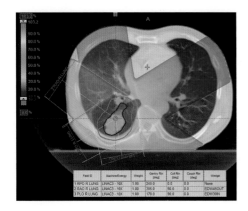

Figure 20.7 Beam arrangement and dose colourwash for a T2N0 lung cancer situated posteriorly in the right lower lobe. Lung windowing is used to demonstrate the primary tumour more clearly.

For larger tumours, in particular those crossing the midline in the mediastinum, it is more difficult to cover the medial extent of the tumour with ipsilateral beams. Adding a contralateral beam will significantly increase the dose to normal lung. Such tumours can be treated in two phases. In phase 1, an arrangement of opposing MLC-shaped photon beams ensures all the mediastinal extent is treated and also reduces lung dose, at the expense of a poorly conformal plan with oesophagus and cord within the treated volume. Phase 2 uses a conformal three- or four-beam plan which will give a higher lung dose. By varying the number of fractions in each phase it can be possible to deliver adequate dose to the PTV and remain within cord, lung and oesophageal tolerance (Fig. 20.8).

Primary tumours close to the spinal cord may have a PTV that is very close to, or even overlaps the spinal cord PRV. Rather than miss some of the PTV throughout a course, it is preferable to use two phases for treatment accepting full dose to the cord for phase 1 with the addition of MLCs to shield the cord from at least two beams in phase 2. Again, the number of fractions in each phase is varied until the sum of the two plans is within to cord tolerance.

In SCLCs or NSCLCs with N2 disease, the PTV will often be very close to the oesophagus. The risk of grade 3 acute toxicity or long-term oesophageal stricture is related to the length of oesophagus in the treated volume and ideally this is kept below 8 cm by choosing beam angles carefully. For some patients it may be appropriate to accept some underdosing of the PTV to achieve this. Concomitant chemotherapy in either non-small cell or small cell disease increases the risk of oesophagitis.

The plan should be assessed carefully by the oncologist using DVHs. We recommend aiming to keep the V20 (volume of lung minus PTV receiving >20 Gy) below 32 per cent. *In vivo*, the risk of radiation pneumonitis depends not only on the dose absorbed but also on the use of concomitant chemotherapy, pre-existing lung disease, the lobe being treated and vascular perfusion. A 3D dose distribution cannot take these points into consideration and is then reduced to a 2D graphic illustration – the DVH. To then base an assessment of pneumonitis solely on whether this curve is above or below one point on the graph is perhaps an oversimplification. Other targets such as minimising V5 and having a mean lung dose lower than 20 Gy have also been shown to correlate with pneumonitis. A V20 of <32 per cent is a useful target but for patients with poor lung function, a lower target may be needed, whereas for those

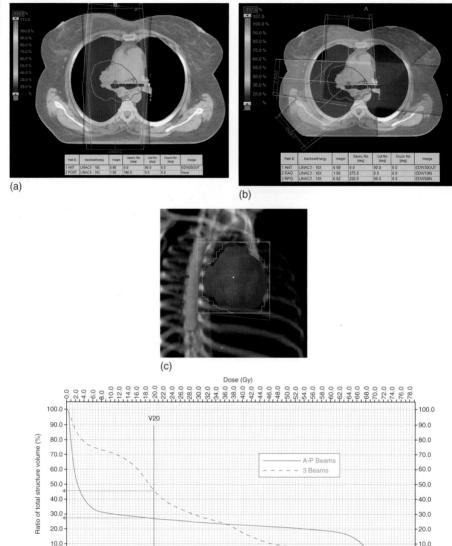

Figure 20.8 Treatment of a large T3N2 NSCLC with a two-phase technique. (a) AP beams to minimise lung dose. (b) Three-beam plan to reduce cord dose. (c) BEV of posterior oblique beam from the three-beam plan. The beam angle is chosen to maximise the gap between the spinal cord PRV and the PTV. (d) DVH for lung-PTV for the AP beams and the three-beam plan. The V20 would be 46 per cent if the three-beam plan were used for the whole treatment (66 Gy in 33 fractions) so a two-phase technique is necessary.

with good lung function a value closer to 40 per cent may be acceptable. It is therefore difficult to use one value in assessing all plans.

Similarly, there are several parameters of the oesophageal DVH identified that correlate with the risk of grade 3 or 4 acute oesophagitis or the risk of strictures.

We recommend aiming to keep the length of oesophagus within the treated volume to less than 8 cm where possible and certainly to less than 12 cm. Other variables including the V40 or V50 have also been shown to correlate with toxicity in some series.

Beam energies above 10 MV should be avoided because secondary electrons have a greater range in lung tissue so higher energy photon beams have a wider penumbra. Modern dose calculation engines such as voxel Monte Carlo will produce more accurate dose calculations within the lung than the older pencil beam convolution algorithms implemented in most planning systems.

■ Complex

The principal challenges in lung cancer radiotherapy are volume definition and accounting for motion. Complex treatment dose solutions should only be used when tumour motion is also accounted for. In such circumstances IMRT may produce more conformal dose distributions, particularly for tumours close to the spinal cord.

Dose-fractionation

■ Curative NSCLC

55 Gy in 20 daily fractions of 2.75 Gy given in 4 weeks.
66 Gy in 33 daily fractions given in 6½ weeks.

■ Adjuvant NSCLC

50 Gy in 20 daily fractions of 2.5 Gy given in 4 weeks.
60 Gy in 30 daily fractions given in 6 weeks.

■ Curative SCLC

40 Gy in 15 daily fractions of 2.67 Gy given in 3 weeks.

Consider

66 Gy in 33 daily fractions given in 6½ weeks
  or
45 Gy in 30 fractions of 1.5 Gy treating twice daily given in 3 weeks.

■ Palliative

10 Gy in 1 fraction.
16 Gy in 2 fractions of 8 Gy a week apart (the dose has been reduced from 17 Gy in 2 fractions to minimise the risk of spinal cord damage if survival is prolonged).

■ If PS 0–1 and life expectancy >6 months, consider

20 Gy in 5 fractions of 4 Gy given in 1 week
  or
36 Gy in 12 fractions of 3 Gy given in 4 weeks (39 Gy in 13 fractions if spinal cord not in treated volume).

■ Prophylactic cranial irradiation

24 Gy in 10 daily fractions of 2.4 Gy given in 2 weeks.

Treatment delivery and patient care

Patients should be reviewed weekly by a trained radiographer or physician so that acute side effects are treated proactively. A mild increase in dyspnoea or cough is common but rarely needs treatment though intercurrent infections should be excluded. Advice on skin care is given. When the oesophagus is within the treated volume, pain on swallowing and dysphagia usually begin in the third week of treatment. Systemic analgesia, topical local anaesthetic agents and advice on soft and high calorie diets from a dietician should be available.

Verification

Ideally the treatment isocentre on a DRR from the CT simulation is compared with portal images of the isocentre on the treatment machines using electronic portal imaging. Off-line correction protocols are used for standard conformal treatment. Images are taken on days 1–3 and weekly thereafter with a correction made if the mean error in any one plane is >5 mm. If stereotactic radiation or IGRT is used, online correction protocols are necessary.

Other points

A single fraction of HDR brachytherapy can provide useful palliation in NSCLC. Other local treatments such as stent insertion, laser debulking and cryotherapy can produce similar results and the choice of treatment depends largely on local expertise. EBRT is likely to be more effective in patients who have not had radiation before, but brachytherapy can offer good palliation after curative radiotherapy.

key trials

Saunders M, Dische S, Barrett A *et al.* (1999) Continuous, hyperfractionated, accelerated radiotherapy (CHART) versus conventional radiotherapy in non-small cell lung cancer: mature data from the randomised multicentre trial. CHART Steering Committee. *Radiother Oncol* 52: 137–48.

Slotman B, Faivre-Finn C, Kramer G *et al.* (2007) Prophylactic cranial irradiation in extensive small-cell lung cancer. *N Eng J Med* 357: 644–72.

Turrisi AT 3rd, Kim K, Blum R *et al.* (1999) Twice-daily compared with once daily thoracic radiotherapy in limited small-cell lung cancer treated concurrently with cisplatin and etoposide. *N Engl J Med* 340: 265–71.

Information sources

Alberts WM (2007) Diagnosis and management of lung cancer executive summary: ACCP evidence-based clinical practice guidelines, 2nd edition. *Chest* 132(3 suppl): S1–19.

Auperin A, Arriagada R, Pignon JP *et al.* (1999) Prophylactic cranial irradiation for patients with small-cell lung cancer in complete remission. Prophylactic Cranial Irradiation Overview Collaborative Group. *N Engl J Med* **341**: 476–84.

Cancer Care Ontario Lung Cancer Evidence-based Series and Practice Guidelines (2005) *Postoperative Adjuvant Radiation Therapy in Stage II or IIIA Completely Resected Non-Small Cell Lung Cancer: Cancer Care Ontario Practice Guidelines Initiative.* Available at: www.cancercare.on.ca/english/home/toolbox/qualityguidelines/diseasesite/lung-ebs/ [cited 2008 October 11] (accessed 26 September 2008).

Chapet O, Kong FM, Quint LE *et al.* (2005) CT-based definition of thoracic lymph node stations: an atlas from the University of Michigan. *Int J Radiat Oncol Biol Phys* **63**: 170–8.

De Ruysscher D, Pijls-Johannesma M, Bentzen SM *et al.* (2006) Time between the first day of chemotherapy and the last day of chest radiation is the most important predictor of survival in limited-disease small-cell lung cancer. *J Clin Oncol* **24**: 1057–63.

Lester JF, Macbeth FR, Toy E *et al.* (2006) Palliative radiotherapy regimens for non-small cell lung cancer. *Cochrane Database Syst Rev* (**4**): CD002143.

National Collaborating Centre for Acute Care, London. Available at: www.nice.org.uk/Guidance/Topic/Cancer/Lung (accessed 8 December 2008).

National Institute for Health and Clinical Excellence (2005) *Lung Cancer: Diagnosis and Treatment.* Clinical guideline 24. Available at: www.nice.org.uk/guidance/CG24 (accessed 5 December 2008).

Pignon JP, Arriagada R, Ihde DC *et al.* (1992) A meta-analysis of thoracic radiotherapy for small-cell lung cancer. *N Engl J Med* **327**: 1618–24.

Rowell NP, Williams CJ (2001) Radical radiotherapy for stage I/II non-small cell lung cancer in patients not sufficiently fit for or declining surgery (medically inoperable). *Cochrane Database Syst Rev* (**2**): CD002935.

Rowell NP, O'Rourke NP (2004) Concurrent chemoradiotherapy in non-small cell lung cancer. *Cochrane Database Syst Rev* (**4**): CD002140.

Scottish Intercollegiate Guidelines Network Guidance 80 (2005) *Management of Patients with Lung Cancer.* National Clinical Guideline 80. Available at: www.sign.ac.uk/guidelines/published/index.html (accessed 5 December 2008).

Senan S, De Ruysscher D, Giraud P *et al.* (2004) Literature-based recommendations for treatment planning and execution in high-dose radiotherapy for lung cancer. *Radiother Oncol* **71**: 139–46.

21 Mesothelioma

Indications for radiotherapy

For many years mesothelioma has been regarded as relatively resistant to radiotherapy. The increasing incidence of this disease and interest in new therapeutic strategies with curative intent has led to more patients with mesothelioma receiving radiotherapy.

■ Adjuvant radiotherapy

A few patients with good PS (WHO 0–1), low comorbidity and early stage disease confined to the thoracic pleural surface are treated with combined modality therapy with curative intent. This comprises chemotherapy, surgery (extrapleural pneumonectomy [EPP] – *en bloc* removal of the parietal pleura, lung, diaphragm and pericardium) and adjuvant radiotherapy. Published single centre series in highly selected patients support this intensive approach with median survival rates of 20–30 months, but there is no confirmatory phase III evidence. Eligible patients should be included in phase III studies where possible or at least treated at centres with experience of this programme. To irradiate one hemithorax while minimising dose to critical structures (heart, spinal cord, liver, kidneys and contralateral lung) presents a major radiotherapeutic challenge. The lowest local recurrence rates with acceptable toxicity have been achieved by treating the hemithorax to 54 Gy. Comparative series suggest that lower doses are less effective.

■ Prophylactic radiotherapy

Radiotherapy has been given to prevent painful subcutaneous masses forming at sites of trans-thoracic interventions such as pleural biopsies or chest drains. Seeding of malignant cells along such needle tracts is reported to occur in 15–50 per cent of sites, but there is no good evidence that such masses are symptomatic in most patients. There are a number of phase III studies comparing prophylactic radiotherapy with no radiation but all are small and underpowered. Interventions such as CT-guided fine needle biopsies may pose less risk of seeding than large-bore chest drains used for treatment of pleural effusions. In the absence of evidence either in favour of or against this practice, we recommend considering prophylactic radiotherapy for patients of PS 0–1 who have had a chest drain or thoracotomy (Fig. 21.1). Ideally it is performed within 2 weeks of the intervention.

■ Palliative radiotherapy

Palliative radiotherapy can help alleviate chest wall pain in mesothelioma. Several small single centre series suggest response rates of 20–70 per cent but the doses

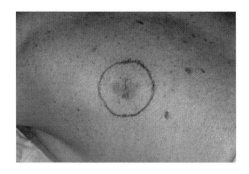

Figure 21.1 Prophylactic radiotherapy with 12 MeV electrons to the site of a chest drain. The beam edge is marked in pen – 2 cm from the drain site.

used and methods of response evaluation were very variable. There is no good evidence of a dose–response relationship. Mesothelioma often presents as diffuse pleural disease and it can be difficult to decide which part of the pleural disease should be targeted with palliative radiotherapy. Radiotherapy is best considered as one method of pain control alongside opiates, antineuropathic agents and cordotomy.

Sequencing of multimodality therapy

If radiotherapy is used as part of multimodality therapy, it should follow neoadjuvant chemotherapy and EPP, ideally commencing 8–10 weeks after surgery. There is no evidence that high dose hemi-thoracic radiation has any benefit outside this protocol.

Clinical and radiological anatomy

Mesothelioma usually spreads locally within the pleural space on the parietal and mediastinal pleural surfaces and can invade the chest wall and mediastinum.

A contrast-enhanced CT scan of the thorax and upper abdomen is used to assess the degree of pleural space involvement and mediastinal lymphadenopathy.

Assessment of primary disease

If multimodality therapy is to be attempted careful patient selection is very important. All such patients should have a mediastinoscopy to evaluate mediastinal lymph nodes, and a staging PET scan to exclude patients with inoperable disease. Patients should be assessed by a multidisciplinary team including medical oncologist, surgeon and radiation oncologist before commencing the treatment programme to ensure they are eligible for all modalities involved.

If palliative radiotherapy is to be of value, it needs to be targeted to a site likely to be causing pain and this can be difficult to assess given the diffuse nature of mesothelioma. A careful history and clinical examination are most useful but chest radiographs or CT scans can show rib or vertebral destruction, which may correlate with sites of pain.

Data acquisition

■ Immobilisation

For adjuvant radiotherapy patients should be supine with arms above the head in a comfortable and reproducible position. A head rest, knee pillow and arm support may be helpful, and a vacuum bag for the thorax should be considered.

Patients for prophylactic or palliative electron treatment should be placed in a comfortable position on the simulator couch which allows skin apposition of the electron applicator.

■ CT scanning

For adjuvant radiotherapy, drain sites and all chest incisions other than the median sternotomy scar are marked with radio-opaque wire. CT slices no more than 5 mm thick are obtained from the cricoid cartilage to the iliac crests. A treatment isocentre is tattooed at the time of CT scanning in order to reduce systematic set-up errors.

■ Simulator

Palliative radiotherapy can be planned on a simulator if a single electron beam or parallel opposing photon beams are used. Painful chest wall masses or sites of origin of pain are marked with radio-opaque wire before screening.

Target volume definition

■ Adjuvant radiotherapy

The entire pleural cavity should be marked with radio-opaque clips at the time of surgery to facilitate CTV definition. Clips at the insertion of the diaphragm and on the pleural reflections are especially useful. Volumes are defined after consultation with the surgeon and pathologist to identify high risk sites in the hemithorax such as residual macroscopic or microscopic disease or locations where there was tumour on the mediastinal pleural surface.

The GTV is residual macroscopic disease if present. The CTV1 (54) comprises the GTV with a minimum 10 mm margin in each plane and any sites of microscopic residual disease (positive resection margins). The CTV2 is defined as the entire ipsilateral thoracic cavity from lung apex to insertion of the diaphragm, ipsilateral mediastinal pleura, mediastinal tissues at sites where there was evidence for tumour invasion, the ipsilateral pericardial surface, and full thickness of the thorax at the sites of thoracotomy and chest tube incisions. It is very challenging to treat all the CTV2 to 54 Gy so some dose compromise to this large volume may be unavoidable. It can be very helpful to review the CTVs with the thoracic surgeon once they have been defined.

The CTVs are grown by at least 10 mm to produce the PTVs, but this margin should be adjusted according to measured departmental errors for hemithoracic radiation.

The spinal cord with a 5 mm margin, contralateral lung, heart, liver, oesophagus and kidneys are contoured as OAR volumes.

■ Prophylactic radiotherapy

As electrons or 300 kV photons are used and the beam border marked onto the patient's skin, GTV, CTV and PTV are not defined. A 2 cm margin from the edge of the scar being treated to the 50 per cent electron beam edge is recommended to account for the shape of isodoses at depth. This will usually mean a 6 cm circle-shaped field for simple drain sites with larger fields for patients who have had a thoracotomy for a video-assisted thoracoscopic pleurodesis or a decortication.

■ Palliative radiotherapy

As beams are usually defined on the simulator, GTV, CTV and PTV are not defined. A 1 cm margin from the edge of any masses to the beam edge is recommended.

Dose solutions

■ Conformal – adjuvant radiotherapy

It is a major challenge to produce a conformal plan to treat the PTV uniformly to 54 Gy while maintaining critical organ tolerance (Fig. 21.2). Table 21.1 gives suggested OAR tolerance doses when the dose prescribed to the PTV is given in 1.8 Gy fractions.

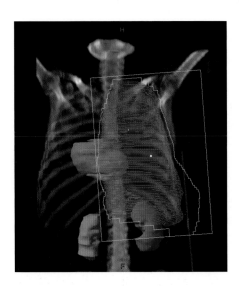

Figure 21.2 Target volume for adjuvant radiotherapy after extrapleural pneumonectomy. A DRR showing the overlap of PTV2 (red) with the kidney, spinal cord and heart. It is impossible to treat this volume to 54 Gy with conventional photon fields while keeping to critical organ tolerance doses.

Dose to the PTV2 can be compromised to achieve target doses to the spinal cord, contralateral lung, contralateral kidney and liver. The minimum dose to PTV2 should be 45 Gy and the PTV1 should receive the prescribed dose of 54 Gy.

The large circumferential CTV and multiple OAR mean the best conformal solution is a pair of anterior and posterior photon beams with MLC shielding to the liver, kidneys, heart and spinal cord added during the treatment course depending on their tolerance. The shielded areas within the target volume are then treated with electrons matched as well as possible to the photon fields.

Table 21.1 Suggested tolerance doses for OAR in adjuvant radiotherapy for mesothelioma*

OAR	Target
Spinal cord + 5 mm	50 Gy
Contralateral lung	V20 ≤15 per cent. Some centres also recommend constraints on mean lung dose (e.g. MLD <9.5 Gy) and V5 (e.g. V5 <60 per cent)
Contralateral kidney	D80 per cent <15 Gy
Ipsilateral kidney	As low as possible
Heart	D70 per cent <45 Gy and D_{max} <60 Gy. These limits may be exceeded if residual disease is present close to the heart
Liver	Mean dose <35 Gy
Oesophagus	Less than 12 cm length in treated volume

*Taken from the MARS trial with permission of Dr Senan.

■ Complex – adjuvant radiotherapy

In view of the difficulties of producing a conformal plan that adequately treats the PTV while achieving the dose constraints in Table 21.1, IMRT has been used in this setting. A potential disadvantage of IMRT is the increased dose to the remaining lung with small single centre series reporting death rates from pneumonitis as high as 50 per cent. To reduce this risk, the gantry angles for IMRT should be chosen to minimise exit through the contralateral lung.

The IMRT beams can also be restricted so that the superior part of the PTV is treated with just a few beams thus avoiding exit doses to the contralateral lung and reducing pulmonary toxicity. The inferior portion near the heart or liver is treated with all beams to maximise the advantage of highly conformal dose in this part of the volume.

Another possible solution is to use combined photon IMRT and electron beams – using the electrons to produce a conformal dose at depth to the more superficial part of the PTV and IMRT to produce conformality in other planes.

■ Conventional – prophylactic and palliative radiotherapy

In prophylactic treatment electrons are preferred, with the energy chosen to treat from the skin surface down to the pleura within the 90 per cent isodose. The depth of the pleura is best measured on diagnostic CT scans but can be estimated clinically. In practice, 9–12 MeV electrons with 5 mm tissue equivalent bolus are frequently used. While standard cut-outs are used for drain sites, a patient-specific cut-out is usually required for larger scars that follow more complex procedures. If electrons are not available, 300 kV photons can be used, but this technique will not produce adequate coverage of the tract close to the pleural surface.

Palliative radiotherapy for painful masses can be achieved with a direct electron beam or with parallel opposed photon beams. Photons are often more appropriate given the depth of painful lesions, particularly when the mass extends around the curved chest wall.

Dose-fractionation

■ Adjuvant

PTV1

54 Gy in 30 daily fractions of 1.8 Gy given in 6 weeks.

The plan chosen must deliver a minimum dose of 45 Gy to PTV2.

Prophylactic

21 Gy in 3 daily fractions of 7 Gy given in 3 days.

Palliative

8 Gy in 1 fraction.
20 Gy in 5 fractions of 4 Gy given in 1 week.

Treatment delivery and patient care

■ Adjuvant radiotherapy

Cardiac function (ejection fraction must be >40 per cent) and contralateral renal function (serum creatinine or glomerular filtration rate [GFR] estimation and evaluation of differential renal function) should be assessed before treatment. A dietetic assessment before radiotherapy is desirable to initiate high calorie supplements if necessary. Patients should be advised about good skin care (gentle washing with simple soap, and application of aqueous cream) and management of oesophagitis (see Chapter 19). Codeine linctus or oral opiates may help alleviate cough. 5-HT antagonists may be required to prevent emesis.

A careful discussion with the patient about the potential benefits and possible late effects of radiotherapy is essential. Patients are treated daily with no compensation for missed days.

■ Palliative/prophylactic radiotherapy

Patients should be instructed in skin care – the use of simple soaps and aqueous cream to keep the skin moisturised. Bright erythema is usual when 21 Gy in 3 fractions over 3 days is used, and some long-term pigmentation of the skin is common.

Verification

Treatment is verified using the protocol described for lung cancer in Chapter 19.

key trials

Boutin C, Rey F, Viallat JR (1995) Prevention of malignant seeding after invasive diagnostic procedures in patients with pleural mesothelioma. *Chest* **108**: 754–8.

MARS (Mesothelioma and Radical Surgery) trial. *Three Cycles of Chemotherapy Followed Either by EPP and Radiotherapy or by No Surgery or Radiotherapy.* ICR, Scientific Principal Investigator Prof Julian Peto. Closed 2008.

O'Rourke N, Garcia JC, Paul J *et al.* (2007) A randomised controlled trial of intervention site radiotherapy in malignant pleural mesothelioma. *Radiother Oncol* **84**: 18–22.

SAKK 17/04 study. *Neoadjuvant Chemotherapy and Extrapleural Pneumonectomy of Malignant Pleural Mesothelioma With or Without Hemithoracic Radiotherapy.* A randomised multicentre phase II trial. Swiss trial aiming to recruit over 150 patients.

Information sources

Allen AA, Schofield D, Hacker F *et al.* (2007) Restricted field IMRT dramatically enhances IMRT planning for mesothelioma. *Int J Radiation Oncology Biol Phys* **69**: 1587–92.

Waite K, Gilligan D (2007) The role of radiotherapy in the treatment of malignant pleural mesothelioma. *Clinical Oncology* **19**: 182–7.

Breast

22

Indications for radiotherapy

■ Breast radiotherapy

Adjuvant radiotherapy given following surgery for primary carcinoma of the breast has been shown to reduce the incidence of locoregional recurrence from 30 per cent to 10.5 per cent at 20 years and breast cancer deaths by 5.4 per cent at 20 years.

Radiotherapy is standard treatment after complete local excision of ductal carcinoma *in situ* (DCIS) and current trials are evaluating its role in 'low risk' patients compared with surgery alone.

Clinical T1, T2 less than 3 cm, N0 invasive breast cancers are treated by wide local excision (WLE) followed by radiotherapy with comparable local control rates to mastectomy, both combined with axillary surgery. The tumour site, size, histological type, grade and extent of *in situ* disease, as well as the size of the breast, all influence choice of treatment, as does consideration of the expected cosmetic result and patient preference. Radiotherapy is indicated for all patients after conservative surgery. As yet no 'low risk' group has been identified where surgery alone gives adequate local control, but ongoing trials are addressing this issue. Contraindications to conservative surgery include multifocal breast tumours, extensive DCIS, central tumours in a small breast and incomplete excision. Significant pre-existing cardiac or lung disease, scleroderma and limited shoulder mobility may prevent the use of radiotherapy. Patients with operable tumours which are 3–4 cm or more in diameter have a higher local recurrence rate with conservative surgery and radiotherapy, and may be offered primary systemic therapy. Long-term results of this strategy, which aims to downstage the tumour and avoid mastectomy in many patients, are awaited. After primary chemotherapy, indications for locoregional radiotherapy are determined by high risk factors at presentation and preoperative clinical staging rather than postoperative pathological staging.

Primary lymphoma of the breast is commonly high grade and treated by primary chemotherapy followed by local radiotherapy. For malignant phylloides tumours and sarcomas of the breast, mastectomy is the treatment of choice.

Patients with bilateral tumours are treated according to the indications for each individual tumour site.

■ Tumour bed boost radiotherapy

After complete excision, the decision to use a 'boost' dose to the tumour bed should balance the individual's risk of local recurrence (dependent on factors such as age, tumour grade and size, lymphovascular invasion, margin status, endocrine receptor status, and use of systemic therapy) against the risk of late effects (e.g. cardiac or lung damage because of shallow breast tissue over heart or ribs). EORTC 22881 showed that in patients younger than 40, a boost dose of 16 Gy resulted in a greater reduction of local failure than for other age groups, but the relative risk reduction was similar for all ages. All patients who have microscopic tumour present at a resection margin, and where re-excision or mastectomy is declined, should be considered for boost radiotherapy.

■ Post-mastectomy radiotherapy

More patients are having immediate breast reconstruction after mastectomy using either microvascular techniques or an implant. Subsequent radiotherapy may lead to a risk of late fibrosis and outcomes are being monitored. Post-mastectomy radiotherapy is recommended for patients with T3, T4 tumours and those with four or more positive axillary nodes who have a high risk of local recurrence (around 30 per cent), which is reduced by at least two-thirds. The Danish Breast Cancer Trials Group (DBCG) reported a 9 per cent absolute increase in survival rate at 15 years after post-mastectomy locoregional radiotherapy in all groups of node positive patients. Therefore patients with one to three nodes, and for example, young patients and those with large T2–3 tumours, grade III, oestrogen receptor negative, lymphovascular invasion or lobular histology with an estimated 10–20 per cent local recurrence risk at 10 years, may also be considered for locoregional radiotherapy. Local guidelines must be developed with a threshold chosen for the level of risk of local recurrence that merits treatment until further trial data are available.

For inoperable T3 and T4 tumours, primary systemic therapy is given before combined local treatment with surgery and locoregional radiotherapy, the sequence depending on tumour regression, staging and prognostic factors.

■ Lymph node irradiation

If no axillary surgery has been performed and prognostic factors are good, axillary radiotherapy may not be indicated.

Sentinel node biopsy allows selective axillary dissection for patients with a positive node biopsy. Current EORTC trials are comparing axillary dissection with axillary radiotherapy after positive sentinel node biopsy. Where sentinel node biopsy is not available, lymph node irradiation is unnecessary if an axillary dissection up to the lateral border of the pectoralis minor (level I) is negative.

Retrospective meta-analyses have shown that in high risk patients, axillary radiotherapy is as effective as axillary surgery in preventing axillary recurrence.

If level I axillary nodes are involved, there is a >5 per cent risk of subsequent supraclavicular fossa (SCF) recurrence, so irradiation may be given to levels II and III axillary and SCF nodes. When four or more nodes, a single node >2 cm or level III nodes are involved, the risk of SCF involvement is 15–20 per cent and radiotherapy is indicated. After axillary dissection to level III with positive nodes, axillary radiotherapy is associated with considerable morbidity and should be avoided unless there is known residual disease, but SCF treatment is given. Nodal radiotherapy is indicated for locally advanced disease after primary systemic treatment, where surgery is not possible.

Radiotherapy to the internal mammary nodes is not recommended outside a clinical trial because of the risk of cardiac toxicity and results of EORTC trial 22922/10925 are awaited.

Improved adjuvant systemic therapies such as anthracyclines, taxanes and trastuzumab alter the risk versus benefit analysis of breast and lymph node irradiation because of the risk of cardiac toxicity. Gene expression profiling of primary breast cancer will be used to individualise indications for radiotherapy in the future, based on predictions of risk of locoregional recurrence.

■ Palliative radiotherapy

Radiotherapy has a major role in the palliation of locally advanced and fungating breast tumours as well as in treating symptomatic metastases at sites such as bone, brain, skin, lymph nodes, choroid and meninges.

Prognostic factors, PS and patient preference all affect the final decision made by the multidisciplinary team.

Sequencing of multimodality treatment

In the adjuvant setting, chemotherapy is given before radiotherapy to reduce side effects. This may mean that radiotherapy is delayed by 4–6 months and it is not yet known whether this will compromise local control. The optimal sequencing of chemo- and radiotherapy was the subject of the SECRAB trial where treatment was randomised to a sequential versus synchronous schedule of chemo- and radiotherapy, and these results are awaited. Primary chemotherapy for operable breast cancer is followed by surgery and then subsequent radiotherapy. For locally advanced disease, primary chemotherapy or endocrine therapy may be followed by surgery if technically feasible or further downstaging using locoregional radiotherapy may be attempted, reserving surgery for excision of residual disease if restaging is clear.

Clinical and radiological anatomy

Breast cancer spreads locally by direct infiltration of the surrounding parenchyma and may extend to underlying muscle and overlying skin, including the nipple. A dense network of lymphatics in the skin may facilitate widespread cutaneous permeation by tumour.

Lymphatics drain laterally to the axilla, medially to internal mammary nodes and superiorly to the supraclavicular fossa (Fig. 22.1). Lymphatic vessels from the whole breast drain to the internal mammary nodes, which communicate with the contralateral chain superiorly. The internal mammary nodes lie on the internal surface of the anterior chest wall closely applied to the internal mammary artery. Although the anatomical drainage pattern is complex, involvement by tumour is most commonly found in the axillary lymph nodes. These are divided into levels I–III, which are used to guide surgical axillary node dissection. Levels are described in relation to the pectoralis minor muscle. Level I nodes lie inferolateral to its lateral border, level II posteriorly between its medial and lateral borders, and level III medial to the medial border of pectoralis minor adjacent to the axillary vein and first rib. Level III nodes are continuous with the supraclavicular nodes medially and anteriorly and also with the infraclavicular nodes.

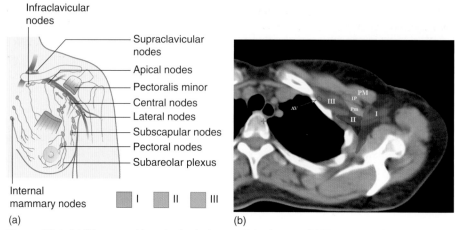

Figure 22.1 (a) Diagram of lymphatic drainage of the breast. (b) Transverse CT scan of the left axilla (patient with arms up) both showing position of levels I–III axillary lymph nodes. AV, axillary vessels; Pm, pectoralis minor; PM, pectoralis major; IP, inter-pectoral nodes.

Assessment of primary disease

Ideally the radiation oncologist should examine the patient preoperatively. Breast examination includes inspection for nipple or skin retraction, discharge, ulceration or asymmetry, and palpation for size and site of the lump and fixation to adjacent structures. Glandular drainage areas are also assessed and TNM staging recorded on an accurate diagram. A photograph may be used to show the exact position of the lesion. Mammography is performed to demonstrate the tumour and to detect calcification, multifocal or *in situ* disease and bilateral involvement. Ultrasound is used to measure the size of the lesion and to guide fine needle aspiration cytology and/or core biopsy for histology. MRI can be used to exclude multifocal disease prior to conservative surgery, particularly for large tumours in a radiographically dense breast and for lobular cancers. MRI is also used to monitor response to therapy where primary chemotherapy is used. Axillary node status may be assessed using ultrasound and guided fine needle aspiration (FNA), or, where there is palpable disease, with CT as part of a staging procedure for more advanced disease. Examination of the surgical specimen should define the size, site and local extent of the primary lesion with macroscopic margins and the number and position of axillary nodes in the specimen. Histological review determines size, type of tumour, grade, microscopic assessment of excision margins, lymphovascular invasion, oestrogen, progesterone and HER2 receptor status, number of lymph nodes involved and removed, and any extracapsular extension. Many oncoplastic techniques place the surgical scar at a distance from the tumour bed and this relation should be shown in an accurate operative diagram. Details of the level of any axillary dissection, any residual disease and the placement of titanium clips or gold seeds in the tumour bed should all be recorded. When inoperable primary tumours remain palpable after systemic therapy, they can be assessed by palpation and ultrasound, the dimensions marked on the skin, and a photograph taken.

All patients are discussed in multidisciplinary meetings, with review of imaging and histopathology. If the radial or superficial margins are incomplete, re-excision is advised, although usually the deep margin has been cleared down to pectoral fascia. Extensive DCIS is an indication for mastectomy, but minor focal margin involvement by DCIS may be dealt with by re-excision or a tumour bed boost, according to risk factors. Severe lung or cardiac disease, scleroderma, other significant comorbidity or immobility that would contraindicate radiotherapy should be identified so that mastectomy can be considered instead of conservative surgery.

Data acquisition

■ Immobilisation

The position of the patient must remain identical for localisation on a CT scanner or simulator and during subsequent treatment. Most commonly the patient is treated supine using an immobilisation device which secures both arms above the head, as this lifts the breast superiorly, reducing cardiac doses, and also provides symmetry if contralateral breast irradiation is required later. A headrest, elbow and armrests, knee supports and a footboard provide stability. Care must be taken at data acquisition to adapt all the supporting devices to the individual patient's size and shape to maximise comfort, and so aid reproducibility for subsequent treatment. These recorded parameters, with a system of medial and lateral tattoos and orthogonal laser lights, ensure alignment of the patient and consistency of set-up (Fig. 22.2). Often an inclined plane is used with fixed angle positions. This brings the chest wall parallel to the treatment couch and may reduce the need for collimator angulation. The inclination is limited to a 10–15° angle for 70 cm, and 17.5–20° for larger 85 cm aperture CT scanners or simulator planning. Some centres treat the patient lying flat on the couch top, without an incline, with a similar immobilisation system but using collimator rotation.

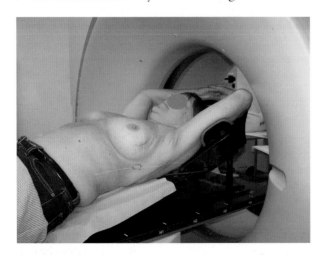

Figure 22.2 Large-bore CT scanner with patient immobilised on system using inclined plane, arms up, with reference points outlined with radio-opaque material and aligned with laser lights.

Patients with large or pendulous breasts treated supine require a breast support, either with a thermoplastic shell, or breast cup which can be used to bring the lateral and inferior part of the breast anteriorly away from the heart, lung and abdomen. It is important to avoid displacing the breast too far superiorly over the neck. Increased erythema due to loss of skin sparing by the shell may be offset by reduced severity of skin reaction in the inframammary fold. Alternatively, patients with pendulous breasts can be treated in the prone position, which reduces mean lung and cardiac doses and produces a more homogeneous dose distribution (Fig. 22.3). This may improve cosmesis, but risks under dosage at the medial and lateral borders of the PTV close to the chest wall, and should be avoided for primary tumours in these situations. This technique cannot be combined with lymph node irradiation but can be used to treat bilateral tumours.

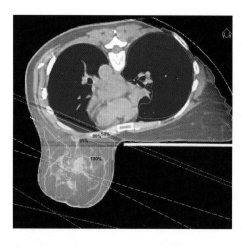

Figure 22.3 CT dose distribution to right breast with patient in the prone position (6 MV, [gantry 296° and 107°, weighting 100 per cent lat/105 per cent med. 15.6 [W] × 19 [L]). Courtesy of Greg Rattray, Royal Brisbane and Women's Hospital.

Whole breast

CT scanning

Where available, CT scanning has become standard for planning breast radiotherapy. After palpation, the breast CTV and surgical breast scar are marked with radio-opaque material before scanning. The upper and lower limits of the CT scan are chosen so that CT data are acquired superiorly from above the shoulder to include the neck and inferiorly to include all of the ipsilateral lung and 5 cm below breast tissue. CT data of the whole breast and critical structures such as lung and heart are needed for DVH calculations and to position lymph node beams. Slice thickness should be sufficient (usually 2–3 mm but dependent on agreed local CT protocols) to produce good quality images for target volume and OAR definition and to create DRRs for accurate portal image comparison. Three reference tattoos are placed on the central slice and in the medial and lateral positions on right and left sides so that measurements can be made to subsequent beam centres.

The volumetric CT data are exported to the treatment planning system (TPS) and a virtual simulation package can be used to define medial and lateral tangential beams to encompass the breast CTV. These can be adapted by viewing the posterior border of the CTV on all CT slices to ensure coverage of the tumour bed as delineated by titanium clips or gold seeds on CT. CLD should be less than 2 cm to avoid symptomatic pneumonitis. The heart, especially the left anterior descending artery, should be excluded. Where this is impossible, maximum heart distance (MHD) must be kept to less than 1 cm. CT also helps distinguish glandular from adipose tissue, especially at the posterolateral aspect of the breast. If the heart cannot be excluded completely from the target volume without compromising the tumour bed CTV, localised cardiac shielding can be introduced at the dose planning stage. The final virtual simulation is performed by a radiographer, usually with an oncologist, and diagrams, DRRs and virtual simulation rendered images are created before the dose plan is produced (Fig. 22.4). Alternatively, the breast CTV and PTV can be outlined on each CT image with full 3D delineation of the target volume. This is more time consuming but has advantages where more advanced or inoperable tumours are visualised or when inverse planned IMRT is used. The lung is contoured in its entirety for all 3D dose planning and DVHs.

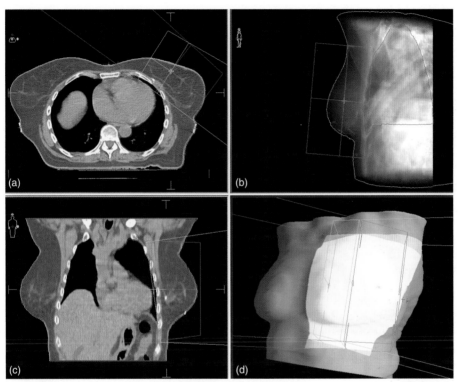

Figure 22.4 Virtual simulation of breast with clips in tumour bed showing (a) axial scan with adjustment of beam border anteriorly from skin markers to avoid heart, (b) sagittal, (c) coronal and (d) rendered image of tangential beams.

Target volume definition

■ CTV breast

For adjuvant radiotherapy after surgical excision of tumour there is no GTV and the whole breast is the CTV. The aim is to treat all the glandular breast tissue down to deep fascia, but not the underlying muscle, rib cage, overlying skin or excision scar. A CTV-PTV margin is added to account for respiration, variations in patient position, both intra- and inter-fractionally, breast swelling and set-up uncertainties. Each department should measure its systematic and random errors using a verification programme comparing simulator or DRR images with EPIs. Most departments record standard deviations for systematic errors of around

2–5 mm and an additional margin of 5 mm is reported as sufficient to account for respiratory motion. This gives a CTV-PTV margin of 1 cm for a standard breast target volume. When implanted clips are viewed in the tumour bed at CT, the proposed CTV and PTV margins may need to be repositioned to ensure adequate coverage of the tumour bed. During virtual simulation, the tangential beams can be redesigned to encompass the CT-derived CTV and PTV and to reduce the amount of lung and heart included in the treatment volume.

■ GTV breast

For inoperable tumours and following partial regression after primary systemic therapy where surgery is still not feasible, the gross tumour is present. This can be defined with the patient in the treatment position using palpation, CT or ultrasound to design boost volumes.

■ CTV-reconstructed breast or chest wall

The target volume is the skin flaps and scar and any subcutaneous tissues down to the deep fascia overlying muscles. In locally advanced breast cancer with skin infiltration, skin is included in the target volume. The extreme ends of the surgical scar may be excluded medially or laterally to reduce dose to underlying heart and lung to tolerance limits. It is important to know the site of the primary tumour within the breast at presentation and histological details of the surgical specimen when adjusting beams in this way at virtual simulation.

■ Simulator

Conventionally, a simulator has been used to localise the breast with the immobilisation system described above and the patient aligned with two laterals and a sagittal laser light. Field borders rather than target volumes are defined by palpating the entire breast and adding a 1.5 cm margin which includes penumbra. The superior border covers as much of the breast as possible and lies at about the level of the suprasternal notch medially, and just below the level of the abducted arm laterally to allow beam entry. The inferior border lies 1.5 cm below the breast, or more if the tumour bed is situated very inferiorly. The medial border is usually in the midline and the lateral border 1.5 cm from the lateral border of the breast. However, these borders should be modified, both to ensure good coverage of the tumour bed and also to reduce heart (MHD <1 cm) and lung doses (CLD <2 cm), even if in some patients this means compromising coverage of peripheral breast tissue sited away from the tumour bed (Fig. 22.5).

Using the simulator, an isocentric technique of medial and lateral tangential fields is constructed. The anterior border of the field in free air should be at least 1.5 cm from the skin surface to ensure a satisfactory dose distribution. The borders of the medial and lateral fields are then marked on the skin. Two reference tattoos are made at medial and lateral field centres over reproducible stable sites with a third one made on the contralateral side of the body to align with lasers to prevent rotation. An external contour of a transverse cross-section of the patient is taken in 2D through the centre of the fields. Where a simulator CT is available, three CT outlines may be taken at different levels for lung correction and superior–inferior dose compensation.

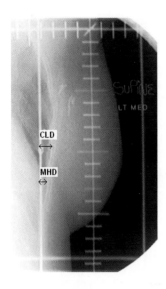

Figure 22.5 Simulator film of left medial tangential field with CLD, MHD and clips in the tumour bed.

Beam divergence into the lung at the posterior border of the field can be reduced by using either independent collimators to block the posterior half of the beam, or an appropriate gantry angle to align the opposing posterior field borders.

■ Breast tumour bed

Target volume

Using CT data, the tumour bed can be visualised in 3D by using clips placed in pairs (to identify migration) at surgery around the wall of the surgical cavity to mark its posterior, lateral, medial, superior and inferior borders (Fig. 22.6). The anterior border of the cavity should also be marked with clips if the surgical scar is not located anterior to the tumour bed. The CTV (tumour bed) then includes the tumour bed and any seroma and a 1.5 cm margin in all directions, editing 5 mm from the skin and lung surfaces. The CTV may be increased in any radial dimension if excision margins are less than 5 mm. The CTV-PTV margin is chosen as 5 mm for tumour bed boost irradiation, making a total 2 cm margin around the tumour bed. Both CT scanning and the use of clips have been shown to improve accuracy of localisation of the volume, depth of the tumour bed and choice of electron energy compared with clinical assessment alone.

Commonly, boost radiotherapy to the tumour bed is given with electron therapy. To aid treatment delivery, rendered images can be produced to show the position of the electron beam in relation to the surface scar.

When partial breast EBRT is given, a CTV-PTV margin of 1 cm is used for the boost with an additional 5 mm added for penumbra, and treatment is delivered using small ('mini') tangential beams.

■ Axillary and supraclavicular lymph nodes

CT scanning

A CT protocol is used similar to that described for whole breast. Axillary surgical clips may aid localisation, but uninvolved nodes are not seen on CT. CT scanning

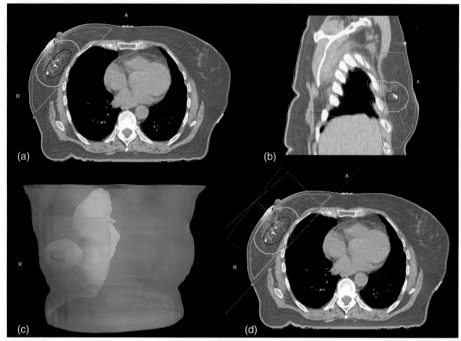

Figure 22.6 (a) Axial CT scan with clips in the tumour bed (dark blue), boost CTV (cyan) and whole breast PTV (red). (b) Sagittal view. (c) 3D image (lung in green). (d) Axial CT scan with beams for whole breast EBRT (6 MV, gantry 221° and 47°, 9.5[W] × 20[L]).

can be used to design a mono-isocentric technique for combined breast and lymph node irradiation where a single isocentre is set up at depth on the match line of the tangential and anterior nodal fields (Fig. 22.7).

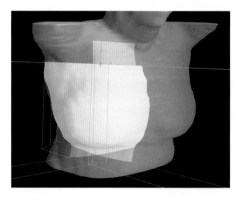

Figure 22.7 Single isocentric technique for EBRT to treat breast, axillary and supraclavicular lymph nodes shown with 3D rendered CT image.

Target volume

The lymphatic drainage to the axillary and supraclavicular nodes forms an irregular volume with its upper border lying anteriorly in the supraclavicular fossa, and extending more posteriorly at the lower border to include all groups of axillary nodes (see Fig. 22.1, p. 268).

CT studies have shown that axillary nodes lie at a mean depth of 3–5 cm and are anterior to the mid-axillary line. Supraclavicular nodes lie at a mean depth of 4 cm.

Internal mammary lymph nodes lie 2–4 cm lateral and deep to the midline in the first three intercostal spaces. CT scanning can be used to locate the internal mammary arteries which are closely applied to the nodes to help delineate the target volume. Studies show that level I axillary nodes may not be routinely included in the standard breast CTV and great care must be used to delineate these nodes marked with surgical clips in the axillary tail of the breast CTV when treatment is indicated.

The irregular target volume of the breast or chest wall and regional lymph nodes makes it technically difficult to deliver an equal and adequate dose to all areas and to spare the lungs, heart, brachial plexus and spinal cord.

■ Simulator

Immobilisation, patient positioning and alignment are as described for breast radiotherapy. An anterior field is used to include level II and III axillary and supraclavicular nodes in the target volume. The medial border is placed 1 cm lateral to the midline or at the midline with a 10° gantry angle away from the larynx and spinal cord. The lateral border lies at the outer edge of the head of the humerus. The superior border extends at least 3 cm above the medial end of the clavicle, but laterally leaves a 1–2 cm margin of skin clear superiorly to avoid excessive skin reaction. Using a mono-isocentric technique to treat breast and lymph nodes, the inferior border is on line with the superior border of the tangential fields through the match line with the isocentre at depth. Shielding of the acromioclavicular joint and humeral head is important to avoid fibrosis and maintain shoulder mobility. Shielding to the apex of the lung should be applied with care as it may shield level II and/or III nodes which may be part of the target volume. Where level III nodes have been removed, an anterior field to the supraclavicular fossa nodes only is used, with the lateral border altered to lie at the coracoid process (see Fig. 8.7, p. 104). Placement of surgical clips may mark the level II and III axillary lymph node areas and should be used to design the nodal field borders.

Dose solutions

■ Breast and reconstructed breast

For most patients, 6 MV (range 4–8 MV) photons are chosen as optimal. However, with increased breast volume and separation, higher energies (commonly 10 MV) may produce better homogeneity. Because of the increased skin sparing of higher energy beams, care should be taken to check that superficial cavity wall margins and scars of reconstructed breasts receive adequate dose.

■ Conformal or complex

Using virtual simulation, beams have been optimised and CT data are used to correct for lung density. A significant number of plans fail to achieve a homogeneous 3D dose distribution (–5 per cent, +7 per cent) when the 2D tangential technique is calculated in 3D (Fig. 22.8). Forward planned 3D dose compensation can be achieved using a variety of methods. A randomised clinical trial has shown that patients treated with IMRT and improved 3D dose homogeneity have significantly better breast cosmesis (Fig. 22.9). Inverse planned dose solutions aim at optimisation to a set of dose volume constraints and may improve homogeneity still further. This is particularly important for the reconstructed breast.

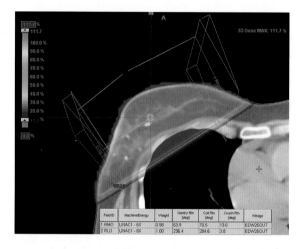

Figure 22.8 Dose colour wash for 3D conventional tangential plan through isocentre, off axis dose maximum 111.7 per cent.

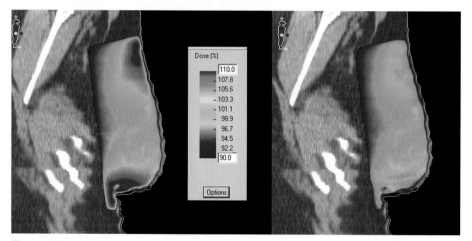

Figure 22.9 Sagittal dose distributions of conventional breast radiotherapy (left) compared with dose-compensated IMRT (right) with dose ranges.

The position of the left anterior descending coronary artery (LAD) can be seen on CT to lie within the target volume for many patients having left sided breast radiotherapy. Full dose to this segment of artery may be the cause of increased cardiac mortality from left breast radiotherapy reported in the literature. Modern planning techniques reduce dose to the heart and it is anticipated that in the future this will translate into decreased cardiac mortality and increase in overall survival with breast radiotherapy. With forward planned dose compensation, MLC leaves can be used to shield the heart (Fig. 22.10) and left anterior descending coronary artery for one or both beams, without shielding the tumour bed site which has been marked with clips and is clearly seen in 3D with CT planning. Doses to the contralateral breast may also be lower, reducing the risk of secondary malignancies.

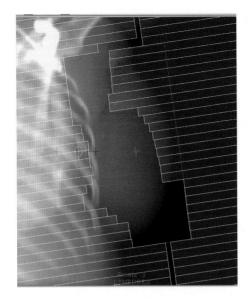

Figure 22.10 Sagittal DRR with segmented fields for dose-compensated IMRT with cardiac shielding. Clips seen in the tumour bed and axilla (within shielding).

Respiratory motion may affect the dosimetry of dynamic MLC/IMRT techniques and hence gated therapy or ABC devices to suspend respiration may have advantages in this situation.

■ Conventional

A 2D outline with centres of field borders marked is used to prepare a dose distribution with opposing medial and lateral tangential fields and wedges used as missing tissue compensators. The presence of lung tissue increases dose to the medial and lateral aspects of the breast and although the amount varies, it is important to incorporate lung corrections. An estimation of lung tissue is marked on the outline from the simulator film and a correction factor (range 0.2–0.3) is applied and a dose solution produced, aiming at a homogeneous dose distribution on a single slice of –5 per cent, +7 per cent (ICRU50). This does not give information at superior or inferior levels of the target volume where dose inhomogeneities of up to 10–15 per cent can occur, especially in large patients. Ideally these patients should have at least three outlines taken through the centre, superior and inferior levels of the volume using a simulator CT facility or camera based outlining system. Dose distributions can then be produced at multiple levels and tissue compensators used to improve homogeneity. Cardiac shielding using blocks or MLC leaves can be used in both beams, although care must be taken with inferior quadrant tumours where the tumour bed may overlie the heart. A risk versus benefit analysis then has to be made, and the MHD reduced to less than 1 cm by altering the posterior field border or partial shielding if possible.

■ Chest wall

Conventional planning uses opposing tangential fields but dosimetry is rarely optimal because of the thin target volume of the chest wall surrounded by air and lung. Skin doses cannot be calculated or measured accurately and the role of bolus to the skin remains controversial. Selective use of bolus in high risk disease after excision of local recurrence or extensive lymphovascular invasion may be considered, usually for the first half of the treatment so that it can be removed if the skin reaction is excessive.

Electron fields have the advantage of avoiding the lung and heart, but CT or ultrasound should be used to measure thickness of the chest wall which may vary throughout its volume, making choice of electron energy difficult. If the chest wall is very convex in shape, standoff may occur at the medial and lateral field edges with reduction of dose at these sites. Electrons to the chest wall may be combined with photons to the axilla and supraclavicular nodes, as used in the Danish Breast Cancer Group studies.

Where immediate breast reconstruction has taken place, conformal or IMRT techniques should be used to optimise homogeneity of dose and bolus should be avoided if possible to maintain good cosmesis. Higher energies (e.g.10 MV) should be avoided because of the risk of low skin dose due to increased skin sparing.

■ Tumour bed

Electron beams are commonly used for tumour bed boost irradiation. The target volume should be delineated and is usually 5–8 cm in diameter requiring an electron applicator of 7–10 cm to allow for lateral penumbra. The electron energy is chosen using CT, simulator-CT or ultrasound to measure depth of the target volume, which should be encompassed by the 90 per cent isodose (ICRU71).

Electrons of 4–15 MeV may be required but exit doses to the heart should be avoided. For larger volumes or where gross tumour is present, small tangential beams with CT planning or interstitial brachytherapy may be preferable.

■ Axillary and supraclavicular lymph node irradiation

A single anterior beam alone is recommended for adjuvant radiotherapy to supraclavicular and axillary lymph nodes. For advanced palpable axillary disease, extensive extranodal involvement or residual axillary disease, an additional posterior axillary beam may be needed to give adequate tumour dose. When the axillary separation exceeds 15 cm, the MPD to the axilla for a single anterior beam falls below 80 per cent for 6 MV photons. An adequate MPD to the axilla can be achieved using a posterior axillary beam every day and weighted according to the separation in the axilla (e.g. for 16–18 cm, 1:10 weighting of posterior: anterior beam applied doses). However, the dose to D_{max} increases for larger separations to 110 per cent and care must be taken to stay within the tolerance of the brachial plexus situated at 2–3 cm depth. A dose distribution must be produced for each patient when this technique is used. Placement of the posterior axillary beam is difficult and should be by CT and/or clinical palpation for macroscopic tumour and the use of surgical clips marking residual or extranodal extension of disease. 3D conformal treatment volumes may prove optimal.

■ Internal mammary node irradiation

Megavoltage anterior beams are no longer used to treat internal mammary lymph nodes because of the exit dose to the heart. For medial quadrant disease, the tumour bed may lie so close to the internal mammary nodes that it is impossible to treat both target volumes homogeneously. Treatment may then have to be given to the primary tumour alone, by moving the tangential beam further across the midline on to the contralateral side. Studies show that standard fields do not encompass internal mammary nodes consistently and often overtreat normal tissues. CT planning is therefore mandatory for internal mammary node irradiation. Electron or combined electron/photon beams can be used to treat internal mammary nodes as in the EORTC 22922/10925 trial protocol. Alternatively, wide tangential fields with cardiac and lung shielding may be used, as in the NCIC CTG MA20 trial. Care must be taken to ensure homogeneity of dose to the primary tumour bed and a match must be made of the internal mammary node fields to adjacent tangential breast fields.

■ Combined breast/chest wall and nodal irradiation

The inferior border of the nodal beam has to be matched to the superior border of the tangential beams, to avoid underdosage or overdosage. This can be achieved by half beam blocking the inferior border of the nodal beam and rotating the collimator and couch to eliminate the divergence of the superior border of the tangential beams at the match line.

A technique with a single isocentre at depth on the match plane uses asymmetric collimation, but restricts the maximum wedged length of the breast tangential beams. However, it is the preferred technique as it avoids couch and collimator rotations with risk of collisions and errors and reduces treatment time. When nodal irradiation is required for relapse after breast radiotherapy, a gap can be left between fields to allow for divergence of the superior tangential beams.

■ Bilateral breast irradiation

When bilateral breast irradiation is indicated, both arms are immobilised above the head as illustrated in Fig. 22.2 (p. 269). An appropriate gap of 1–1.5 cm should be left in the midline between the tangential fields to avoid overlap.

When radiotherapy is later required for a primary tumour in the contralateral breast, it is important to use the same immobilisation device as for the first tumour treatment to keep the patient position constant. Previous radiotherapy should be reconstructed to avoid overlap of treatment, especially in the midline and supraclavicular regions, and dose to the underlying spinal cord should be estimated.

■ Partial breast irradiation (within clinical trials)

Studies show that around 85 per cent of local recurrences after surgery and radiotherapy for operable breast cancer occur in the same quadrant as the primary tumour. A risk-adapted strategy for breast radiotherapy has led to the investigation of partial breast irradiation (PBI) treating the volume around the primary tumour site only. Techniques include external beam radiotherapy with or without concomitant IMRT boost, low and high dose brachytherapy, balloon catheter brachytherapy (Ammonite device), kV X-ray applicators (Intrabeam) and intraoperative electron therapy. Clinical trials are being carried out to test PBI using these different modalities. Protocols defining the tumour bed, CTV and PTV for PBI use radio-opaque markers and a careful quality assurance programme which will ensure accurate treatment delivery. PBI should at present be restricted to treating patients within the setting of a clinical trial.

Dose-fractionation

■ Breast, reconstructed breast and chest wall

40 Gy in 15 daily fractions of 2.67 Gy given in 3 weeks.
42.5 Gy in 16 daily fractions of 2.66 Gy given in 3½ weeks.
50 Gy in 25 daily fractions given in 5 weeks.

All these regimens have been tested in randomised trials with good results. The same fractionation regimens can be used treat to DCIS, as there is no evidence that it has a different radiosensitivity from invasive disease.

■ Breast boost irradiation

Tumour bed

16 Gy in 8 daily fractions given in 1½ weeks.
10 Gy in 5 daily fractions given in 1 week.

Doses are prescribed using electron therapy to D_{max} or using photons to the ICRU point at the centre of the target volume; 16 Gy in 8 daily fractions has been shown in the EORTC trial 22881 to reduce local failure by a factor of 2 compared with no boost. 10 Gy in 5 daily fractions may be used in patients with lower risk of local recurrence.

Incomplete excision or residual primary tumour

20–26 Gy in 10–13 daily fractions given in 2–2½ weeks.

Interstitial implantation may also be considered for tumour bed boost irradiation.

Lymph node irradiation

40 Gy in 15 daily fractions of 2.67 Gy given in 3 weeks.
50 Gy in 25 daily fractions given in 5 weeks.

Doses are prescribed at D_{max} (e.g. at 1.5 cm for 6 MV photons).

■ Palliative radiotherapy

Patients with breast cancer often live many years with metastatic disease, especially in bone. Care must be taken to check sites of previous irradiation and to match fields carefully to avoid overdosage and unwanted toxicity.

8 Gy single fraction for most bone metastases for relief of pain.
20 Gy in 5 daily fractions of 4 Gy given in 1 week may be used for sites such as cervical spine, meningeal disease, and nodal masses.
36 Gy in 6 fractions of 6 Gy once or twice weekly, given in 6 weeks for fungating primary tumours, especially in frail patients.

Treatment delivery and patient care

Treatment delivery will vary according to available technology. Where manual wedges, physical compensators or couch rotation are used, the overall time for each treatment fraction is longer. IMRT with wedged tangential beams and additional MLC shaped dose compensating segments has been shown to take very little longer to deliver than conventional tangential fields.

Patients are instructed to avoid abrasion of the irradiated skin when washing and to use simple soap. Aqueous cream is applied twice daily at least 2 h before or after treatment to keep the skin moisturised. One per cent hydrocortisone cream may be used to relieve the irritation of dry desquamation. If moist desquamation occurs, treatment is temporarily stopped and Atrauman gauze with a pad or hydrogel sheet or foam dressing applied until healing occurs. Tight fitting clothes should be avoided as much as possible to reduce friction and abrasion of the skin. Loose cotton garments are recommended. Gentle arm exercises started after surgery are continued.

Later side effects may include breast oedema, shrinkage, pain and tenderness, rib fracture, skin telangiectasia, symptomatic lung fibrosis, cardiac morbidity or late malignancy when radiotherapy is combined with chemotherapy. After nodal radiotherapy, there is a risk of arm lymphoedema, shoulder stiffness or nerve complications.

Verification

The immobilisation device, room laser lights, set-up instructions and rendered images are all used to ensure an identical patient position and accurate treatment delivery. Portal imaging should be undertaken using locally agreed evidence-based imaging protocols. This typically consists of imaging the first three daily fractions and then weekly checks, with images being compared with the CT-generated DRR or simulator films and a ± 5 mm tolerance accepted in the CLD/isocentre position. Consideration should be given to any change in soft tissue contour where forward planned IMRT is used to ensure the delivery of a homogeneous dose distribution. *In vivo* dosimetry using a diode or TLD measurement is carried out on day 1 in all patients to ensure delivery of the planned dose to each field/segment. To ensure true readings, consideration should be given to the positioning of the diode/TLD for the smaller dose compensation segments used in forward planned techniques. IGRT can be used to match the position of titanium clips in the tumour bed for pretreatment verification.

key trials

- EORTC 22922/10925: Breast ± internal mammary-medial SCF node irradiation for selected high risk group patients. http://astro2005.abstractsnet.com/handouts/000156_ASTRO_Meeting__September_2005.pdf (accessed 5 December 2008).
- EORTC 22881/10882: Boost versus No Boost tumour bed RT. See Antonini *et al.* below (www.ncbi.nlm.nih.gov/pubmed/17126434).
- IMPORT LOW and HIGH (Intensity Modulated and Partial Organ RadioTherapy). Whole v partial breast IMRT in two risk groups. www.icr.ac.uk/research/research_sections/clinical_trials/trials_by_disease/breast_cancer/index.shtml (accessed 5 December 2008).
- SECRAB: Sequencing of chemotherapy and radiotherapy in adjuvant breast cancer. See Bowden *et al.* below.
- START Trials A and B: Fractionation study of breast RT (see below).
- SUPREMO (Selective Use of Post Operative Radiotherapy after Mastectomy): mastectomy ± chest wall RT for intermediate risk patients. www.supremo-trial.com/ (accessed 5 December 2008).

Information sources

Adlard JW, Bundred NJ (2006) Radiotherapy for ductal carcinoma in situ. *Clin Oncol* **18**: 179–84.

Antonini N, Jones H, Horiot JC *et al.* (2007) Effect of age and radiation dose on local control after breast conserving treatment: EORTC trial 22881-10882. *Radiother Oncol* **82**: 265–71.

Bowden SJ, Fernando IN, Burton A (2006) Delaying radiotherapy for the delivery of adjuvant chemotherapy in the combined modality treatment of early breast cancer: is it disadvantageous and could combined treatment be the answer? *Clin Oncol* **18**: 247–56.

Dobbs HJ, Greener AJ, Driver D (2003) Geometric uncertainties in radiotherapy of breast cancer. In: *Geometric Uncertainties in Radiotherapy: Defining the Planning Target Volume.* BIR Report, BIR Publications Dept, London, UK.

Donovan E, Bleakley N, Denholm E *et al.* (2007) On behalf of the Breast Technology Group (UK) Randomised trial of standard 2D radiotherapy versus intensity modulated radiotherapy in patients prescribed breast radiotherapy. *Radiother Oncol* **82**: 254–64.

Early Breast Cancer Trialists' Collaborative Group (EBCTCG) (2005) Effects of radiotherapy and of differences in the extent of surgery for early breast cancer on local recurrence and 15 year survival: an overview of the randomised trials. *Lancet* **366**: 2087–106.

Goodman RL, Grann A, Saracco P *et al.* (2001) The relationship between radiation fields and regional lymph nodes in carcinoma of the breast. *Int J Radiat Oncol Biol Phys* **50**: 99–105.

Hurkmans CW, Borger JH, Pieters BR *et al.* (2001) Variability in target volume delineation on CT scans of the breast. *Int J Radiat Oncol Biol Phys* **50**: 1366–72.

Lievens Y, Poortmans P, Van den Bogaert W (2001) A glance on quality assurance in EORTC study 22922 evaluating techniques for internal mammary and supraclavicular lymph node chain irradiation in breast cancer. *Radiother Oncol* **60**: 257–65.

Overgaard M, Nielsen HM, Overgaard J (2007) Is the benefit of postmastectomy irradiation limited to patients with four or more positive nodes, as recommended in international consensus reports? A subgroup analysis of the DBCG 82 b and c randomised trials. *Radiother Oncol* **82**: 247–53.

Owen JR, Ashton A, Bliss JM *et al.* (2006) Effect of radiotherapy fraction size on tumour control in patients with early breast cancer after local excision: long term results of a randomised trial. *Lancet Oncol* **7**: 467–71.

Ragaz J, Olivotto IA, Spinelli JJ *et al.* (2005) Loco regional radiation therapy in patients with high risk breast cancer receiving adjuvant chemotherapy: 20 year results of the British Columbia randomised trial. *J Natl Cancer Inst* **97**: 116–26.

Recht A, Edge SB, Solin LJ *et al.* (2001) Post mastectomy radiotherapy: clinical practice guidelines of the American Society of Clinical Oncology. *J Clin Oncol* **19**: 1539–69.

Special Issue: Radiotherapy of breast cancer (2007). *Radiother Oncol* **82**: 243–357.

The START Trialists' Group (2008) The UK Standardisation of Breast Radiotherapy (START) Trial B of radiotherapy hypofractionation for treatment of early breast cancer: a randomised trial. *Lancet* **371**: 1098–107.

The START Trialists' Group (2008) The UK Standardisation of Breast Radiotherapy (START) Trial A of radiotherapy hypofractionation for treatment of early breast cancer: a randomised trial. *Lancet Oncol* **9**: 331–41.

Whelan T, Mackenzie R, Julian J *et al.* (2002) Randomised trial of breast irradiation schedules after lumpectomy for women with lymph node-negative breast cancer. *J Natl Cancer Inst* **94**: 1143–50.

Lymphomas

23

Indications for radiotherapy

■ Hodgkin lymphoma

Results of treatment for Hodgkin lymphoma have improved greatly over the past three decades, with 80 per cent of patients now achieving long-term cure. Favourable prognostic factors include stage I disease, lymphocyte predominant or nodular sclerosing histology, age <40, low erythrocyte sedimentation rate (ESR) and no B symptoms. Higher stage, age and ESR, involvement of the mediastinum, tumour bulk, increasing number of nodes involved, male gender, anaemia and extranodal sites are all indicators of a worse prognosis.

For patients with early and intermediate stage disease, original treatment regimens were based on primary extended field radiotherapy, often combined early or at relapse with extensive and prolonged chemotherapy. Using these strategies, 15–20-year survival figures were high but mortality from second malignancies and cardiac deaths exceeded that from the disease itself. However, results from more recent randomised trials have shown that the use of shorter periods of chemotherapy combined with involved field radiotherapy (IFRT) gives equivalent survival rates to that of extended field radiotherapy with reduction of late toxicity. Radiotherapy remains a key part of combined modality treatment to ensure locoregional control.

For early stage I and II disease, treatment with two to four cycles of chemotherapy, depending on prognostic factors, followed by local radiotherapy, gives 5-year survival rates of 90–95 per cent. Studies have shown that after chemotherapy alone, sites of relapse are predominantly in initially involved nodes. Current data using advanced imaging techniques suggest that involved lymph node radiotherapy (INRT) may be as effective as IFRT, and would further reduce doses to normal tissues such as the lung, heart and breast. Smaller target volumes and lower radiation doses are improving the therapeutic index for patients with early stage disease. Confirmation is awaited from trials as to whether radiotherapy can be omitted in patients who have a negative PET scan after short course chemotherapy.

For more advanced stages, intensive chemotherapy is the mainstay of treatment, combined with radiotherapy for selected patients who do not achieve complete remission. Relapsed Hodgkin lymphoma is treated with high dose chemotherapy and autologous stem-cell transplantation, when possible, with 50 per cent long-term survival rates. For other patients who relapse, combined chemotherapy and radiotherapy can produce worthwhile responses. Radiotherapy may also be used to palliate symptoms from lymph node or other tumour masses that are causing pain, obstruction or bleeding.

■ Non-Hodgkin lymphoma

Low grade follicular lymphoma presents as localised stage I or II disease in 20–30 per cent of cases. INRT alone gives 50–60 per cent 15-year survival rates and these results have not yet been improved by the addition of chemotherapy. Stage IE and IIE MALT lymphomas of the stomach, which are *Helicobacter pylori* negative or do not respond to antibiotic therapy, are treated with local radiotherapy, with very high local control and cure rates. Other MALT sites include thyroid, salivary glands, skin, breast, lung and orbit and, when presenting as stage IE or IIE disease, are treated with local radiotherapy, with 70–80 per cent 10-year survival rates.

Patients with stage III and IV low grade follicular lymphoma may be asymptomatic, so treatment with chemotherapy may be deferred until disease progression. Response rates with conventional chemotherapy are around 60 per cent but the disease is not curable, and more aggressive regimens with stem cell support are considered at relapse for fit patients. The monoclonal antibody rituximab, given in combination with chemotherapy or as maintenance after initial treatment, has improved response rates and progression-free survival.

Diffuse aggressive B or T cell lymphomas are treated with initial chemotherapy, combined if they are CD20 positive with monoclonal antibody therapy. This is followed in early stage disease by radiotherapy localised to initial bulky sites of involvement. Five-year survival rates for stage I and II disease are 80–90 per cent. Patients with adverse prognostic factors such as increasing stage, high lactate dehydrogenase, B symptoms and extensive or bulky disease are treated with more intensive and prolonged chemotherapy. Radiotherapy is used for those with residual nodal masses.

Extranodal lymphomas are usually diffuse large B cell lymphomas in type and occur at a wide variety of sites such as the CNS including extradural tissue, head and neck, breast, stomach, skin and bone. They are commonly treated with initial chemotherapy followed by localised radiotherapy to the initial and/or bulky sites of disease. When treating CNS lymphoma, care must be taken with whole brain irradiation after chemotherapy and high-dose methotrexate. Radiotherapy may then be omitted in older patients (>60) because of the increased risk of neurological toxicity, particularly dementia.

Splenic irradiation is rarely used now as involvement of the spleen usually represents systemic disease, best treated by chemotherapy. Where hypersplenism due to myelofibrosis cannot be treated by surgical splenectomy, radiotherapy may be given.

Radiotherapy is also used sometimes in the following situations:

- prophylactic cranial irradiation in lymphoblastic lymphoma and acute lymphocytic leukaemia (Chapter 18)
- total body irradiation (TBI) before allogeneic and selected autologous transplants (Chapter 38)
- post-transplant salvage for residual PET visualised disease
- immune modulation with single fraction (2 Gy) for reduced intensity conditioning
- irradiation for CSF/CNS involvement (Chapter 18)
- prophylactic testicular irradiation in testicular lymphoma (Chapter 38).

Skin lymphomas and their management are discussed in Chapter 7. Palliative local radiotherapy is useful for relieving symptoms in patients with large uncontrolled nodal masses or in patients who are unfit for chemotherapy.

Clinical and radiological anatomy

The WHO histological classification separates nodular lymphocyte predominant Hodgkin lymphoma from other classical Rye subtypes and divides non-Hodgkin lymphoma into B and T/NK cell types.

Lymphomas can affect any lymph node site in the body as well as extranodal sites such as Waldeyer's ring, thyroid, gastrointestinal tract, CNS, testes, breast, bone and skin. The staging system used for lymphomas is the Ann Arbor classification, with the Cotswolds' modification for Hodgkin lymphoma. This is based on number of anatomical sites of involved lymph nodes above or below the diaphragm, splenic or extranodal disease, B symptoms and the addition of bulky disease for Hodgkin lymphoma in the Cotswolds' modification. Spread occurs to contiguous lymph nodes and by the bloodstream to spleen, liver, lungs, bone marrow or skin, with extranodal sites being much more common with non-Hodgkin lymphoma. Sites such as paranasal sinuses, testicular and vitreous lymphomas have a predilection for CNS spread.

Assessment of primary disease

Clinical examination should include all nodal sites with measurement of any palpable involved lymph nodes by the radiation oncologist at diagnosis. This is especially important for INRT and should be done before any chemotherapy is given. Excision biopsy of an entire lymph node is required for accurate histological diagnosis with fresh and fixed material. Image guided needle core biopsies are used for inaccessible lymphadenopathy to avoid mediastinoscopy and laparotomy whenever possible. Chest X-ray identifies gross mediastinal lymphadenopathy. CT scan of the chest, abdomen, pelvis and neck is needed for full staging of the primary site as well as to assess other lymph node sites and organ spread. MRI is indicated for CNS tumours and extradural lymphomas, as well as for primary lymphoma of bone. Radioisotope bone scans or PET scans are performed for primary lymphoma of bone to exclude other bone lesions, as multifocal disease is common. Bone marrow aspiration and trephine is performed in all patients with non-Hodgkin lymphoma and selected patients with Hodgkin lymphoma.

[^{18}F]2-fluoro-2-deoxy-D-glucose (FDG) PET-CT scanning has a sensitivity of greater than 90 per cent for the detection of most types of non-Hodgkin lymphoma, except MALT and small lymphocytic lymphomas where sensitivity is less. PET-CT has the highest rate of disease detection of any imaging modality for Hodgkin lymphoma and should be performed whenever possible in the radiotherapy treatment position so that scans can be used for subsequent image registration for planning radiotherapy. PET scanning changes initial staging in 10–20 per cent of patients with Hodgkin lymphoma, and if it is repeated after two or three cycles of chemotherapy, response can be used to predict overall long-term

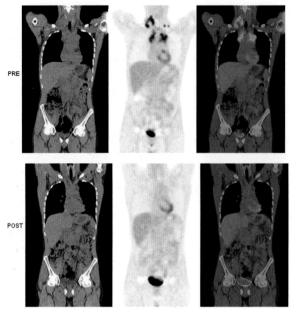

PRE

POST

Figure 23.1 PET scan of patient with stage IIA (bilateral lower neck and mediastinum) Hodgkin lymphoma pre- and post-chemotherapy.

survival (Fig. 23.1). PET is more sensitive at detecting residual disease than CT, which cannot differentiate post-treatment fibrotic mediastinal masses from active disease. However, it should be used in combination with CT for target volume delineation as PET – avid areas have been shown to represent only 25 per cent of the total tumour mass seen on CT.

Data acquisition

To minimise toxicity to normal organs, and optimise dose distribution for the target volume, 3D CT planning is used. Patients are scanned lying supine with appropriate immobilisation devices for the anatomical site to be treated, with a system of skin tattoos. For axillary radiotherapy, the arm is abducted and supported using an arm pole or other restraint. For cervical nodal irradiation, a thermoplastic or vacuum shell is used with reference marks on the shell for alignment with lasers.

As lymphomas occur at a wide variety of anatomical sites, general principles should be applied and decisions made about the proposed treatment technique before CT scanning to ensure that the most appropriate CT protocol is used. If palpable masses are present, these are marked with radio-opaque material before scanning with the patient in the treatment position. The scan should include the whole volume of critical organs such as lung, liver, and kidneys for DVH assessment. CT scans of 3 mm slice thickness are taken using intravenous contrast to aid delineation of lymph nodes adjacent to vascular structures.

PET-CT and CT scans taken in the treatment position before chemotherapy are co-registered with the post-chemotherapy CT planning scans for target volume delineation. In addition, diagrams showing the initial lymph node measurements at diagnosis are used.

Target volume definition

Traditionally, wide or extended field radiotherapy treatments such as 'Mantle' and 'Inverted Y' were used as primary treatment for lymphomas with good cure rates but late toxicity, particularly to the heart, lungs and breasts. With treatments now combining chemotherapy and adjuvant radiotherapy, data have accumulated to support the use of local radiotherapy instead of extended fields, to reduce toxicity by sparing normal tissues.

There are three possible approaches to using smaller volume treatments. Since lymphatic spread involves nodes adjacent to the primary site of disease first, locoregional treatment that includes elective adjuvant irradiation of the first node stations may be given (IFRT). The CTV includes the GTV, which is the primary site, and adjacent nodes as CTV (a situation analogous to treatment of uninvolved nodes in head and neck cancer). Alternatively, only the initial macroscopic volume of disease (GTV), whether in lymph node (involved nodal INRT), or an organ (sometimes called involved site ISRT) is treated with a GTV-CTV margin. Finally, the residual GTV following chemotherapy, defined by PET-CT, could be the basis of the target volume. In published reports the target volumes used may combine aspects of these different conceptual approaches.

■ IFRT

When primary radiotherapy without chemotherapy is given (e.g. stage I follicular non-Hodgkin lymphoma or nodular lymphocyte predominant Hodgkin lymphoma), IFRT is used to include the uninvolved first node station in the CTV as well as the macroscopically involved GTV (Fig. 23.2).

The CTV is designed using the initial volume of involved lymph nodes, i.e. the initial GTV as shown on staging CT, MRI and FDG-PET-CT scans. These scans need to be taken in the radiotherapy treatment position, whenever possible, for accurate co-registration with subsequent CT planning scans which are taken after chemotherapy. When primary radiotherapy is given, the GTV is present both clinically and on imaging. After chemotherapy there may be a complete response (PET and CT negative) with no GTV, or a partial response with a residual GTV.

The original GTV is outlined on the post-chemotherapy CT planning scan using the co-registered initial CT and PET scans. The patient's anatomy will have altered with response to chemotherapy, and the principle is to cover the site of original disease, but to reduce toxicity by excluding wherever possible normal tissues that were displaced, but not involved by tumour. Anatomical planes act as boundaries and the volume should not extend into adjacent bone, air or viscera.

For both IFRT and INRT of the mediastinum, the pre-chemotherapy volume is used for the superior–inferior extension and the post-chemotherapy volume for the axial to reduce dose to blood vessels, heart, coronary arteries and lung which may have returned to their normal position (Fig. 23.3). Where there was definite tumour infiltration into adjacent tissues at diagnosis, the whole volume should still be included.

The CTV for IFRT includes the clinically and radiologically involved lymph nodes as imaged at presentation (GTV) with the adjacent lymphatics and uninvolved first node station. CT outlining of lymph nodes uses the Ann Arbor staging system and is aided by atlases such as those published by Gregoire for the head and neck and Taylor for pelvic nodes.

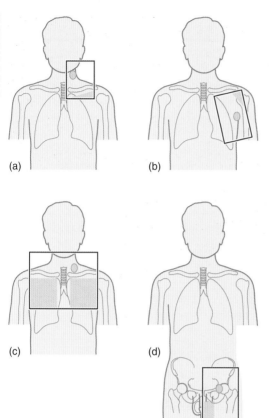

Figure 23.2 Diagrams of opposing fields for IFRT.
(a) Unilateral cervical field for stage IA high cervical node with shielding to lung apex. (b) Axillary field with shielding of humeral head.
(c) Neck and mediastinum with lung shielding. (d) Groin with shielding of testes and small bowel.

A CTV-PTV margin is added to allow for organ motion which will vary for different sites, for example it should be 5 mm for mediastinal nodes. A further 5–10 mm margin is used for daily variations in set-up, the exact value determined according to individual departmental protocols, making a total CTV to PTV margin of 10–15 mm.

■ INRT or ISRT

This target volume is based on initial macroscopic disease pre-chemotherapy (GTV), rather than on lymph node region, and is defined using initial CT and PET scans co-registered with subsequent CT planning scans. If the initially involved nodes are no longer visible after a complete response, the CTV is the initial site of involvement.

For neck, mediastinum and para-aortic nodes, a GTV-CTV margin of 20 mm in the cranio-caudal and 10 mm in other dimensions is used. For hilar, SCF and common iliac nodes, a GTV-CTV margin of 10 mm in the anteroposterior (AP) and 20 mm in other directions is used. For axillary, external and internal iliac, inguinal and femoral nodes, a GTV-CTV margin of 20 mm is used in all directions. These variable margins are based on observation and designed to exclude initially displaced normal structures which have returned to their usual position.

A CTV-PTV margin of 5–10 mm in 3D is added according to anatomical site and departmental set-up error measurements.

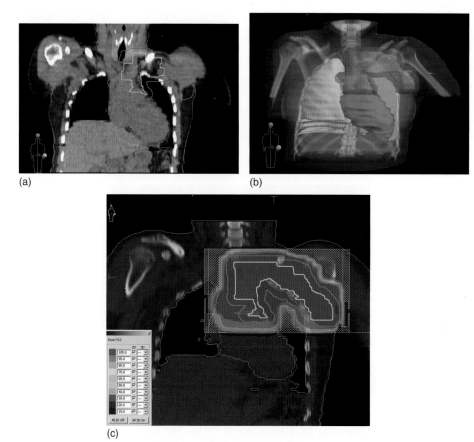

(a)
(b)

Dose (%):

	2D	3D
105.9		
95.0		
85.0		
75.0		
65.0		
50.0		
40.0		
30.0		
20.0		
10.0		

All 2D Off | All 3D On

(c)

Figure 23.3 IFRT for a patient with stage IIA Hodgkin lymphoma (in complete remission after chemotherapy) showing radiotherapy to the mediastinum, left SCF and left axilla. (a) Coronal CT scan with target volumes. (b) 3D image. (c) Dose distribution using anterior and posterior beams with MLC. Lungs green; heart yellow; spinal cord light yellow; (b) and (c) are at different slice level to (a).

INRT may be used for adjuvant radiotherapy after chemotherapy (Fig. 23.4). If only a partial remission is obtained, a residual GTV will be defined on post-chemotherapy CT scans. This is used to create a boost CTV, which is the GTV plus a 10–15 mm margin used to deliver extra irradiation to residual disease.

■ Extranodal sites

When primary radiotherapy is given for stage IE non-Hodgkin lymphoma, the GTV is usually the whole of the involved organ such as stomach, orbit or breast with an appropriate margin for microscopic disease to create the CTV. For a solid organ, the volume is designed using the original GTV with a GTV-CTV margin of 15 mm in the cranio-caudal dimension. In the AP and lateral dimensions the residual, not initial, GTV are included with a 15 mm 3D margin to minimise normal tissue doses. CTV-PTV margins vary according to the mobility of the organ, e.g. for stomach a 20 mm cranio-caudal margin may be used to allow for respiration (Fig. 23.5).

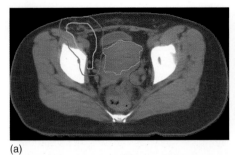
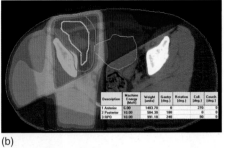

(a)   (b)

Figure 23.4 INRT for patient with stage IA follicular non-Hodgkin lymphoma showing treatment to unilateral right inguinal lymph nodes, showing (a) axial CT scan with target volume and (b) conformal dose plan. Uterus yellow, left; adnexa green.

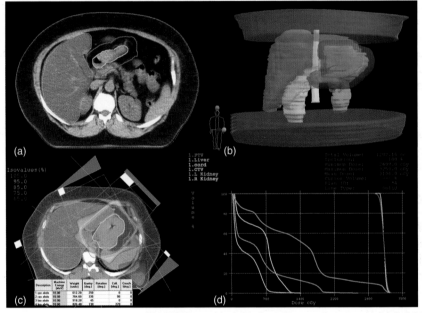

Figure 23.5 Patient with stage IE MALT non-Hodgkin lymphoma of stomach. (a) Axial CT scan showing target volume. (b) 3D image. (c) Conformal plan. (d) DVH with liver (yellow), kidneys (green) and spinal cord (light yellow).

There is no evidence yet to change the established practice of treating the whole of Waldeyer's ring, the parotid gland or whole brain after chemotherapy and large margins may still be allowed (30 mm cranio-caudal) for bone lymphoma. For splenic irradiation, CT scanning is used to localise the target volume (whole spleen) and organs at risk which include the left kidney and stomach although doses are below tolerance. No GTV-PTV margin is needed as even partial organ radiotherapy is effective (Fig. 23.6).

■ Palliative radiotherapy

Gross disease (GTV) is delineated with as small a margin as possible to minimise side effects.

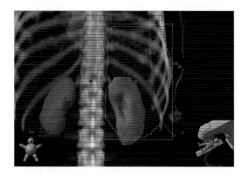

Figure 23.6 DRR showing anterior BEV with spleen outlined for splenic radiotherapy showing relations to left (green) and right (magenta) kidney.

Very occasionally extended field treatments may be used for palliation. Mantle fields include all lymph node areas above the diaphragm and the inverted Y, infra-diaphragmatic nodes. CT scans are performed with the patient immobilised in the treatment position and palpable nodes marked with radio-opaque material. Involved nodes may be contoured on each slice or virtual simulation used to design beams to encompass disease. Shielding to the oral cavity, lungs, humeral heads, spinal cord, breast, kidneys, bladder and bowel is obtained by appropriate MLC configurations. A simple arrangement of anterior and posterior beams is used.

■ OAR

Normal organs such as lungs, heart, spinal cord, major blood vessels and breasts should be outlined and PRVs created. DVH for critical organs are obtained and tolerance restrictions applied to specific organs.

Dose solutions

Using 3D CT planning, the most appropriate conformal multi-beam plan can be prepared. Less often anterior and posterior beams are used, sometimes unequally weighted and shaped using MLC in 3D to spare normal tissues. Inhomogeneity corrections are made to account for lung tissue in the mediastinum. IMRT may have benefit at sites near the spinal cord but care must be taken to avoid increasing dose to lungs, heart and breasts.

Dose-fractionation

■ Hodgkin lymphoma

Early stage, after complete response to chemotherapy
20 Gy in 10 daily fractions given in 2 weeks.

Advanced stage, with residual disease after chemotherapy
30 Gy in 15 daily fractions given in 3 weeks, with additional 6 Gy in 3 fractions depending on bulk of disease.

Palliative treatment
20 Gy in 5 daily fractions given in 1 week.
30 Gy in 10 daily fractions given in 2 weeks.

Extended field 30 Gy in 15 daily fractions given in 3 weeks.
8 Gy given in a single fraction.

■ Non-Hodgkin lymphoma

Primary radiotherapy for stage I, IE, II, IIE low grade disease

24–30 Gy in 12–15 daily fractions given in 2½–3 weeks
(or 4 Gy in 2 daily fractions).

Radiotherapy after chemotherapy for all other histologies

30 Gy in 15 daily fractions given in 3 weeks.

Palliative treatment

20 Gy in 5 daily fractions given in 1 week.
30 Gy in 10 daily fractions given in 2 weeks.
4 Gy in 2 daily fractions.

Splenic irradiation

10–12 Gy in fractions of 0.5–1.5 Gy given up to three times/week.

If blood counts are initially very low, treatment is started cautiously with low doses given once a week with full blood count check before each treatment.

Treatment delivery and patient care

Laser lights, skin markers and immobilisation devices are used exactly as for CT planning. Portal imaging or EPIs are used to verify the treatment and compare with DRRs. *In vivo* dosimetry is performed at the first treatment. Where IGRT is available, this may be useful to optimise daily localisation of the target volume.

Acute side effects depend on the particular anatomical site being treated. Skin reactions are usually mild, unless a shell is used with loss of skin sparing. Brisker reactions are seen in the axilla, groin and perineum. Aqueous or 1 per cent hydrocortisone cream can be used. Temporary occipital epilation and dry mouth may occur with upper cervical treatments, and sore throat, hoarseness and dysphagia with lower cervical radiotherapy. Symptomatic remedies are given such as artificial saliva and soluble analgesia. Groin and pelvic nodal treatment can cause acute cystitis and diarrhoea. Bone marrow suppression may occur especially with large pelvic fields after chemotherapy and blood counts are monitored for neutropenia and thrombocytopenia. Cough due to mild pneumonitis may occur. Lhermitte's syndrome is rarely seen now that spinal cord shielding is used with conformal and IMRT. Loss of fertility and early menopause may occur with pelvic treatment.

Extended mantle radiotherapy was used to irradiate axillae electively and included much of the lateral part of the breasts. This led to an increased incidence of second malignancies, particularly breast cancer in patients treated in young adulthood, and lung cancer in smokers. Ten-year results have confirmed that the use of involved field radiotherapy alone after chemotherapy with reduced dose to breast, heart and lungs leads to fewer second malignancies. Chemotherapy is associated with an increased incidence of leukaemia.

EORTC H9-F. Chemotherapy + IFRT 36 Gy v 20 Gy or no radiotherapy for favourable HL. Available at http://groups.eortc.be/lymphoma – see H9 trial (accessed 10 December 2008).

HD 8 (GHSG). Comparison of IFRT with extended field RT after chemotherapy for early stage Hodgkin lymphoma and HD 10 & 11 (GHSG). Comparison of two versus four courses of ABVD + IFRT 20 Gy v 30 Gy.

Klimm B, Diehl V, Pfistner B et al. (2005) Current treatment strategies of the German Hodgkin Study Group (GHSG). Eur J Haematol 75(S66): 125–34.

key trials

Information sources

Aleman BM, Raemaekers JM, Tirelli U et al. (2003) Involved-field radiotherapy for advanced Hodgkin's lymphoma. N Engl J Med 348: 2396–406.

Bonnadonna G, Bonfante V, Viviani S et al. (2004) ABVD plus subtotal nodal versus involved-field radiotherapy in early-stage Hodgkin's disease: long term results. J Clin Oncol 22: 2835–41.

Dobbs HJ, Barrett A, Rostom AY et al. (1981) Total-body irradiation in advanced non-Hodgkin's lymphoma. Br J Radiol 54: 878–81.

Eich H, Mueller R, Engert A et al. (2005) Comparison of 30 Gy versus 20 Gy involved field radiotherapy after two versus four cycles ABVD in early stage Hodgkin's lymphoma: interim analysis of the German Hodgkin's Study Group Trial HD10. Int J Radiat Oncol Biol Phys 6: S1–2.

Engert A, Schiller P, Josting A et al. (2003) Involved-field radiotherapy is equally effective and less toxic compared with extended-field radiotherapy after four cycles of chemotherapy in patients with early stage unfavourable Hodgkin's lymphoma. Results of the HD 8 trial of the German Hodgkin's Lymphoma Study Group. J Clin Oncol 21: 3601–8.

Girinsky T, van der Maazen R, Specht L et al. (2006) Involved-node radiotherapy (INRT) in patients with early Hodgkin's lymphoma: concepts and guidelines. Radiother Oncol 79: 270–7.

Girinsky T, Ghalibagian M, Bonniaud G et al. (2007) Is FDG-PET scan in patients with early stage Hodgkin lymphoma of any value in the implementation of the involved-node radiotherapy concept and dose painting? Radiother Oncol 85: 178–86.

Kaplan HS, Rosenberg SA (1966) The treatment of Hodgkin's disease. Med Clin North Am 50: 1591–610.

Koontz B, Kirkpatrick J, Clough R et al. (2006) Combined modality therapy versus radiotherapy alone for treatment of early-stage Hodgkin's disease: cure versus complications. J Clin Oncol 24: 605–11.

Lee YK, Cook G, Flower MA et al. (2004) Addition of 18F-FDG PET scans to radiotherapy planning of thoracic lymphoma. Radiother Oncol 73: 277–83.

National Institute for Health and Clinical Excellence (2008) Rituximab for the Treatment of Relapsed or Refractory Stage III or IV Follicular Non-Hodgkin's Lymphoma. Technical appraisal no 137. NICE, London.

Sawyer EJ, Timothy AR (1997) Low dose palliative radiotherapy in low grade non-Hodgkin's lymphoma. Radiother Oncol 42: 49–51.

Shahidi M, Kamangari N, Ashley S et al. (2006) Site of relapse after chemotherapy alone in Stage I and II Hodgkin's disease. Radiother Oncol 78: 1–5.

Sutcliffe SB, Gospodarowicz MK, Bush RS et al. (1985) Role of radiation therapy in localised non-Hodgkin's lymphoma. Radiother Oncol 4: 211–23.

Yahalom J, Mauch P (2002) The involved field is back: issues in delineating the radiation field in Hodgkin's disease. Ann Oncol 13: 79–83.

Yahalom J (2006) Don't throw out the baby with the bathwater: on optimizing cure and reducing toxicity in Hodgkin's lymphoma. J Clin Oncol 24: 544–8.

24 Oesophagus and stomach

Indications for radiotherapy

The oesophagus is arbitrarily divided into the cervical portion (from the lower border of the cricoid cartilage to the thoracic inlet or suprasternal notch) and the intrathoracic portion. The latter can further be divided into upper, middle and lower thirds. Most oesophageal tumours are SCCs.

The term oesophago-gastric junction (OGJ) cancer usually includes adenocarcinomas of the lower oesophagus and gastric cardia as well as the true junction between the two. OGJ cancer is increasing in incidence in the Western world. Most stomach cancers are adenocarcinomas.

The stage and location of the tumour are more important than histology in guiding therapeutic decision making. The presence and number of involved lymph nodes is the most important prognostic factor. In oesophageal cancer survival falls from 70 per cent to 25 per cent when nodes are involved.

■ Oesophagus

Surgery is the principal curative therapy but only 40 per cent of patients survive for 2 years. Preoperative radiation does not improve cure rates but a meta-analysis has shown that preoperative chemoradiation leads to a survival benefit of 13 per cent at 2 years. However, individual phase III studies have often failed to show this benefit and there is concern about perioperative morbidity and mortality. Moreover, preoperative chemotherapy alone has shown a survival benefit in some studies. The role of preoperative chemoradiation therefore remains unclear.

There is no good evidence to support adjuvant radiotherapy for any one group of patients, but it should be considered in selected patients where the risk of local recurrence is particularly high and exceeds that of distant metastases, e.g. with an involved circumferential resection margin in node negative patients.

Non-surgical curative treatment has usually been used when patients are medically inoperable or decline surgery or with T3N1 or T4 disease where surgical cure is felt unlikely. Concomitant radiochemotherapy with cisplatin and 5-fluorouracil (5FU)-based chemotherapy improves survival compared to radiation alone. Most regimens also include two cycles of chemotherapy either before or after the radiochemotherapy. The 2-year survival with combined chemotherapy and radiotherapy is very similar to that of surgery but there have been no large trials comparing the two approaches. If the patient has small (<5 cm length) localised disease but is not able to tolerate surgery or radiochemotherapy, radiation alone is used as potentially curative therapy.

Resection of a cervical oesophageal cancer would require a laryngo-oesophagectomy so radiochemotherapy is the treatment of choice.

Many patients with oesophageal cancer are elderly, of poor PS or have metastases at presentation. Radiotherapy is useful to palliate dysphagia or pain but rarely relieves complete dysphagia. Intraluminal brachytherapy is also used in palliation.

■ Stomach

Surgery is the treatment of choice for localised tumours. The extent of surgery is important. A D2 resection (extensive lymphadenectomy including nodes along the branches of the coeliac axis) produces better local control than a D1 resection (lymphadenectomy of perigastric nodes) though with an increase in postoperative complications and no clear survival benefit. Many patients have a local recurrence after surgery. A large RCT has shown adjuvant radiochemotherapy improves 3-year survival from 41 per cent to 50 per cent but only 10 per cent of patients in the trial had a D2 resection so adjuvant treatment may be compensating for poor surgery. Combined pre- and postoperative chemotherapy has also been shown to improve survival compared with surgery alone and the extra benefit of conformal postoperative radiotherapy when added to chemotherapy is not known. Radiotherapy can be used to palliate obstructive symptoms or persistent bleeding.

Sequencing of multimodality therapy

The optimal combination of surgery, radiotherapy and chemotherapy for potentially curable oesophageal cancer is not clear. Where preoperative chemo-radiation is used there should be a 6-week gap before surgery.

Clinical and radiological anatomy

Oesophageal cancers can invade longitudinally along the oesophageal wall as ulcers best seen at endoscopy. The lack of a serosal barrier means tumours can spread radially to invade adjacent local structures such as the tracheobronchial tree, pleura or recurrent laryngeal nerves.

Skip metastases – intramural tumour deposits distant from the primary – are formed by extravasation from the network of submucosal lymphatics. They can occur as much as 5–6 cm from the primary tumour and are found in up to a third of patients. The lymphatic system enables longitudinal flow of lymph both proximally and distally before it drains into adjacent nodes deep to the muscularis layer.

The submucosal lymphatics also account for the high incidence of involved lymph nodes and allow spread to distant nodes relatively early in the disease. The cervical oesophagus drains first to the deep cervical nodes medial to the internal jugular vein and then to those lateral to the vein in the supraclavicular fossa. The thoracic oesophagus drains first to the para-oesophageal nodes and then to other nodes in the mediastinum (see Fig. 20.2, p. 246). More inferior tumours spread to the para-cardial nodes around the superior branch of the left gastric artery, the left gastric nodes and the lesser curvature nodes before spreading to the coeliac axis. However, surgical series show 28 per cent of upper third tumours have involved gastric nodes and 33 per cent of lower third tumours have already spread to the superior mediastinum. The risk of nodal spread also increases with T stage.

The stomach is divided arbitrarily into the fundus (cardia), body and pylorus (antrum). As in the oesophagus there are extensive submucosal lymphatics that facilitate intramural spread of tumour and make it difficult to predict the location of involved nodes. Lymphatic drainage is initially to the perigastric nodes on the greater and lesser curvatures and then to the nodes along the branches of the coeliac axis (left gastric, hepatic, splenic and coeliac) (Fig. 24.1). Proximal tumours can also spread to the para-oesophageal nodes.

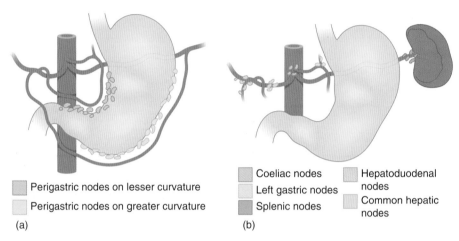

(a)

■ Perigastric nodes on lesser curvature
■ Perigastric nodes on greater curvature

(b)

■ Coeliac nodes
□ Left gastric nodes
■ Splenic nodes
■ Hepatoduodenal nodes
□ Common hepatic nodes

Figure 24.1 Lymphatic drainage of the stomach. (a) Perigastric nodes. (b) Stomach removed to show nodes along the branches of the coeliac axis.

Assessment of primary disease

■ Oesophagus

Most tumours are diagnosed at endoscopy and the superior and inferior extent is usually documented as the distance from the incisor teeth. Assuming an incisor to carina distance of 25 cm may help to register endoscopic information with the planning CT but this distance is more variable than previously thought. All patients should have contrast-enhanced CT scan of the neck, thorax and abdomen to assess the primary tumour and to look for enlarged nodes. Axial CT slices enable radial spread to be assessed. Longitudinal extent can also be estimated with CT, particularly when coronal and sagittal reconstructions are performed. Endoscopic ultrasound (EUS) is the most accurate way to assess superior and inferior extent of the primary tumour and can detect intramural skip metastases. The EUS information should be described with reference to a point (e.g. carina) that can be seen on the planning CT scan so that the position of the tumour can be accurately defined.

A bronchoscopy or vocal cord assessment should be performed if invasion of the tracheobronchial tree or recurrent laryngeal nerves is suspected.

Curative treatment volumes should ideally cover all lymph node sites at significant risk of harbouring microscopic metastases and would necessarily be very large. However, much of the evidence for lymphatic spread comes from relatively old surgical series. Modern staging with EUS, which has high sensitivity, and with PET-CT, which has high specificity, enables high risk nodes to be identified more accurately. A combination of CT, EUS and PET-CT will perhaps produce the most accurate nodal staging.

■ Stomach

The surgeon, oncologist and pathologist should meet to discuss the most likely sites of recurrence if adjuvant radiotherapy is to be considered, in view of its complexity.

Data acquisition

■ Simulator

For palliation, treatment volumes can be defined in the simulator. The patient lies supine with arms by their sides as lateral or oblique beams are not used. The GTV is defined from endoscopic and CT information. Barium can be used to determine the superior extent of the tumour on fluoroscopy. No CTV is defined. The PTV is the GTV with a 2 cm superoinferior margin and a 1 cm axial margin. In effect, the beam edges are defined as 2–3 cm proximal and distal to the GTV with a 2 cm lateral margin.

A similar technique is used for palliative radiotherapy for stomach cancer with barium and CT information used to define the position of the tumour.

■ Immobilisation

Patients undergoing conformal radiotherapy are planned and treated lying supine with arms above the head, ideally immobilised with a vacuum-formed polystyrene bag. For cervical oesophagus tumours, a thermoplastic or Perspex shell should be created in the same way as for hypopharyngeal tumours.

■ CT scanning

CT slices 3–5 mm thick are obtained from the hyoid bone to the inferior border of the kidneys with intravenous contrast if possible. For adjuvant stomach radiation the volume scanned should extend from the carina to the iliac crests.

Target volume definition

■ Oesophagus

First, the superior and inferior extent of the GTV is defined by the bulk of disease seen on the diagnostic and planning CT scans and by the information from EUS and endoscopy. If these two modalities produce discordant results, the GTV should encompass the greatest apparent extent of tumour superiorly and inferiorly from all investigations. The axial extent of the GTV is defined using CT information although EUS may help to indicate enlarged nodes that need to be included. If the GTV is more than 10 cm long, a palliative approach should be strongly considered.

A CTV is then produced by expanding the GTV by 2 cm longitudinally and 1 cm axially. This is edited in the axial plane to take account of possible routes of spread (e.g. edited off the spinal column and aorta). The superior and inferior slices are edited to ensure they reflect possible spread along the axis of the oesophagus.

The para-oesophageal nodes in the superior mediastinum are posterior to the trachea and to the left and right of the oesophagus, and more inferiorly they include nodes adjacent to the thoracic duct and aorta. In practice they will be included in the CTV as defined above.

There is no consensus about the inclusion of clinically negative nodes in the CTV although there are now data to support a low rate of recurrence in adjacent nodes when there is no prophylactic nodal radiotherapy. Many centres still recommend irradiating high risk nodal sites particularly in N1 disease and would include nodes in the supraclavicular fossae bilaterally for cervical oesophageal tumours, adjacent mediastinal nodes for mid-oesophageal tumours, and the left gastric nodes (along the lesser curve of the stomach) and coeliac nodes for OGJ tumours.

The CTV is grown isotropically by 5 mm axially and 10 mm superoinferiorly to produce the PTV, although these margins can be individualised in each centre if the internal margin and set-up errors have been measured (Fig. 24.2).

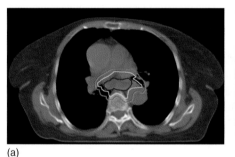
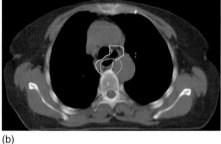

(a)   (b)

Figure 24.2 Volume definition for a T3N1 carcinoma of the thoracic oesophagus. (a) GTV, CTV and PTV. (b) Superior axial slice to show the isotropically expanded CTV (orange) which does not cover the oesophagus and the edited CTV (cyan) which does.

■ Stomach

For adjuvant treatment the CTV should include the tumour bed with a 2 cm margin proximally and distally, and the perigastric nodes on the greater and lesser curvature. The phase III trial which showed a survival advantage for chemoradiation included the coeliac, local para-aortic, splenic, hepato-duodenal and pancreatico-duodenal nodes and most authors therefore recommend these are treated. For tumours of the fundus, the lower para-oesophageal nodes should be included but the pancreatico-duodenal nodes can be omitted. For antral tumours the splenic nodes can be omitted. A 10 mm margin is added isotropically to produce the PTV.

The liver, kidneys and heart are contoured as OAR.

Dose solutions

■ Conformal

Oesophagus

Thoracic oesophageal volumes are best treated with an anterior and two posterior oblique beams or with four equispaced beams. Both these arrangements spare the spinal cord but deliver more dose to the lung than opposing AP beams (Fig. 24.3). Angles for the lateral beams are chosen to avoid dose to the spinal cord PRV. The weight applied to each beam is altered until a plan is produced which adequately covers the PTV while not exceeding tolerance doses to the spinal cord PRV, lungs or heart. The plan can be individually tailored depending on comorbidity. For example in a patient with respiratory disease it may be appropriate to choose a solution that further minimises lung dose at the expense of being closer to (but not exceeding) tolerance of spinal cord PRV and heart. A superoinferior wedge may be required in the anterior and posterior beams when more proximal tumours are being treated to compensate for the inclined plane of the oesophagus which is closer to the anterior chest wall in the upper thorax.

In some patients a two-phase technique is used with opposing AP beams for half to two-thirds of the treatment and a three- or four-beam arrangement for the remainder. This reduces the mean lung dose and can be especially useful if surgery is planned after chemoradiation because respiratory complications are common with tri-modality therapy.

Tumours of the cervical oesophagus are much more anterior so the anterior beam is supplemented by right and left anterior oblique beams. A superoinferior wedge is again required.

The spinal cord PRV dose should be kept below 40 Gy in view of the likely length of cord adjacent to the PTV and the use of concomitant chemotherapy. The heart V40 should be less than 30 per cent and the lung V20 less than 25 per cent.

Stomach

Anterior and posterior opposing beams were used to cover the target volume in the Macdonald trial but more conformal volume-based techniques are now also described using five coplanar or four non-coplanar beams. In addition to the critical organ doses specified for oesophageal cancer, the liver V30 should be below 60 per cent and two-thirds of one kidney (and ideally both) should be below 20 Gy.

■ Complex

IMRT has been used in both oesophageal and adjuvant stomach cancer. IMRT with seven coplanar beams has significant theoretical advantages in sparing normal tissues in stomach cancer but there is little published clinical data to support its use compared with conformal radiotherapy for either tumour type.

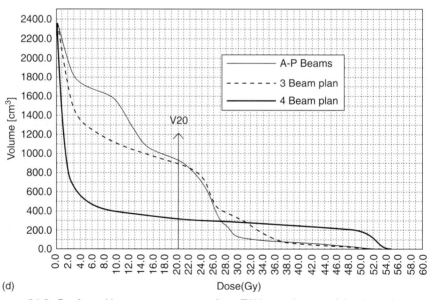

Figure 24.3 Conformal beam arrangements for a T3N1 carcinoma of the thoracic oesophagus. (a) Plan with anterior and posterior beams – minimal lung dose but high dose to the cord and heart. (b) Three-beam plan for the same volume – low cord dose, higher lung dose than a four-beam solution. (c) Four-beam plan for the same volume. (d) DVHs for both lungs minus PTV for each plan treated to 50 Gy in 25 fractions.

Dose-fractionation

■ Oesophagus

Definitive radiochemotherapy

50 Gy in 25 daily fractions with cisplatin-5FU given in 5 weeks reduced to 45 Gy in 25 daily fractions if radiochemotherapy is given preoperatively.

Curative radiotherapy

55 Gy in 20 daily fractions of 2.75 Gy given in 4 weeks.

Palliative radiotherapy

30 Gy in 10 fractions of 3 Gy given in 2 weeks.
or 20 Gy in 5 fractions of 4 Gy given in 1 week.

■ Stomach

Adjuvant radiotherapy

45 Gy in 25 daily fractions of 1.8 Gy given in 5 weeks with concomitant 5FU and leucovorin.

Treatment delivery and patient care

Mucositis is the predominant symptom in patients undergoing oesophageal radiotherapy and should be proactively managed with analgesia and dietary advice. High calorie supplement drinks are useful to maintain adequate oral intake.

Many patients receiving adjuvant radiotherapy for stomach cancer experience grade 3 or 4 toxicity and nausea, lethargy and haematological effects are common. Patients should be weighed and assessed weekly throughout treatment and should be given prophylactic antiemetics (5-HT antagonist). It is essential to ensure adequate nutritional intake before treatment begins.

Verification

Ideally the treatment isocentre on a DRR from the CT simulation is compared with portal images of the isocentre on the treatment machines using electronic portal imaging. Off-line correction protocols are used for standard conformal treatment. Images are taken on days 1–3 and weekly thereafter with a correction made if the mean error in any one plane is >5 mm.

Brachytherapy

High dose rate brachytherapy can be used to palliate dysphagia although expandable metal stents are the treatment of choice for this symptom. A single fraction of 10–15 Gy is prescribed at 1 cm from the central axis of the source.

Brachytherapy has also been advocated in addition to curative radiation or for local recurrence after definitive radiotherapy.

key trials

Cooper JS, Guo MD, Herskovic A *et al.* (1999) Chemoradiotherapy of locally advanced esophageal cancer: long-term follow-up of a prospective randomized trial (RTOG 85–01). Radiation Therapy Oncology Group. *JAMA 5* **281**: 1623–7.

Macdonald JS, Smalley SR, Benedetti J *et al.* (2001) Chemoradiotherapy after surgery compared with surgery alone for adenocarcinoma of the stomach or gastroesophageal junction. *N Engl J Med* **345**: 725–30.

Randomized Phase III Trial of Adjuvant Chemotherapy or Chemoradiotherapy in Resectable Gastric Cancer (CRITICS) (currently recruiting patients). Dutch colorectal cancer group/Netherlands Cancer Institute. M Verheij, principal investigator.

Information sources

Arnott SJ, Duncan W, Gignoux M *et al.* (2005) Oesophageal Cancer Collaborative Group. Preoperative radiotherapy for oesophageal carcinoma. *Cochrane Database Syst Rev* (**4**): CD001799.

Button MR, Morgan CA, Croydon ES *et al.* (2008) Study to determine adequate margins in radiotherapy planning for esophageal carcinoma by detailing patterns of recurrence after definitive chemoradiotherapy. *Int J Radiat Oncol Biol Phys*. **73**: 818–23.

Cancer Care Ontario Gastrointestinal Cancer Evidence-based Series and Practice Guidelines. Available at: www.cancercare.on.ca/english/home/toolbox/qualityguidelines/diseasesite/ gastro-ebs/ [cited 2008 October 11] (accessed 28 July 2008).

Gebski V, Burmeister B, Smithers BM *et al.* (2007) Survival benefits from neoadjuvant chemoradiotherapy or chemotherapy in oesophageal carcinoma: a meta-analysis. *Lancet Oncol* **8**: 226–34.

Scottish Intercollegiate Guidelines Network (2006) *Management of Oesophageal and Gastric Cancer*. National Clinical Guideline no. 87. Available at: www.sign.ac.uk/pdf/sign87.pdf (accessed 4 December 2008).

Smalley SR, Gunderson L, Tepper J *et al.* (2002) Gastric surgical adjuvant radiotherapy consensus report: rationale and treatment implementation. *Int J Radiat Oncol Biol Phys* **52**: 283–93.

Wong RK, Malthaner RA, Zuraw L *et al.* (2003) Cancer care Ontario practice guidelines initiative gastrointestinal cancer disease site group. Combined modality radiotherapy and chemotherapy in nonsurgical management of localized carcinoma of the esophagus: a practice guideline. *Int J Radiat Oncol Biol Phys* **55**: 930–42.

Pancreas and liver

25

Pancreas

■ Indications for radiotherapy

Cancer of the pancreas is the fifth (USA) or sixth (UK) commonest cause of cancer death. With locally advanced disease (40 per cent), median survival is 6–10 months, and after successful complete resection (R0) alone for early stage disease, 11–15 months. After surgery, locoregional relapse occurs in 75 per cent. Forty per cent of patients have metastases at presentation and untreated, median survival is 3–6 months and at 1 year is only 1 per cent.

Most tumours are adenocarcinomas (90 per cent). They usually present late because of an insidious and asymptomatic onset, especially those in the body (15 per cent) or tail (10 per cent). Lesions in the head (75 per cent) may cause obstruction of the bile ducts with jaundice but usual presenting symptoms are anorexia, nausea and vomiting, fatigue and weight loss. CA19.9 is a useful biochemical marker for monitoring treatment but it is not useful for screening as it is negative in 10–15 per cent of cases.

Surgical resection is a prerequisite for long-term control but is only feasible in about 20 per cent of patients, of whom only 30 per cent will actually have an adequate R0 resection margin of >1 mm. Surgery can only be considered if there is no evidence of metastatic disease (commonly in the liver or peritoneum), no involvement of the coeliac, hepatic or superior mesenteric arteries, no obstruction of the confluence of the superior mesenteric and portal veins, and minimal portal vein involvement ($<180°$ involvement over <1 cm). The general PS of the patient must be good.

Adjuvant chemotherapy with 5FU or gemcitabine after resection has been shown to improve 5-year survival in this group by 10–20 per cent. The addition of adjuvant radiotherapy has not yet improved outcomes.

For patients with borderline resectable tumours, neoadjuvant chemotherapy or chemoradiotherapy are currently recommended to try to achieve resectability. For locally advanced, unresectable tumours, initial chemotherapy with good evidence of response may be followed by chemoradiotherapy.

For patients with metastatic or progressive disease in spite of adjuvant or neoadjuvant treatment, palliation with gemcitabine and/or short course radiotherapy is given. The evidence for these treatments is based on small phase I and II trials with poor methodology and quality control (especially for radiotherapy). New trials with neoadjuvant or adjuvant treatment using complex and conformal radiotherapy in combination with drugs with a radiosensitising effect, such as 5FU, and new agents such as bevacizumab are underway.

■ Sequencing of multimodality treatment

After complete resection, chemotherapy is given adjuvantly. For other patients there are various regimens for combining chemotherapy with radiotherapy. Commonly, high dose radiotherapy is given with chemotherapy (5FU, gemcitabine/bevacizumab) but since there are no studies which have yet shown statistically significant benefit in terms of overall survival, it is recommended that patients should be entered into collaborative clinical trials, with accurate staging, standardised chemotherapy and carefully defined and optimised radiotherapy, organised from centres with special expertise in the management of these rare tumours.

■ Clinical and radiological anatomy

The pancreas is a retroperitoneal structure lying within the four parts of the duodenum. Developmentally, it forms from ventral and dorsal outgrowths of the foregut which fuse around the vessels that become the superior mesenteric artery and vein. The head of the pancreas lies anterior to the inferior vena cava overlying the first to third lumbar vertebral bodies. The body passes obliquely to the left overlying the aorta, the left psoas muscle and the splenic artery and vein, while the tail extends in front of the left kidney to the hilum of the spleen (Fig. 25.1).

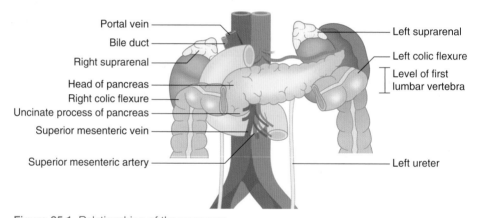

Figure 25.1 Relationships of the pancreas.

■ Assessment of primary disease

The patient's general medical condition and performance must be assessed. Significant adverse prognostic factors which should be taken into account in planning treatment are haemoglobin <12 g/dL and weight loss of >5 per cent in the previous 3 months. Risk factors for pancreatic cancer, which will also increase the complication rate after treatment, include smoking and alcohol use, obesity and poor diet, chronic pancreatitis and previous peptic ulcer disease.

EUS, contrast-enhanced CT scanning and MRI can all be used to demonstrate the primary tumour. CT and MRI are equivalent for assessing extent of local disease, but neither is good at assessing margins of extension accurately, detecting peritoneal spread or predicting lymph node involvement. Percutaneous biopsy should be avoided if resection is planned, and EUS is preferred to investigate and biopsy small tumours. Transabdominal ultrasound is performed if the patient presents with biliary obstruction. Otherwise a contrast-enhanced CT scan with water (1 L orally) and intravenous contrast is used for staging with images acquired with a 1–1.25 mm slice thickness, to determine involvement of visceral arteries or the portal vein, lymph node enlargement, bile duct obstruction and metastases. Dynamic contrast-enhanced MRI can also be used to delineate primary tumour, vascular involvement and liver metastases. FDG-PET-CT has limited usefulness as it cannot distinguish between tumour and inflammation at the tumour margins where the main uncertainty in GTV definition occurs, due to a surrounding desmoplastic stromal reaction and infiltrating growth pattern.

■ Data acquisition

Immobilisation

The patient lies supine in a vacuum moulded bag with arms above the head in arm rests.

CT scanning

CT scans are acquired as described above with a slice thickness of 5 mm at 2–5 mm interslice intervals from the top of the liver or top of T11 to cover lymph nodes, to the lower border of L3 and/or kidneys. Appropriate marks on the bag and the patient's skin are used to align lasers. CT images are usually used for planning (Fig. 25.2) although CT-MRI fusion may be appropriate in some cases if additional information is derived from an MR scan.

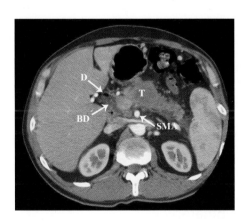

Figure 25.2 Axial CT scan showing tumour of pancreatic body. T, tumour; SMA, superior mesenteric artery; BD, bile duct; D, duodenum.

■ Target volume definition

Because of the difficulty in determining tumour margins, radiologist and radiation oncologist should consult closely to delineate from scans the GTV which includes any enlarged regional lymph nodes of >1.5 cm (GTV-T and -N).

The CTV should include visible tumour and surrounding oedema. This is an area of considerable uncertainty and margins must be individually designed.

PTV margins are anisotropic with 5–10 mm in the AP direction, 2–4 mm in the transverse plane and 15–30 mm cranio-caudally to take account of organ movement with respiration or gut motion, as well as set-up variations. If breath holding techniques or gating are used, cranio-caudal margins may be reduced.

OAR include the spinal cord, kidneys, liver and small bowel. Dose-limiting small bowel tolerance is reflected in the recommended dose-fractionation. These OAR should be outlined on all slices for DVH assessment. A PRV may be added, but in the transverse plane compromise may be needed to maintain these dose limits to OAR.

■ Dose solutions

Conformal

Using 6–10 MV photons, CT forward planning with volumes shaped with MLC may be used to minimise dose to kidneys, liver, spinal cord and small bowel (Fig. 25.3).

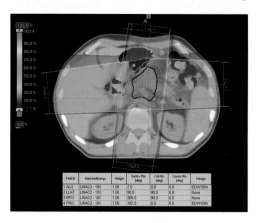

Figure 25.3 Dose distribution for treatment of tumour of pancreatic body (shown in Fig. 25.2).

Complex

Complex plans may not be cost-effective at present outside trials because of poor tumour outcomes, but full inverse planning using dose constraints to OAR and IMRT with a five- (three anterior/two lateral) or seven-beam plan may be optimal to reduce dose to the small bowel.

Conventional

For palliative or simple low dose treatments, AP/PA beams may give a satisfactory dose distribution, or a plan with an anterior and two lateral wedged beams may be used.

■ Dose-fractionation

Radical (in combination with chemotherapy with gemcitabine or 5FU)

45–50.4 Gy in 25–28 fractions of 1.8 Gy given in 5–5½ weeks.

Palliative

30 Gy in 10 daily fractions of 3 Gy given in 2 weeks.

This dose may be used to palliate pain or in association with more intensive chemotherapy.

■ Treatment delivery and patient care

A 5-HT antagonist antiemetic should be prescribed before treatment begins. Decline in performance status may be noted within 14 days of the start of treatment and nausea, diarrhoea and pain may continue to cause problems, or, if there is a tumour response, may improve during treatment. Antacids and analgesics may also be needed. Severe mucositis or even ulceration of the stomach or duodenum may occur. Special attention must be given to maintaining adequate nutrition and hydration. Concomitant chemotherapy may result in bone marrow suppression. It is sometimes difficult to separate side effects from treatment from those due to progressive disease. Patients should be seen weekly for close monitoring and symptom management.

■ Verification

EPIs should be taken on the first 5 days of treatment, for comparison with DRR images obtained after CT planning, and then repeated once weekly after any necessary adjustments have been made. *In vivo* dosimetry with TLD or diodes should be used to ensure treatment dose is delivered as planned.

Liver and biliary tumours

■ Indications for radiotherapy

Primary liver tumours are the fifth commonest cancers in the world, being four times more frequent in Asia than in Europe and the USA. Chronic liver infection, an ageing population and increasing obesity contribute to an increasing incidence.

Liver tumours

Radical removal of liver tumours, where feasible, is the treatment of choice. For early small volume disease (<3 cm), resection may be possible. More widespread involvement by tumour may necessitate liver transplantation.

For inoperable disease, thermal ablation by various means or chemotherapy may be used. Response rates of 25 per cent can be achieved but there is no improvement in survival, although intrahepatic chemotherapy with embolisation may produce a slightly higher response rate.

Conventional and conformal EBRT have shown some responses which increase with dose given, but radiation hepatitis is a dose limiting factor. This may be partially overcome with complex treatment planning and stereotactic delivery of radiation, and leads to 5–10 per cent long-term control.

Treatment with iodine-131 labelled antiferritin antibodies or lipiodol has shown no survival benefit. Yttrium-90 is being investigated.

Cholangiocarcinoma

Gall bladder cancer has also been treated with EBRT with or without intraoperative radiotherapy (IORT) (15 Gy) and 5FU, with good outcomes for patients with previous complete resection or microscopic residual disease (80 per cent 2-year local control).

For inoperable disease, EBRT may be followed by a boost from IORT or brachytherapy if feasible, with prolongation of time to recurrence of 4 months and 2-year survival of 21 per cent. There is conflicting evidence about whether increasing dose improves outcomes. Stereotactic radiotherapy is now being studied for localised inoperable disease.

Liver metastases

Whole liver irradiation doses must not exceed 30 Gy if radiation-induced liver disease (radiation hepatitis) is to be avoided.

Advances in conformal EBRT and IMRT have made it possible to deliver focal high dose radiotherapy treatments to individual metastases in patients with good prognosis disease when surgical excision is not feasible. Response rates may exceed 50 per cent with high doses of EBRT (>60 Gy) or stereotactic radiosurgery (26 Gy) giving 80 per cent local control at 18 months.

The use of helical tomotherapy may make it possible to give highly focused IMRT to metastases at the same time as the primary tumour.

■ Assessment of primary disease

Primary hepatic tumours may be classified as unifocal expansive, infiltrating or multifocal (50 per cent). They invade the portal vein and spread thence to the lungs. They present commonly with non-specific symptoms of abdominal pain, malaise, fever and weight loss, although rupture and haemorrhage may occur. Staging is by contrast-enhanced ultrasound, CT or MRI. Characteristically in the arterial phase there is hypervascularity with wash-out in the portal venous phase which must be seen in two different techniques of imaging to confirm the diagnosis. Biopsy is only done if scans are not characteristic.

Expected toxicity from treatment can be predicted from the Child–Pugh classification of cirrhosis which takes into account levels of bilirubin, prothrombin time, albumin, and presence of ascites and encephalopathy to classify into grades A, B and C (worst).

■ Target volume definition

Liver tumours or metastases

The GTV may be defined using PET-CT scans or MR images taking into account all respiratory phases. A CTV margin of 5 mm and CTV-PTV margin of a further 5 mm are contoured.

Cholangiocarcinoma

GTV is determined by preoperative CT. CTV should include the gall bladder fossa and adjacent liver and regional nodal areas. To allow for movement with respiration, margins for CTV to PTV should be about 20 mm cranio-caudally, 8 mm AP and 9 mm left to right.

■ Dose solutions

These treatments require complex solutions with stereotaxis or tomotherapy and should be carried out in centres with appropriate equipment and expertise.

■ Dose-fractionation

Cholangiocarcinoma

Inoperable disease
54 Gy in 30 daily fractions of 1.8 Gy given in 6 weeks
±15 Gy as IORT boost.

or

EBRT 36–55 Gy + brachytherapy 15 Gy in 3 daily fractions of 5 Gy HDR or 25 Gy at 1 cm LDR.

Stereotactic radiotherapy is now being studied for localised inoperable disease.

Liver metastases

20–30 Gy in 13–20 daily fractions of 1.5 Gy may occasionally be used to relieve painful hepatomegaly.

Stereotactic radiosurgery of 26 Gy or tomotherapy delivering 40 Gy in 5 fractions of 8 Gy are being investigated for single or few liver metastases and for treatment of primary tumours.

■ Treatment delivery and patient care

Nausea and vomiting are controlled with 5-HT antagonist antiemetics with or without steroids. Bilirubin, prothrombin time and albumin must be monitored.

Whole liver irradiation doses must not exceed 30 Gy if radiation induced liver disease (radiation hepatitis) is to be avoided. This presents 2 weeks to 2 months after radiotherapy with ascites, hepatomegaly, confusion and jaundice with raised levels of alkaline phosphatase, prothrombin time and thrombocytopenia. The pathological basis is veno-occlusive disease and the outcome is fatal in 10–20 per cent of patients.

■ Verification

DRRs derived from CT planning are compared with EPIs or on board imaging, which is recommended for these complex treatments.

---

key trials

Pancreas

Neoptolemos JP, Stocken DD, Friess H *et al.* (2004) European Study Group for Pancreatic Cancer. A randomised trial of chemoradiotherapy and chemotherapy after resection of pancreatic cancer. *N Eng J Med* **350**: 1200–10.

Neuhaus P, Riess H, Post S *et al.* (2008) CONKO-001: Final results of the randomised, prospective, multicenter phase III trial of adjuvant chemotherapy with gemcitabine versus observation in patients with resected pancreatic cancer (PC). *J Clin Oncol* **26**(20 suppl): abstract LBA4504.

Oettle H, Post S, Neuhaus P *et al.* (2007) Adjuvant chemotherapy with gemcitabine vs. observation in patients undergoing curative-intent resection of pancreatic cancer: a randomised controlled trial. *JAMA* **297**: 267–77.

Regine WF, Winter KA, Abrams RA *et al.* (2008) Fluorouracil vs. gemcitabine chemotherapy before and after fluorouracil-based chemoradiation following resection of pancreatic adenocarcinoma: a randomised controlled trial. *JAMA* **299**: 1019–26.

Information sources

■ Pancreas

Ghaneh P, Costello E, Neoptolemos JP (2007) Biology and management of pancreatic cancer. *Gut* **56**: 1134–52.

Small W Jr, Berlin J, Freedman GM *et al.* (2008) Full-dose gemcitabine with concurrent radiation therapy in patients with nonmetastatic pancreatic cancer: a multicenter phase II trial. *J Clin Oncol* **20**: 942–7.

Sultana A, Tudur-Smith C, Cunningham D *et al.* (2007) Meta-analyses of chemotherapy for locally advanced and metastatic pancreatic cancer. *J Clin Oncol* **25**: 2607–15.

Van Laethem J, Van Cutsem E, Hammel P *et al.* (2008) Adjuvant chemotherapy alone versus chemoradiation after curative resection for pancreatic cancer: feasibility results of a randomised EORTC/FFCD/GERCOR phase II/III study (40013/22012/0304). ASCO Meeting Abstracts: 4514.

■ Liver and biliary tract

Graco C, Catalano G, Grazie AD *et al.* (2004) Radiotherapy of liver malignancies. From whole liver irradiation to stereotactic hypofractionated radiotherapy. *Tumori* **90**: 73–9.

Lawrence TS (2008) Radiotherapy for intrahepatic cancers: the promise of emerging sophisticated techniques. *J Support Oncol* **6**: 14–15. Available at www.SupportiveOncology.net.

Pugh RN, Murray-Lyon IM, Dawson JL (1973) Transection of the oesophagus for bleeding oesophageal varices. *Br J Surg* **60**: 646–9. (Child–Pugh classification).

Tse RV, Hawkins M, Lockwood G (2008) Phase 1 study of individualised stereotactic body radiotherapy for HCC and intra-hepatic cholangiocarcinoma. *Clin Oncol* **26**: 657–64.

Rectum

26

Indications for radiotherapy

Colorectal cancer is the second most common cancer in the UK in terms of incidence and mortality. Both incidence and cure rates are increasing. One-third of colorectal tumours arise in the rectum, more commonly in men.

Most rectal cancers are adenocarcinomas which are discussed here. Subtypes which have a poorer prognosis include signet ring, and mucinous adenocarcinomas (associated with microsatellite instability and hereditary non-polyposis colorectal cancer [HNPCC]). Medullary carcinoma may be associated with a better prognosis. Rare types of rectal cancer include small cell carcinoma, carcinoids, lymphoma, sarcoma and squamous cell carcinoma. Squamous cell carcinomas arising from the transitional area between rectum and anal verge are classified and treated as anal cancer.

■ Curative radiotherapy

Surgery is the mainstay of treatment and gives 5-year overall survival rates of 93 per cent (stage I), 72–85 per cent (stage II), 44–83 per cent (stage III) and 8 per cent (stage IV). The 5-year survival in stage IV disease with resection of liver metastases after primary treatment is 36 per cent. The most significant improvement in treatment has been the widespread use of total mesorectal excision (TME) which has reduced local recurrence rate to less than 10 per cent, compared with 30 per cent with older surgical techniques.

In selected T1,N0,M0 tumours <3 cm in diameter that are not poorly differentiated, endocavitary local contact radiotherapy with the Papillon technique using a low energy 50 kV machine has produced good results and new equipment for this technique is being developed. HDR brachytherapy can also be used for small, localised rectal tumours.

■ Adjuvant radiotherapy

Pre- and postoperative adjuvant therapies are used in high-risk cases to improve resectability, reduce local recurrence, increase sphincter preservation, and improve overall survival. Based on the same evidence, practices differ. In North America, resectable cancers are treated with postoperative chemoradiotherapy if they are found to be T3/4 or node positive. Some centres in Europe advocate short course preoperative radiotherapy for all resectable rectal cancers as it provides a quick, effective, practical and cheap method of delivering neoadjuvant radiotherapy. Alternatively long course preoperative chemoradiotherapy can be given to selected patients with non-resectable tumours or resectable tumours with MRI features predictive of subsequent incomplete excision:

- primary tumour or lymph node is threatening the circumferential resection margin (CRM) i.e. within 1–2 mm of mesorectal fascia
- involvement or extension beyond the mesorectal fascia
- involved lymph nodes outside the mesorectal fascia
- extramural vascular invasion (EMVI).

Additional high risk factors for local recurrence are:

- tumours in the lower third of the rectum which often require abdominoperineal resection (APER) with risk of poor lateral margin clearance with consequent higher local recurrence rates
- large anterior quadrant tumours, where sphincter-preserving surgery may be difficult.

Preoperative chemoradiotherapy is the subject of ongoing studies but it is used more often in these poor risk tumours. All patients are discussed in a multidisciplinary team meeting between surgeons, pathologists, radiologists and oncologists to plan multimodality treatment for each individual patient on the basis of risk factors.

■ Palliative radiotherapy

Palliation may be achieved for unresectable and locally advanced T4 tumours with radiotherapy alone. Alternatively long course chemoradiotherapy may be given to try to downstage the tumour for resection. Hypofractionated weekly radiotherapy may be used to palliate local symptoms in patients unfit for longer chemoradiotherapy schedules. Local recurrence is less of a problem with widespread use of TME and preoperative radiotherapy. It may cause neuropathic sacral and sciatic pain with bladder and bowel dysfunction. Chemoradiotherapy or radio-therapy alone may offer effective short-term palliation for patients with local recurrence who have not previously been irradiated. Patients who have received radiotherapy previously may be considered for re-irradiation, but long-term toxicity data are lacking and small bowel toxicity may occur.

An algorithm for the management of rectal cancer is shown in Figure 26.1. The type of surgical resection needed depends on the site of the cancer. Upper third rectal tumours can be removed by a high anterior resection and TME, mid and lower third tumours can be removed by anterior resection with TME, and low rectal tumours less than 5 cm from the anal verge or those with sphincter involvement require an APER. TME and sphincter-preserving surgery can only be performed if the surgical resection margin below the tumour is 1 cm away from the sphincter.

The main RCTs that have influenced practice are shown in Table 26.1.

Sequencing of multimodality therapy

Surgery is performed 1 week after short course preoperative EBRT. Surgery is delayed until 6–10 weeks after long course preoperative chemoradiotherapy. After 12 weeks, radiation fibrosis presents problems at surgery. The standard chemotherapy used with radiotherapy for rectal cancer is 5FU as bolus, continuous

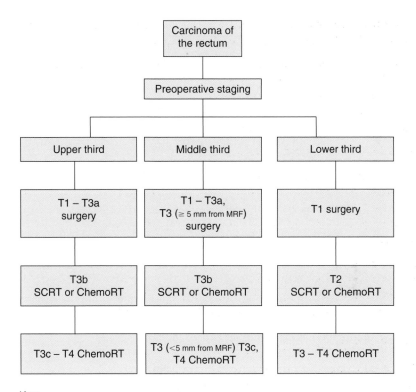

Key:
T3a,<5mm extramural tumour invasion
T3b, 5–10mm
T3c, >10mm
MRF, Mesorectal fascia
SCRT, Short course preop Radiotherapy
ChemoRT, Long course preop Chemoradiotherapy

Figure 26.1 Algorithm for management of rectal cancer.

Table 26.1 Main RCTs which have influenced management of rectal cancer

Trial	Randomisation	Results
GTSG Study; *N Engl J Med* (1985)	Surgery	9-year OS 27 per cent, LR 25 per cent
	Surgery + POCRT	9-year OS 54 per cent*, LR 10 per cent*
Mayo NCCTG; *N Engl J Med* (1991)	S + PORT	5-year OS 40 per cent, LR 25 per cent
	S + POCRT	5-year OS 55 per cent*, LR 15 per cent*
Swedish Rectal Trial; *N Engl J Med* (1997)	Surgery	5-year OS 48 per cent, CSS 65 per cent, LR 27 per cent
	Preop SCRT + S (25 Gy/5#)	5-year OS 58 per cent*, CSS 74 per cent*, LR 11 per cent*
Dutch Rectal Trial; *N Engl J Med* (2001)	S (TME)	2-year OS 81.8 per cent, LR 8.2 per cent
	Preop SCRT + S(TME) (25 Gy/5#)	2-year OS 82.0 per cent, LR 2.4 per cent*

(Continued)

Table 26.1 Continued

Trial	Randomisation	Results
German Rectal Trial; *N Engl J Med* (2004)	Pre-op LCCRT + S (TME)	5-year OS 76 per cent, LR 6 per cent*
	S (TME) + POCRT	5-year OS 74 per cent, LR 13 per cent
CR07 Rectal Trial; ASCO 2006	Preop SCRT + S (TME)	3-year OS 80.8 per cent, DFS 79.5 per cent, LR 4.7 per cent*
	S (TME) + selective POCRT	3-year OS 78.7 per cent, DFS 74.5 per cent, LR 11.1 per cent
Polish Study; *Br J Surg* (2006)	Preop SCRT + S(TME)	4-year OS 67.2 per cent, DFS 58.4 per cent, LR 9 per cent
	Preop LCCRT + S(TME)	4-year OS 66.2 per cent, DFS 55.6 per cent, LR 14.2 per cent

*p <0.05.

S, surgery; PORT, postoperative radiotherapy; POCRT, postoperative chemoradiotherapy; preop LCCRT, preoperative long course chemoradiotherapy; preop SCRT, preoperative short course radiotherapy; TME, total mesorectal excision; OS, overall survival; CSS, cause-specific survival; DFS, disease-free survival; LR, local recurrence.

infusion or orally. Studies are underway comparing different combination regimens with new agents such as capecitabine and oxaliplatin.

Clinical and radiological anatomy

The rectum extends from the external sphincter to the recto-sigmoid junction. It is divided into a lower third 3–6 cm, middle third 5–6 cm to 8–10 cm, and upper third 8–10 to 12–15 cm from the anal verge (Fig. 26.2). The upper third of the rectum is surrounded by peritoneum on the anterior and lateral surfaces and is retroperitoneal posteriorly. At the recto-vesical or recto-uterine pouch, the rectum becomes completely retroperitoneal and follows the curve of the sacrum entering the anal canal at the level of the levator ani. The mesorectum contains the blood supply and lymphatics for the upper, middle and lower rectum. The location of a rectal tumour is defined by the distance from the lower edge of the tumour to the anal verge.

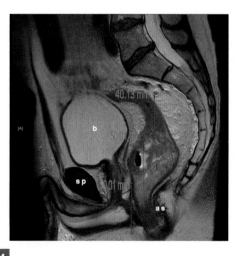

Figure 26.2 Sagittal T2-weighted MRI of a middle third rectal cancer showing division of the rectum into lower, middle and upper thirds. b, bladder; sp, symphysis pubis; as anal sphincter.

Flexible endoscopes can overestimate this distance compared with measurements with rigid endoscopes, which therefore may be preferred since the distance from the anal sphincter to the tumour is critical for planning sphincter sparing surgery.

Rectal carcinomas arise in the mucosa and may be exophytic, ulcerated or annular, when they may produce obstruction of the lumen. Tumours extend through the wall of the serosa to invade surrounding organs such as the bladder, prostate and vagina, with direct extension into the presacral region in advanced cases. The lymphatic drainage of the rectum is to the mesorectal lymph nodes (contained in mesorectal fascia), mesenteric lymph nodes (along inferior mesenteric artery), lateral lymph nodes (along middle rectal, obturator and internal iliac vessels) and external iliac lymph nodes. There is also drainage to hypogastric and presacral lymph nodes as shown in Fig. 26.3. Spread toward the anal margin may be associated with inguinal lymph node involvement.

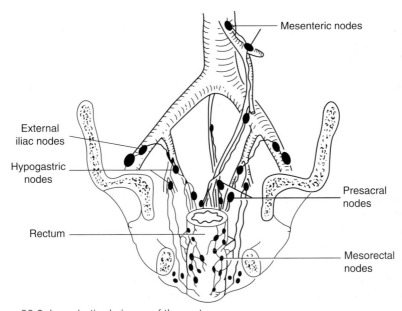

Figure 26.3 Lymphatic drainage of the rectum.

Assessment of primary disease

The standard staging procedure includes a history, examination and digital rectal examination (DRE) to determine the distance of the tumour from the anal verge, sphincter involvement and clinical fixation. Full blood count, renal and liver function tests and CEA are performed. A raised CEA suggestive of metastases predicts a poor prognosis. Examination of the entire colon with a barium enema or colonoscopy to exclude a synchronous primary is essential. CT scanning is used to assess the pelvis, abdomen and liver, with CT or CXR to assess the lungs. Endorectal ultrasound or MRI are used to stage the primary rectal tumour. The European multi-institutional MERCURY study has shown the central role of MRI in staging rectal cancers. Accuracy (92 per cent), specificity (98 per cent), positive and negative predictive values (73 and 93 per cent, respectively) confirm its usefulness. In patients in whom an MRI predicts a clear CRM, 94 per cent will have a clear margin at surgery. If it predicts probable involvement or shows tumour less than 1 mm from the CRM, it is highly likely that there is involvement.

The AJCC and UICC 6th edition TNM staging system 2002 is currently used for evaluating rectal cancer. Patients are staged clinically and radiologically before surgery to define the need for neoadjuvant therapy, and pathologically staged postoperatively to define the need for adjuvant therapy. Nodal involvement carries a poorer prognosis but it is recognised in the staging system that patients with T1–T2, N1 rectal cancer have a better prognosis than other stage III rectal cancers. Disease staged N0 after surgery has a better prognosis when 12–14 lymph nodes are identified. A close or positive CRM is a poor prognostic indicator.

Data acquisition

Patients lie in the prone position. The small bowel can be displaced anteriorly by the use of devices such as a bellyboard, which allows it to fall forwards into the bellyboard aperture (Fig. 26.4). Modern bellyboard devices are more comfortable, improve immobilisation and reduce set-up errors in the prone position. A full bladder protocol is used for planning and treatment as this displaces small bowel superiorly. A radio-opaque marker is placed on the anal verge and a DRE performed to determine the distance from the anal verge marker to the inferior edge of the tumour. The anterior border of the vagina can be identified using a radio-opaque tampon. Oral contrast may be used to help identify small bowel. Treatments are planned using CT-based virtual simulation or conformal CT planning. A planning CT scan is performed with 3 mm slices from the level of L5 to 2 cm below the anal marker. Low rectal tumours are better defined on MRI than on CT. However at present staging MRI is performed with the patient supine. In the future there may be a role for co-registration of planning CT with prone MR scans. The use of FDG-PET for rectal cancer planning is currently being investigated. If a simulator has to be used, bony landmarks help to define the target volumes.

Target volume definition

■ Preoperative radiotherapy

The target volume includes the primary tumour, adjacent lymph nodes and the presacral region. The inferior mesenteric nodes are not included because they are removed at later surgery. It has been shown that extension of the treatment volume above L5 increases late complications significantly. Treatment may be planned by CT defined target volumes or using standard bony landmarks as in the CR07 trial.

CT defined target volumes

Target volumes are based on the known patterns of local recurrence in rectal cancer. The GTV includes all gross tumour seen on the planning CT scan with reference to information from diagnostic endoscopy, MRI and DRE. Any involved lymph nodes, extrarectal extension, or extranodal deposits seen on MRI should be included. The CTV includes the primary tumour, mesorectum from the sacral promontory to insertion of levator ani into the rectal wall, and the posterior

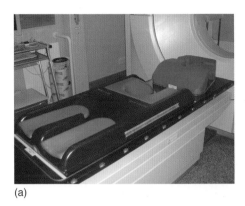

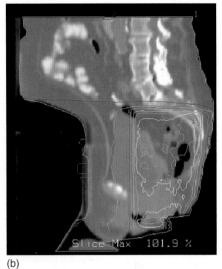

(a)

(b)

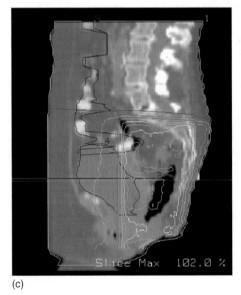

(c)

Figure 26.4 (a) Bellyboard for prone immobilisation. (b) CT plan with bellyboard. (c) CT plan without bellyboard.

presacral space. The inferior pelvic subsite, including the anal perineum, anal sphincter, perianal and ischiorectal space, is included if the tumour is <6 cm from the anal margin or if the tumour invades the anal sphincter. The mesorectal and lateral lymph nodes are included in all patients. The obturator nodes are included when the tumour is <10 cm from the anal margin, and the external iliac lymph nodes included if there is anterior organ involvement. The inguinal lymph nodes may be included if tumour invades the lower third of the vagina, or if there is major tumour extension into the internal and external anal sphincter.

In principle, the PTV is created by adding a margin of 1–1.5 cm to the CTV. In practice, a margin may be added to the GTV to create the PTV directly ensuring the above CTV sites are included. The margins used to grow the GTV to PTV are 3–5 cm superiorly (limited by the L5/S1 junction), 2–3 cm inferiorly, 2 cm anteriorly, and posteriorly to cover the sacrum.

A boost to the primary tumour can be added. The phase 2 PTV then includes the tumour mass with a 2 cm 3D margin. Small bowel is demonstrated by oral contrast and contoured as an OAR.

Conventional planning

The following bony landmarks can be used to define field borders:

- lateral: 1 cm outside bony pelvis
- posterior: 1 cm behind sacrum to include sacral hollow and presacral lymph nodes
- superior: sacral promontory, L5/S1 border as defined on lateral sagittal view
- anterior: 2–3 cm anterior to sacral promontory and including the anterior vaginal wall in females. Care must be taken to include the whole rectum which may be more anteriorly placed. This can be seen on CT, at virtual simulation or on diagnostic MR scans
- inferior: 3 cm below the inferior edge of the tumour. For lower third tumours the border should lie below the anal marker to cover the perineum.

■ Postoperative radiotherapy

Close collaboration with the surgical team and pathologists is essential to aid planning with a full description of the extent of residual tumour, anatomical location of clips demarcating the tumour bed, and sites of close margins. The target for postoperative radiotherapy is the tumour bed, adjacent lymph nodes, presacral region and any residual tumour. Clinical examination is used to localise the level of the anastomosis in patients after anterior resection or the perineal scar following APER. Surgical procedures such as reconstruction of the pelvic floor and absorbable mesh slings can be used to reduce the amount of small bowel in the pelvis.

Because the GTV has been removed and the CTV is large, complex solutions and conformal CT planning are used to minimise the amount of normal tissue (especially small bowel) in the target volume, but the target volume is planned with reference to standard bony landmarks:

- lateral: 1 cm outside bony pelvis
- posterior: 1 cm behind sacrum to include sacral hollow and presacral lymph nodes
- superior: sacral promontory, L5/S1 border as defined on lateral sagittal view
- anterior: 2 cm anterior to sacral promontory and including the anterior vaginal wall
- inferior: 3 cm below the inferior edge of the anastomosis or to the inferior obturator foramen, whichever is lower. For patients who have had an APER the perineal scar is marked to ensure it is covered.

An optional phase 2 volume is individualised to target the tumour bed and any residual tumour with a 2 cm 3D margin. This is best defined on CT using all the operative and pathological information available.

Dose solutions

Dose distributions with high energy beams (10 MV) are often better than with lower energies. A three- or four-beam arrangement includes a direct posterior beam with reduced weighting, and either two lateral or posterior oblique wedged beams depending on the shape of the patient (Fig. 26.5).

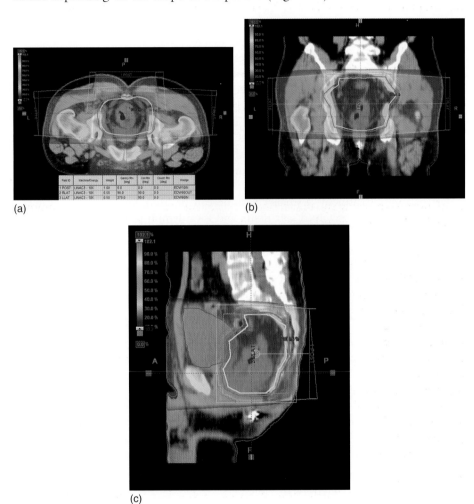

(a)   (b)

(c)

Figure 26.5 Conformal plan using direct posterior and lateral beams shown on CT slice: (a) axial, (b) coronal and (c) sagittal.

Posterior oblique beams at a gantry angle of 45–60° will produce a rounded volume with some anterior spread of dose, whereas lateral beams will give a sharp cut off anteriorly, reducing small bowel dose. Angles of less than 45° are not used as this causes overlap of the beams posteriorly, increasing the skin reaction in the natal cleft. With advanced disease where there is bladder or anterior abdominal wall involvement, a four-beam arrangement or AP opposing beams may need to be used to increase the dose anteriorly.

3D conformal CT planning allows for DVH assessment of the normal tissues and conformal shielding with MLC to reduce the dose to normal tissues, most importantly the small bowel. The TD 5/5 for one-third of the small bowel volume is 50 Gy. This is based on data showing a 3 per cent incidence of late small bowel obstruction with doses of $\geqslant$45Gy delivered to 664 cm^3, about one-third of the small bowel volume. When planning conformally, the volume of small bowel receiving over 45 Gy should be kept to the minimum possible and no small bowel should receive over 50 Gy. Care must be taken to identify small bowel that may be stuck in the sacral hollow postoperatively.

When planning radiotherapy for low rectal tumours or postoperatively following APER, the target volume includes the perineum or perineal scar. External bolus over these areas may be needed to ensure adequate dose inferiorly.

Where possible the anal canal should be excluded from the radiation beams to preserve function of the anal sphincter. The ano-rectal junction can be identified using 3D conformal planning or virtual CT simulation.

IMRT planning has limited value at present. In the future, better definition of volumes with the possibility of dose escalation may make it useful if stage-dependent CTV targets can be defined.

For palliative treatment, a smaller volume can be used which covers the rectal tumour, sacrum and involved soft tissue and local lymph nodes only to minimise the amount of small bowel treated. Treatment can be planned in the same way as described above using CT planning or diagnostic films to identify bony landmarks to create a target volume.

Dose-fractionation

■ Preoperative radiotherapy

Short course
25 Gy in 5 daily fractions of 5 Gy given in 1 week.

Long course
Phase 1
45 Gy in 25 daily fractions of 1.8 Gy given in 5 weeks.

Phase 2 (optional)
5.4–9 Gy in 3–5 daily fractions of 1.8 Gy.

■ Postoperative radiotherapy

Phase 1
45 Gy in 25 daily fractions of 1.8 Gy given in 5 weeks.

Phase 2 (optional)
5.4–9 Gy in 3–5 daily fractions of 1.8 Gy.

■ Palliative radiotherapy

Palliative long course chemoradiotherapy may be used for maximal local control for inoperable rectal cancers where prolonged survival is possible.

Phase 1
45 Gy in 25 daily fractions of 1.8 Gy given in 5 weeks.

Phase 2 (optional)
5.4–14.4 Gy in 3–8 daily fractions of 1.8 Gy
or a hypofractionated regimen can be used
30–36 Gy in 5–6 fractions of 6 Gy once weekly given in 5–6 weeks.

Treatment delivery and patient care

The patient is treated each day in the prone position with a full bladder. A low residue diet is advised and the patient seen weekly to assess toxicity. Erythema and desquamation of the skin can occur in the perineal and sacral areas. Nursing assessment, hydrocolloid dressings, nutritional support and analgesia are important. Diarrhoea should be treated with loperamide hydrochloride as appropriate. If small bowel acute radiation toxicity is suspected with abdominal pain and localised peritonism, the patient should be rested from treatment and the radiotherapy plan and sites of small bowel reviewed. A minority of patients receiving short course preoperative radiotherapy develop an acute sensory neuropathy, which can be alleviated by reduction in the treatment volume to the level of S2/3.

Verification

Patients are set up daily, using sagittal and lateral tattoos (over the iliac crests) and lasers to prevent lateral rotation.

Electronic portal imaging is used to verify the treatment set-up and the EPIs are compared with the DRRs to ensure the isocentre, beams and MLC shielding configuration are correct. Set-up can be monitored with EPIs according to local protocols during treatment with correction for displacements outside tolerance levels of 5–8 mm. With future advances, image guided radiotherapy with kV and cone beam CT may play a greater role in rectal cancer radiotherapy planning.

key trials

Bosset JF, Calais G, Mineur L (2005) Enhanced tumorocidal effect of chemotherapy with preoperative radiotherapy for rectal cancer: preliminary results – EORTC 22921. *J Clin Oncol* **23**: 5620–7.

Braendengen M, Tveit KM, Berglund A *et al.* (2008) Randomised phase III study comparing preoperative radiotherapy with chemoradiotherapy in nonresectable rectal cancer. *J Clin Oncol* **26**: 3687–94.

Bujko K, Nowacki MP, Nasierowska-Guttmejer A *et al.* (2006) Long-term results of a randomised trial comparing preoperative short-course radiotherapy with preoperative conventionally fractionated chemoradiation for rectal cancer. *Br J Surg* **93**: 1215–23.

Gastrointestinal Tumor Study Group (1985) Prolongation of the disease-free interval in surgically treated rectal carcinoma. *N Engl J Med* **312**: 1465–72.

Kapiteijn E, Marijnen CA, Nagtegaal ID *et al.* (2001) Dutch Colorectal Cancer Group. Preoperative radio therapy combined with total mesorectal excision for resectable rectal cancer. *N Engl J Med* **345**: 638–46.

Krook JE, Moertel CG, Gunderson LL *et al.* (1991) Effective surgical adjuvant therapy for high-risk rectal carcinoma. Mayo NCCTG. *N Engl J Med* **324**: 709–15.

MERCURY Study Group (2006) Diagnostic accuracy of preoperative magnetic resonance imaging in predicting curative resection of rectal cancer: prospective observational study. *BMJ* **333**: 779.

Sauer R, Becker H, Hohenberger W *et al.* (2004) German Rectal Cancer Study Group. Preoperative versus postoperative chemoradiotherapy for rectal cancer. *N Engl J Med* **351**: 1731–40.

Sebag-Montefiore D, Quirke P, Steele RJ *et al.* (2006) CR07: Pre-operative radiotherapy vs. selective post-operative chemo-radiotherapy for patients with rectal cancer. ASCO abstract. Pro ASCO 24, 18S, abstract 3511.

Swedish Rectal Cancer Trial (1997) Improved survival with preoperative radiotherapy in resectable rectal cancer. *N Engl J Med* **336**: 980–7.

Information sources

Borger JH, van den Bogaard J, de Haas DF *et al.* (2008) Evaluation of three different CT simulation and planning procedures for the preoperative irradiation of operable rectal cancer. *Radiother Oncol* **87**: 350–6.

Elective Clinical Target Volumes in Anorectal Cancer: An RTOG Consensus Panel Contouring Atlas. Available at www.rtog.org.

Letschert JG, Lebesque JV, Aleman BM *et al.* (1994) The volume effect in radiation-related late small bowel complications: results of a clinical study of the EORTC Radiotherapy Cooperative Group in patients treated for rectal carcinoma. *Radiother Oncol* **32**: 116–23.

MRC Clinical Trials Unit. Results of CR07. Available at www.ctu.mrc.ac.uk/studies/CR07.

Myint AS (2007) Radiotherapy for early rectal cancer. *Clin Oncol* **19**: 637–8.

Nagtegaal ID, Quirke P (2008) What is the role for the circumferential margin in the modern treatment of rectal cancer? *J Clin Oncol* **26**: 303–12.

National Institutes of Health Consensus Conference (1990) Adjuvant therapy for patients with colon and rectal cancer. *JAMA* **264**: 1444–50.

National Institute for Health and Clinical Excellence. *Improving Outcomes in Colorectal Cancer*. Available at: www.nice.org.uk/csgcc.

Nicholls J (2008) The multidisciplinary management of rectal cancer. *Colorectal Dis* **10**: 311–13.

Roels S, Duthoy W, Haustermans K *et al.* (2006) Definition and delineation of the clinical target volume for rectal cancer. *Int J Radiat Oncol Biol Phys* **65**: 1129–42.

Anus

27

Indications for radiotherapy

Anal cancer is rare with approximately 500–600 new cases diagnosed each year in the UK. It is more common in women and the median age at diagnosis is 60. Anal margin tumours, however, are more common in men and at an earlier age. Primary chemoradiotherapy is the current treatment of choice.

Eighty per cent of all anal cancers are epidermoid squamous cell carcinomas, which are discussed here. Most cases are preceded by high grade anal intraepithelial neoplasia (AIN), but only 1 per cent per year of patients with AIN develop invasive cancer. Anal margin tumours are often keratinising and well differentiated while canal tumours are usually non-keratinising and poorly differentiated. Upper canal tumours may be mixed squamous cell and adenocarcinoma of transitional, basaloid or cloacogenic type. Rare types of primary anal cancer include adenocarcinomas, small cell carcinomas, melanoma, lymphoma and leiomyosarcoma.

The risk factors associated with anal cancer are human papillomavirus (16, 18) infection (found in over 80 per cent of cases), genital warts, other sexually transmitted diseases, immunosuppression, ano-receptive intercourse and tobacco smoking. It is associated with human immunodeficiency virus (HIV) infection but not correlated with degree of immunosuppression and is not considered an acquired immune deficiency syndrome (AIDS) defining illness.

With radical chemoradiotherapy, 5-year survival rates are >90 per cent for T1, >80 per cent for T2, 45–55 per cent for T3/4 and 65–75 per cent overall.

■ Curative radiotherapy

The initial studies of Nigro demonstrated the curative potential of chemoradiotherapy for anal cancer. Further studies confirmed the benefit of adding mitomycin C (MMC) and 5FU to radiotherapy for anal cancer and three large RCTs in the1990s confirmed benefits (Table 27.1).

Radical chemoradiotherapy can be considered for all patients with non-metastatic anal cancer who are fit for radical treatment. It is associated with an increased risk of toxicity in patients with HIV infection, inflammatory bowel disease and after previous pelvic surgery or renal transplantation. Patients with HIV and immunosuppression with a CD4 count <200 develop significant toxicity and morbidity with chemoradiotherapy. The dose of radiotherapy and chemotherapy may have to be modified but this reduces control rates. Patients with inflammatory bowel disease tolerate pelvic radiotherapy poorly with a high risk of late toxicity. Patients who have had previous pelvic surgery often have adhesions and risk increased dose to small bowel and late complications. The

Table 27.1 RCTs of chemoradiotherapy for anal cancer

Trial	Randomisation	Results
UKCCR ACT 1 (n = 585)	RT alone	3-year LC 39%, CSS 61%, OS 58%
	RT + 5FU/MMC	3-year LC 61%,* CSS 72%,* OS 65%
EORTC (n = 103)	RT alone	3-year LC 55%, OS 65%
	RT + 5FU/MMC	3-year LC 65%,* OS 70%
RTOG (n = 291)	RT + 5FU	4-year LC 64%, DFS 50%, OS 65%
	RT + 5FU/MMC	4-year LC 83%,* DFS 67%*, OS 67%

*p <0.05.

RT, radiotherapy; OS, overall survival; LC, local control; CSS, cause-specific survival; DFS, disease-free survival.

multidisciplinary team should carefully consider the risks and benefits of radical surgical resection versus radical chemoradiotherapy.

■ Postoperative radiotherapy

Surgery is now most commonly performed for failure after chemoradiotherapy. Local excision may be considered for node negative anal margin tumours less than 2 cm in diameter without anal canal involvement providing the tumour can be completely excised without damage to the sphincter. After incomplete excision, adjuvant chemoradiotherapy is advised.

■ Palliative radiotherapy

Palliative radiotherapy can be considered for patients who present with metastatic disease or have such poor performance status that they will not tolerate radical chemoradiotherapy.

Sequencing of multimodality therapy

Current chemoradiotherapy protocols recommend that the first fraction of radiotherapy should be given after commencement of an intravenous infusion of 5FU chemotherapy. This is given in the first and last weeks of radiotherapy with other agents such as MMC or cisplatin. Trials are studying the best combination of drugs with radiotherapy and whether maintenance chemotherapy is advantageous.

Clinical and radiological anatomy

The anal canal is 3–4 cm long and extends from the anorectal ring (top of 'surgical' anal canal), composed of upper fibres of the internal sphincter, to the anal margin as shown in Fig. 27.1. The anal margin consists of the area of skin around the anal orifice. Tumours of the anal margin are slow growing and tend to infiltrate locally within the perineum, with late spread to lymph nodes. Tumours of the anal canal most commonly arise in the transitional zone just above the dentate line, and tend to spread proximally in the submucosa to the distal rectum. Tumours invade anteriorly into the vagina and uncommonly to the prostate, laterally to the ischio-rectal fossa, and posteriorly along the ano-coccygeal ligament to the coccyx. Anterior spread to the prostate may be limited by Denonvilliers' fascia, and inferior spread may be limited by the suspensory ligaments.

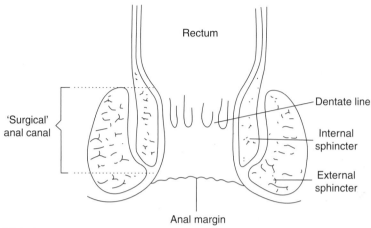

Figure 27.1 Anatomy of the anus.

Lymphatic drainage from the anal margin and perianal skin is to the superficial inguinal and femoral lymph nodes, and thence to the external iliac nodes. The lymphatic drainage of the anal canal, proximal to the dentate line, is to the superior rectal, superior haemorrhoidal, hypogastric, obturator, internal iliac and presacral lymph nodes (Fig. 27.2). Tumours distal to the dentate line drain to superficial inguinal nodes as well as to pararectal nodes.

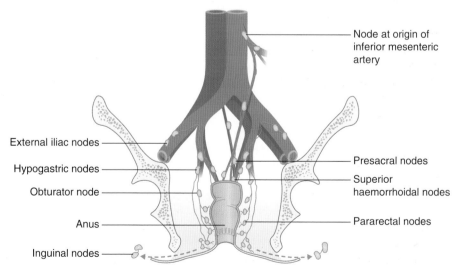

Figure 27.2 Lymphatic drainage of the anus.

Assessment of primary disease

A full history should elicit symptoms of local tumour and possible spread, and record comorbidities, PS and fitness for radical treatment. Clinical examination includes inspection of the perineal skin, DRE to assess the site and extent of the primary tumour, and vaginal examination to detect involvement of the posterior vaginal wall. Endoscopy may be performed to exclude a synchronous rectal or colonic tumour. HIV testing should be done in patients at risk. EUA allows detailed assessment, and biopsies of the tumour and of any enlarged inguinal lymph nodes >1 cm.

Thirty per cent of patients have enlarged inguinofemoral lymph nodes, of which 50 per cent are involved and 50 per cent show reactive inflammatory change only. Further local staging is performed with endorectal ultrasound and MR scan of the pelvis, and CT scan of the chest and abdomen to exclude distant metastases. FDG-PET scanning is useful in primary tumour staging and to assess residual, recurrent and metastatic disease.

Tumours of the anal canal and margin are staged according to the TNM and AJCC 2002 classification. The terms anal margin and perianal skin are synonymous and cancers at this site are classified as skin tumours. Poor prognostic factors are metastases, lymph node spread, higher T stage, older age, poor PS and anaemia (haemoglobin <10 g/dL).

Data acquisition

Patients are treated in the prone position, which displaces small bowel superiorly to reduce toxicity and allows easy visualisation of the anal verge for the application of radio-opaque markers and perianal bolus. The small bowel can also be displaced anteriorly by the use of devices such as a bellyboard, which allows it to fall forwards into the bellyboard aperture (Fig. 26.4, p. 317). Modern bellyboard devices are more comfortable, improve immobilisation and reduce set-up errors in the prone position. The AP separation is less in the prone position than supine.

Treatment is planned with CT scanning, virtual simulation or conventional simulator films. Oral contrast is used to delineate small bowel on CT scans or simulator films. Thin lead wire or a soft flexible catheter containing contrast delineates the anal canal. All palpable disease in the anal margin or lymph nodes is marked with radio-opaque material for identification on CT scans or simulator films. Surface boundaries of the inguinal region are marked on the skin with wire for simulation.

Target volume definition

Current trials such as the RTOG 0529 trial of IMRT for anal cancer define CT-based target volumes for anal cancer (see website below). In the UK the ACT II RCT defines the target volumes in terms of field borders for a two-phase shrinking field technique, which has ensured consistency of treatment between cancer centres.

■ CT planning

The phase 1 target volume includes all macroscopic primary tumour (GTV-T) and involved lymph nodes (GTV-N), and all microscopic disease at risk in the pelvis, inguinal and femoral regions (CTV-TN). The phase 2 target volume includes all macroscopic primary tumour (GTV-T) and involved lymph nodes if present (GTV-N) with a 10–15 mm margin for the CTV. Both these target volumes should be planned at the initial planning visit as the initial macroscopic disease may respond rapidly to treatment.

The extent of tumour in the anal canal is often difficult to determine on planning CT images or simulator films. It may be necessary to use the clinical information about the size of the tumour, its length and distance of the inferior limit from the anal verge to contour the GTV. Using radio-opaque wire on the anal verge and rectal contrast, the distance of the superior extent of the anal tumour from the anal verge can be confirmed. Diagnostic MR scans which show the extent of tumour in three dimensions can be fused with the planning CT scan, or measurements from MRI can be transferred onto the CT planning scan or simulator films.

CTV-PTV margins of 10–15 mm allow for patient positioning and set-up errors. OAR include the small bowel, bladder and vagina. Transplanted kidneys may lie in the pelvis and should be excluded from the treatment volume or repositioned.

■ Conventional planning

Phase 1 volume (all tumours):

- Superior border: 2 cm above inferior aspect of the sacroiliac joints is the standard border. However, the superior border should be enlarged to include a minimum margin of 3 cm above the upper extent of GTV-T or GTV-N.
- Lateral border: to include both inguinal nodal regions – in practice this border lies lateral to the femoral head.
- Inferior border: 3 cm below the anal margin (for disease confined to the anal canal only) or 3 cm below the most inferior extent of tumour (for anal margin tumours)

These borders are shown in Fig. 27.3.

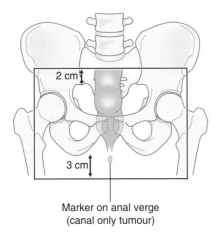

2 cm

3 cm

Marker on anal verge
(canal only tumour)

Figure 27.3 Phase 1 treatment borders for all anal tumours (from ACT II). Reproduced with permission from Dr D Sebag-Montefiore on behalf of the ACT II triallists.

Phase 2 volume

The volume depends on the presence or absence of positive nodes in the inguinofemoral or pelvic regions and is defined from CT scanning. Lymph nodes that are likely to contain tumour should be treated to the full phase 2 dose.

Phase 2 volume for lymph node negative cases (N0)

All borders allow 3 cm around the GTV defined at initial planning as shown in Fig. 27.4 for anal canal tumours and Fig. 27.5 for anal margin tumours.

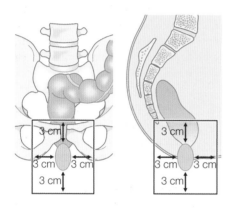

Figure 27.4 Phase 2 treatment borders for N0 anal canal tumours (ACTII). Reproduced with permission from Dr D Sebag-Montefiore on behalf of the ACT II triallists.

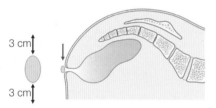

Figure 27.5 Phase 2 treatment borders for N0 anal margin tumours (ACTII). Direct field with 3 cm margins superiorly, inferiorly and lateral to GTV. Reproduced with permission from Dr D Sebag-Montefiore on behalf of the ACT II triallists.

Phase 2 volume for lymph node positive disease (N+)

Figure 27.6 shows borders for treatment of GTV with a 3 cm margin and MLC or lead shielding to exclude normal tissue and reduce toxicity.

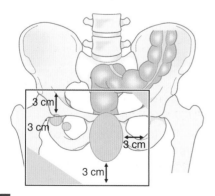

Figure 27.6 Phase 2 treatment borders for N+ anal tumours (ACTII). Reproduced with permission from Dr D Sebag-Montefiore on behalf of the ACT II triallists.

Dose solutions

■ Primary radiotherapy

Conformal/conventional

Phase 1

Beam arrangements are chosen to cover the PTV as defined above, but commonly anterior and posterior opposing beams are used with MLC shielding to normal tissues. With conventional planning, standard borders are used as described above.

High photon energies (10–20 MV) give more satisfactory dose distributions, especially for large patients. Bolus is used between the buttocks and over the perineum to ensure adequate dose to anal margin tumours and tumours within 2 cm of the anal verge. Superoinferior dose compensation may be needed to improve dose homogeneity.

Phase 2 (node negative)

A planned volume with three or four beams is used for anal canal tumours with no involved lymph nodes. A posterior and two wedged lateral beams are used to cover the PTV with a fourth anterior beam added if it improves dose distribution. In the future, with better definition of target volumes, IMRT with sparing of normal tissues may be used.

For patients with disease confined to the anal margin only, a direct photon beam, or electron therapy with energy chosen to encompass the CTV within the 90 per cent isodose, is used. Photons may give better coverage at depth with less lateral scatter than with electrons.

This is best planned in the simulator under direct vision. Tumours that extend onto the anal margin and anal canal tumours that extend to within 2 cm of the anal verge require bolus to the perianal skin to ensure they are not underdosed. Small bolus bags or a custom-made wax block can be used.

Phase 2 (node positive)

For anal canal tumours with involved lymph nodes, anterior and posterior opposing beams are used in the same way as for phase 1 with MLC shielding to as much small bowel and bladder as possible. CT virtual simulation can be used to create a 3 cm margin around the GTV-T and involved lymph nodes (GTV-N) with MLC shaping.

■ Postoperative radiotherapy

As discussed above the need for postoperative treatment following surgery is now uncommon.

In cases where there has been incomplete excision or involved circumferential margins, the patient can be treated with chemoradiotherapy in a similar fashion to that described above for lymph node negative cases. The phase 2 borders are based on the site of the tumour bed, using information from the operation notes and preoperative imaging. For small tumours less than 2 cm with close margins or incomplete excision, single-phase conformal planning or interstitial brachytherapy may be used.

■ Palliative radiotherapy

In patients who present with metastatic disease the initial treatment is with systemic chemotherapy if they are fit. If the volume of metastatic disease is small, many patients benefit from additional chemoradiotherapy to achieve local control in the pelvis. This can be planned as outlined above for radical chemoradiotherapy, or as a smaller volume single-phase treatment of GTV plus a 3D margin of 3 cm. In patients who are unfit for radical treatment, small volume radiotherapy to conventional palliative doses may be used.

■ Interstitial brachytherapy

Both LDR iridium wire and HDR afterloading perineal implants can be used to treat anal cancers. Brachytherapy alone can be used for small T1 tumours and as a boost following radical chemoradiotherapy with local control rates of 80–90 per cent. It can also be used for palliative treatment of recurrent or locally advanced tumours.

Dose-fractionation

■ Curative or adjuvant chemoradiotherapy

Phase 1

30.6 Gy in 17 daily fractions of 1.8 Gy given in 3½ weeks.

Phase 2

19.8 Gy in 11 daily fractions of 1.8 Gy given in 2½ weeks
or

Single phase

50.4 Gy in 28 daily fractions of 1.8 Gy given in 6 weeks.

■ Palliative radiotherapy

8 Gy single fraction.
20 Gy in 5 daily fractions of 4 Gy given in 1 week.

Low dose chemoradiotherapy

30 Gy in 15 daily fractions given in 3 weeks to GTV + 3 cm margin with continuous 5FU.

Treatment delivery and patient care

Patients are treated prone either flat on the couch or using a bellyboard immobilisation system with a full bladder. It is important that set-up for anal margin tumours is checked on the first day by the radiotherapist to ensure that there is adequate cover of the primary tumour inferiorly.

This is one of the few radical treatments where grade 3 and 4 toxicity is expected. The perineal and inguinal tissues are particularly sensitive to irradiation and skin reactions are often brisk and painful. Regular review and use of hydrocolloid dressings, nutritional support, analgesia and antidiarrhoeal medication are essential.

During concomitant chemotherapy, patients should receive appropriate antiemetics, and prophylactic antibiotic cover is advised for the duration of treatment. Blood tests are monitored regularly for myelosuppression and any sign of infection treated promptly.

Verification

Lasers and skin tattoos are used to align the patient each day and lateral tattoos over the iliac crests help to prevent lateral rotation. Electronic portal imaging is used to verify the treatment set-up and the EPIs are compared with the DRR images. Set-up can be monitored with EPIs according to local protocols during treatment with correction for displacements outside tolerance levels of 5–8 mm. Potential changes to radiotherapy target volumes and dose escalation, IGRT with kV and cone beam CT may come to play a greater role in anal cancer radiotherapy.

key trials

Ajani JA, Winter KA, Gunderson LL *et al.* (2008) Fluorouracil, mitomycin, and radiotherapy vs fluorouracil, cisplatin, and radiotherapy for carcinoma of the anal canal: a randomised controlled trial. *JAMA 23*: **299**: 1914–21.

Bartelink H, Roelofsen F, Eschwege F *et al.* (1997) Concomitant radiotherapy and chemotherapy is superior to radiotherapy alone in the treatment of locally advanced anal cancer: results of a phase III randomised trial of the European Organization for Research and Treatment of Cancer Radiotherapy and Gastrointestinal Cooperative Groups. *J Clin Oncol* **15**: 2040–9.

Flam M, John M, Pajak TF *et al.* (1996) Role of mitomycin in combination with fluorouracil and radiotherapy, and of salvage chemoradiation in the definitive nonsurgical treatment of epidermoid carcinoma of the anal canal: results of a phase III randomised intergroup study. *J Clin Oncol* **14**: 2527–39.

Glynne-Jones R, Meadows H, Wan S *et al.* (2008) EXTRA—A multicenter phase II study of chemoradiation using a 5 day per week oral regimen of capecitabine and intravenous mitomycin C in anal cancer. *Int J Radiat Oncol Biol Phys* **72**: 119–26.

James R, Meadows H, Wan S (2005) ACT II: the second UK phase III anal cancer trial. *Clin Oncol* **17**: 364–6.

Nigro ND, Vaitkevicius VK, Considine B Jr (1974) Combined therapy for cancer of the anal canal: a preliminary report. *Dis Colon Rectum* **17**: 354–6.

UKCCCR Anal Cancer Trial Working Party. UK Co-ordinating Committee on Cancer Research (1996) Epidermoid anal cancer: results from the UKCCCR randomised trial of radiotherapy alone versus radiotherapy, 5-fluorouracil, and mitomycin. *Lancet* **348**: 1049–54.

Information sources

ACT II Trial. Available at: www.ucl.ac.uk/cancertrials/trials/actii/index.htm (accessed 8 December 2008).

Brachytherapy (2005) In: Hoskin P, Coyle C (eds) *Radiotherapy in Practice*. Oxford University Press, Oxford.

Charnley N, Choudhury A, Chesser P *et al.* (2005) Effective treatment of anal cancer in the elderly with low-dose chemoradiotherapy. *Br J Cancer* **92**: 1221–5.

Elective Clinical Target Volumes in Anorectal Cancer: An RTOG Consensus Panel Contouring Atlas. Available at: www.rtog.org/

28 Prostate

Indications for radiotherapy

Prostate cancer is now the commonest cancer in men, accounting for almost 25 per cent of all new male cancer diagnoses and is the second most common cause of cancer related death in men. There has been a huge rise in the recorded incidence of prostate cancer with the use of prostate-specific antigen (PSA) and surgery for benign prostatic hypertrophy (BPH), but this is not reflected in increased mortality rates. There are almost 32 000 new cases and 10 000 deaths from prostate cancer a year in the UK. However, most men die with their prostate cancer rather than from it and management must balance the potential toxicity of active treatment, with the chances of benefit in a disease with a long natural history.

Advances in diagnosis and screening policies with the use of PSA have led to a stage migration so that prostate cancer is now detected at earlier stages with better prognostic features.

The most common type of prostate cancer is adenocarcinoma (95 per cent). Tumours are graded using the Gleason scoring system which evaluates architectural details of individual cancer glands and describes five distinct growth patterns from Gleason 1 (well differentiated) to Gleason 5 (poorly differentiated). The two commonest growth patterns seen are summated to give a final Gleason score (GS) ranging from 2 $(1 + 1)$ to 10 $(5 + 5)$. There are other rarer types of prostate carcinoma such as ductal, intralobular acinar, small cell and clear cell. This chapter focuses on the treatment of the common adenocarcinoma. There is less evidence to guide treatment of other pathological subtypes. Prostate cancer is staged using the AJCC and TNM staging.

Tumours are stratified by T stage, GS and PSA into three prognostic groups of low, intermediate and high risk:

- low risk: T1–T2a and PSA <10 ng/mL and GS ≤6
- intermediate risk: T2b or PSA 10–20 ng/mL or GS 7
- high risk: T2c–T4 or PSA >20 ng/mL or GS 8–10.

The risk is higher in an intermediate risk patient who has GS $4 + 3$ than with GS $3 + 4$.

Patients can be offered appropriate treatment options by a multidisciplinary team, according to stage of disease, prognostic risk group and estimated survival taking into account performance status and comorbidity.

■ Curative radiotherapy

EBRT, interstitial brachytherapy and surgery are options for the curative treatment of localised prostate cancer with equivalent outcomes but different side effects.

The options for treatment of low, intermediate and high risk prostate cancer are listed in Box 28.1. Factors that influence the choice include PS, other medical illnesses, likelihood of progression to symptomatic disease, life expectancy, morbidity of treatment (particularly on sexual function) and patient preference.

Box 28.1 Treatment options for localised prostate cancer

Low risk: (T1–T2a), PSA <10 ng/mL, GS ≤6)

- Active surveillance
- Prostate iodine-125 brachytherapy
- Radical prostatectomy (open/laparoscopic/robotic)
- Radical EBRT ± 6 months HT
- Watchful waiting

Intermediate risk (T2b or PSA 10–20 or GS 7)

- Prostate^{125}I brachytherapy (T2b GS 3+4 [in <50 per cent tumour sample] and PSA <15)
- Radical prostatectomy (open/laparoscopic/robotic)
- Radical EBRT with 6 months HT (±WPRT)
- Watchful waiting

High risk:(≥T2c–T4 or PSA >20 or GS ≥8)

- Radical EBRT with 2–3 years HT (±WPRT)
- Hormone therapy alone
- Watchful waiting

HT, hormone therapy; WPRT, whole pelvis radiotherapy.

In general patients should have a life expectancy of greater than 10 years before radical treatment is recommended. Men younger than 75 with other major illnesses such as ischaemic heart disease and diabetes may not live 10 years and men over 75 with no other illnesses may live into their nineties. There is evidence that radical radiotherapy in fit men over 75 is very well tolerated and just as effective. It is the role of the multidisciplinary team to identify patients who will benefit from radical treatment and counsel the patient on the different options available. Radical treatments with surgery, EBRT or brachytherapy have similar outcomes and the patient should be informed of the different side effects of each treatment. Factors that influence the final choice for an individual patient include lower urinary tract symptoms, sexual function, likelihood of infertility, and risks of anaesthesia and surgery. The benefits and risks of surgery, EBRT and brachytherapy are shown in Table 28.1.

The results of radiotherapy are assessed by monitoring the PSA, DRE and symptoms and signs of metastases. A PSA nadir of <2 within 2 years is associated with long-term control. Biochemical failure is defined by a rise in PSA by 2.0 ng/mL above the nadir level following radiotherapy, according to the international RTOG-ASTRO

Table 28.1 Benefits and risks of radical treatment options for localised disease

Treatment	Advantages	Disadvantages
EBRT	Curative No operation No anaesthetic No hospital admission Maintain usual activities during treatment PSA monitoring to detect recurrence (more difficult to interpret than after surgery)	Daily treatment for 6–8 weeks Combined with hormone therapy with side effects Early side effects: • Cystitis and diarrhoea • Fatigue Late side effects: • Rectal toxicity • RTOG G2 12 per cent G3 1 per cent • Bladder toxicity • RTOG G2 10 per cent • Impotence 50 per cent • Infertility
Brachytherapy	Curative 1–2 day-case visits Quick recovery No hormone therapy PSA monitoring to detect recurrence (can take 2 years for PSA to fall) May remain fertile	Needs anaesthetic Early side effects: • Urinary retention 10 per cent • Local discomfort • Urgency and cystitis • Impotence 25–50 per cent • Proctitis 2–5 per cent Late side effects: • Bladder toxicity • RTOG G2 30 per cent • Urethral stricture 10 per cent • Impotence <25 per cent • Incontinence 1 per cent • Rectal bleeding 24 per cent
Surgery	Curative Also treats BPH and symptoms Pathological assessment of whole prostate PSA falls quickly following surgery allowing monitoring	Risks of major surgery 3–7 days as in-patient 6 weeks recovery May leave cells that have breached the capsule Early side effects: • Incontinence (recovers in 6 weeks) • Risks of PE/DVT • Mortality 0.16–0.66 per cent Late side effects: • Incontinence 2–10 per cent • Impotence 5–60 per cent • Stricture 0.5–9 per cent • Infertility
Active surveillance	Avoid unnecessary treatment No side effects	'Worry' while closely monitored Treatment may be needed at later date Only an option for cancers with a low risk of progression

Phoenix consensus. Published nomograms are very useful for assessing potential benefits from treatment. The Memorial Sloane Kettering pretreatment nomogram gives a 5-year progression-free probability following radical EBRT from 70–90 per cent for low risk to 50–70 per cent for intermediate risk and 20–50 per cent for high risk prostate cancer.

■ Pelvic lymph node radiotherapy

Selected patients may benefit from radiotherapy to the pelvic lymph nodes with the prostate and seminal vesicles. A randomised trial has shown that patients with a risk of lymph node involvement between 15 per cent and 35 per cent may benefit from pelvic lymph node irradiation. However, although pelvic radiotherapy has shown a trend to improved 5-year progression-free survival, but not overall survival, this benefit is only seen in patients receiving neoadjuvant, concurrent and adjuvant hormone therapy. This has to be balanced with the increased toxicity associated with WPRT. With modern techniques, including IMRT and IGRT, this balance may become more favourable.

■ Adjuvant and salvage radiotherapy

Adjuvant radiotherapy is not given routinely when PSA levels are undetectable after surgery to avoid overtreatment of the majority of patients already cured. If the PSA is persistently raised following surgery, it may indicate local or metastatic disease. After negative staging investigations, metastases are still likely if the PSA doubling time is <9 months, and local radiotherapy is therefore not recommended. Seminal vesicle or lymph node involvement, especially with a high Gleason score, also correlates with risk of metastases and makes radical local radiotherapy inappropriate. If there is a persistently raised PSA with a doubling time >9 months and there are positive margins at the site of extracapsular extension, local radiotherapy should be considered. Results are better with early salvage radiotherapy when the PSA is <1.2 ng/mL (or 0.2 with the supersensitive assay). In patients in whom PSA later rises on three consecutive occasions (ASTRO definition of biochemical failure), salvage radiotherapy is also offered. Clinical trials of radiotherapy may be appropriate for patients with high risk factors for local recurrence but undetectable PSA.

■ Palliative radiotherapy

Prostate and pelvis

Patients with extensive local disease in the prostate and/or pelvis may benefit from a course of palliative EBRT to relieve symptoms. Bleeding from the prostate may also be alleviated by EBRT.

Bone and lymph node metastases

EBRT is an excellent treatment for palliation of pain from symptomatic bone metastasis. A single fraction of 8 Gy is very effective with few side effects. A fractionated course of EBRT may be used to treat spinal cord compression, and is given postoperatively following orthopaedic fixation of pathological fractures. Symptoms from lymph node and visceral metastases can also be relieved by EBRT.

Radionuclide therapy

Patients with metastatic bone disease and multiple painful sites can be difficult to treat with EBRT to localised areas. The radionucleotides strontium and samarium have been shown to be beneficial in reducing symptoms from bone metastases. This treatment is only considered for patients with good bone marrow reserve, no imminent risk of cord compression and no nodal or visceral metastases.

Breast buds

Gynaecomastia is a major problem for patients on long-term anti-androgen and oestrogen therapy. Superficial X-ray or electron therapy (9–12 MeV) to the breast bud area using a 7–9 cm diameter circular field has been shown to reduce the incidence significantly when used prophylactically. In established cases, radiotherapy can reduce symptoms.

Sequencing of multimodality therapy

■ EBRT and hormone therapy

Hormone therapy before, during and after EBRT (neoadjuvant, concurrent and adjuvant androgen deprivation [NCAD]) has been proven to increase local control, disease-free survival and overall survival for selected patients with prostate cancer. Androgen deprivation reduces the size of the prostate by 30 per cent and the number of tumour cells, possibly through synergistic apoptotic mechanisms.

Six months NCAD can be used with EBRT for low and intermediate risk disease to reduce the target volume and allow safer dose escalation. Treatment must be started at least 2 months before radiotherapy. NCAD with 2–3 years continuing adjuvant androgen deprivation is beneficial for high risk disease (Table 28.2).

Table 28.2 Summary of EBRT target volumes and duration of hormone therapy according to risk group

Risk group	Low	Intermediate	High
Target volume	Prostate + BSV	Prostate + BSV/SV ±WPRT	Prostate + SV ±WPRT
Duration of hormone therapy	None or 6 months	6 months	2–3 years

BSV, base of seminal vesicle; SV, seminal vesicle; WPRT, whole pelvic radiotherapy. The SV is included if the risk of SV involvement is greater than 15 per cent using the Roach formula: SV risk = PSA + [(GS−6) × 10].

Standard androgen deprivation is achieved by cyproterone acetate 100 mg three times daily or bicalutamide 50 mg once daily for 3 weeks starting 1 week before the first LH-releasing hormone agonist/antagonist (LHRHa) injection. The LHRHa is continued monthly for 6 months and then 3 monthly for 2–3 years in high risk cases.

■ EBRT and brachytherapy boost

HDR and LDR brachytherapy may be used as a boost after EBRT to escalate dose to the prostate.

■ EBRT and chemotherapy

The combination of chemotherapy and EBRT for high risk prostate cancer is currently under investigation.

Clinical and radiological anatomy

The prostate gland lies between the pubic symphysis and the anterior rectal wall and is closely applied to the bladder neck and seminal vesicles (Fig. 28.1). The lymphatics drain from the prostate to the obturator, presacral, internal, external, common iliac and para-aortic lymph nodes (Fig. 28.2).

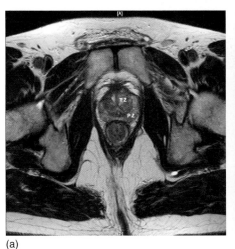
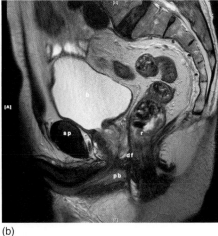

(a)   (b)

Figure 28.1 Anatomy of prostate shown on T2-weighted MRI. (a) Axial (TZ transitional zone, PZ peripheral zone). (b) Sagittal (pb, penile bulb; b, bladder; sp, symphysis pubis; r, rectum; df, Denonvilliers' fascia).

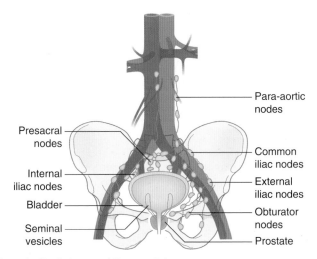

Figure 28.2 Lymphatic drainage of the prostate.

Assessment of primary disease

Prostate cancer is confirmed by multiple biopsies under transrectal ultrasound guidance or transperineally using a perineal template.

The extent of primary disease is assessed by MRI of the prostate and MRI or CT scan of the pelvis and abdomen to detect locoregional and distant spread. Prostate cancer can extend through the prostate capsule, especially posteriorly, at the apex, and at the junctions between the base and bladder neck and seminal vesicles. Denovilliers' fascia reduces spread towards the rectum. Extraprostatic extension is shown on MRI in Fig. 28.3. Spread occurs to the seminal vesicles and lymph nodes with increasing tumour stage and histological grade. The risk of microscopic seminal vesicle and lymph node involvement can be assessed by nomograms or Roach formulae, both based on the Partin data.

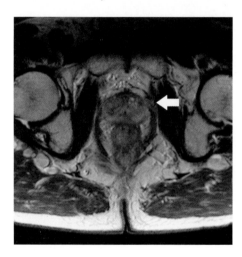

Figure 28.3 T2-weighted MRI showing T3 prostate cancer with extraprostatic extension on left.

Roach formulae:

Percentage risk of seminal vesicle involvement = PSA + [(GS − 6) × 10]

Percentage risk of LN involvement = 2/3 PSA + [(GS − 6) × 10]

Patients in the intermediate and high risk groups also need a bone scan except those with a PSA <20.

Data acquisition

■ Immobilisation

A planning CT scan is obtained in the treatment position. Patients are treated supine rather than prone as this has been shown to produce less prostate motion, reduce doses to normal organs at risk, and is more comfortable for the patient.

A bladder filling protocol should be used to maintain a constant bladder filling – 'comfortably full'. Patients are asked to empty the bladder and drink 200 mL of water 20 min before the scan and before treatment each day. A completely full bladder has been shown to displace small bowel away from the treated volume, but it also leads to greater variation in prostate position and is not recommended. The rectum should be empty for treatment as a full rectum also leads to greater variation in prostate position. Patients should be advised on a low residue diet and if they have a full rectum at the time of planning CT scan should receive further dietary advice before repeating the scan. The use of laxatives, suppositories, enemas and endorectal balloons during treatment continues to be investigated.

An immobilisation system using a head pad combined with individually adjustable knee and ankle supports provides a high degree of accuracy without the need for further pelvic immobilisation (Fig. 28.4).

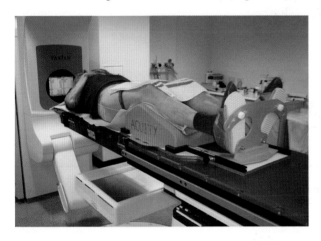

Figure 28.4 Immobilisation for treatment of prostate cancer.

■ CT scanning

With the patient immobilised in the treatment position following bladder and rectal protocols, a radiotherapy planning CT scan is performed. Skin reference tattoos are placed anteriorly on the midline of the symphysis pubis and laterally over the hips and aligned with lasers to prevent lateral rotation. Radio-opaque markers are placed on the skin to locate the tattoos on the CT scans. The CT scan is taken with 3–5 mm slices from the mid sacroiliac joint to 1 cm below the anus/ischium to include the prostate, seminal vesicles, rectum and bladder, and is extended superiorly to L3 if the pelvic lymph nodes are to be treated. No oral or rectal contrast is used, but intravenous contrast may aid delineation of the pelvic lymph nodes. At the time of the planning CT scan, the size of the rectum and bladder should be assessed. If the bladder is empty or the rectum is >4 cm in AP diameter at the level of the prostate base, the scan should be repeated after implementing the bladder and rectal protocols until the desired parameters are met. Inappropriately large rectal volumes have been shown to reduce local control rates by moving the prostate out of the planned PTV.

CT data are then transferred to a radiotherapy planning computer for outlining and target volume definition. To improve target definition, MR scans of the pelvis can be incorporated into radiotherapy planning protocols. Outlining studies have shown that the size of the prostate is overestimated on CT compared with MRI, which defines the apex of the prostate better and is associated with less image degradation with fiducial markers. Solutions to overcome the geometrical distortion and shift artefact seen with MRI are currently being investigated. CT-MRI image registration (Fig. 28.5) is useful for defining the contour of the prostate especially at the apex and for IGRT with fiducial markers.

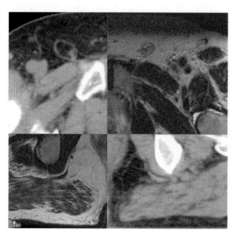

Figure 28.5 Co-registration of CT and MR images for target volume definition.

Target volume definition

■ Prostate ± seminal vesicles

It is not possible to define the GTV accurately with current imaging techniques. It is therefore standard practice to define a CTV that includes the whole prostate and any possible extracapsular extension, with either the base of, or the entire seminal vesicles. The risk of involvement of the seminal vesicles is defined using the Roach formulae and target volume chosen accordingly.

Low risk of seminal vesicle involvement

PSA + [(GS − 6) × 10] <15 per cent
CTV to include prostate + base of seminal vesicles.

Moderate/high risk of seminal vesicle involvement

T3 or (PSA + [(GS − 6) × 10]) >15 per cent
CTV to include prostate and seminal vesicles.

Prostate outlining starts on the mid gland slice along the fat plane between the prostate and pelvic floor muscles and along Denovilliers' fascia posteriorly. Defining the apex can be difficult and this can be aided with reference to diagnostic MR scans or by image registration as discussed above. The base of the seminal vesicles is included in the CTV for all patients. This is defined as 1–2 cm of central seminal vesicles proximal to the base of the prostate often at the same level as the middle lobe that bulges into the bladder. When the entire seminal vesicles are to be included in the CTV, the distal ends may have to be excluded if the seminal vesicles wrap around the prostate, to keep the rectal dose within safe limits. Studies have shown that 90 per cent of seminal vesicle involvement is limited to the proximal 2 cm.

The PTV is defined with a 3D margin around the CTV to include an internal margin accounting for physiological variations in the shape, position and size of the prostate, and a set-up margin to compensate for uncertainties in patient position and set-up during planning and treatment. The set-up margins can be measured with verification studies and quality assurance programmes. The standard margin is 10 mm grown isotropically around the CTV. To limit the dose to the rectum, the posterior margin is reduced to 5 mm if verification studies allow, and is reduced further for a phase 2 volume when needed, to keep within rectal dose constraints. If the rectal volume cannot be reduced to <4 cm in diameter at the base of the prostate, the margins from CTV to PTV may need to be increased posteriorly.

Image guidance techniques discussed later will allow further safe reduction of these margins.

Single phase

CTV 74 = Prostate + base of the seminal vesicles (SV) (or whole SV).
PTV 74 = CTV74 + 10 mm sup/inf/right/left/ant and 5–10 mm post.

Two phase

Phase 1

CTV 56 = Prostate + base SV (or whole SV).
PTV 56 = CTV56 + 10 mm sup/inf/right/left/ant and 5–10 mm post.

Phase 2

CTV 74 = Prostate only.
PTV 74 = CTV74 + 10 mm sup/inf/right/left/ant and 0–5 mm post.

■ Pelvic lymph nodes

Selected patients with a risk of lymph node involvement 15–35 per cent, according to the Roach formula, may benefit from pelvic lymph node irradiation.

Roach formula

Risk of lymph node involvement = 2/3 PSA + [(GS − 6) × 10]

Clinical target volume for these patients includes prostate, seminal vesicles and the common, internal and external iliac, presacral, hypogastric and obturator lymph nodes. The lymph node areas should be outlined according to published guidelines and using contrast-enhanced vessels and a pelvic lymph node atlas (Fig. 28.6).

The prostate and seminal vesicles can be outlined as CTV-T and the lymph node areas as CTV-N as follows.

Phase 1 Pelvis and prostate

CTV T 46 = Prostate and SV.
CTV N 46 = Lymph nodes areas.
PTV TN 46 = CTV T 46 + 10 mm sup/inf/right/left/ant and 5–10 mm post.
CTV N 46 + 5–10 mm.

Phase 2 Prostate + SV

CTV T 56 = Prostate + SV.
PTV 56 = CTV T 56 + 10 mm sup/inf/right/left/ant and 5–10 mm post.

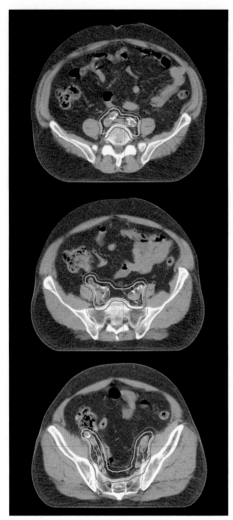

Figure 28.6 CTV and PTV for pelvic node irradiation shown on three level axial CT scans (blood vessels – yellow).

Phase 3 Prostate

CTV T 74 = Prostate only.
PTV 74 = CTV T 74 + 10 mm sup/inf/right/left/ant and 2–5 mm post.

■ Prostate bed

After prostatectomy there is no GTV. The CTV is the prostate bed as best defined on the CT planning scan. The histopathology report of the prostatectomy specimen and preoperative MRI can be helpful. The CTV is based on an estimation of the location of the prostate preoperatively and is centred on the vesico-urethral junction. Surgical clips within the prostate bed are included in the CTV but those in the anatomical position of vessels are not. The preoperative location of the seminal vesicles is included if pathologically involved or the risk of seminal vesicle involvement according to the Roach formula is >15 per cent.

CTV

Inferior border
5 mm cranial to superior border of the penile bulb.

Anterior border
Posterior aspect of symphysis pubis (<2 cm above the vesico-urethral anastomosis).
Posterior 1/3 of bladder wall (>2 cm above anastomosis).

Posterior border
Anterior rectal wall.

Lateral border
Medial border of obturator internus and levator ani muscles.

Superior border
Base of SV if uninvolved and risk <15 per cent.
Distal ends of SV if involved or risk >15 per cent.
The PTV is the CTV + 1 cm isotropically.

■ OAR

The OAR are the rectum, bladder, nerves of the prostatic plexus lying adjacent to the penile bulb, small bowel and femoral heads. The rectum is outlined from the inferior level of the ischial tuberosities and at least 1 cm below the PTV to the recto-sigmoid junction above the PTV to give a length of approximately 12 cm. Consideration of small bowel in the target volume is important when pelvic nodes are treated.

Dose solutions

■ Conformal

Using forward planning, an optimal dose distribution is calculated. Beams with customised MLC shielding are chosen to include the PTV within the 95 per cent isodose and minimise the dose to the OAR. The beams, dose weighting and wedging are optimised. A standard approach is to use a technique with an anterior and two wedged posterior oblique beams as shown in Fig. 28.7. In some cases, wedged lateral beams may spare more normal rectum, and four or six coplanar beam arrangements may reduce doses to the OAR further. When treating the pelvic lymph nodes, an anterior and two wedged lateral beams are used, with a posterior beam if necessary.

The dose to OAR is assessed by DVHs. Plans are reviewed to minimise hot-spots in OAR. The acceptable dose constraints for OAR are shown in Table 4.1 (p. 49).

■ Complex

The increased conformity of IMRT using inverse planning techniques ensures better coverage of the target volume, sparing of OAR, and safer dose escalation. It has significant advantages when irradiating the pelvic lymph nodes with the ability to conform to the nodes and spare normal bowel in the pelvis (Fig. 28.8).

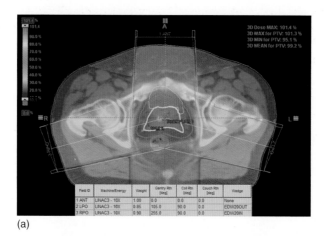

Figure 28.7 (a) Axial and (b) sagittal dose distributions of conformal treatment for prostate cancer. Bladder yellow; rectum brown.

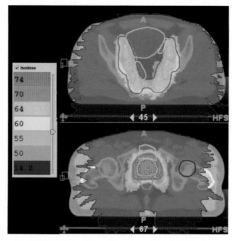

Figure 28.8 Tomotherapy IMRT plan for treatment of (a) pelvic lymph nodes and (b) prostate cancer.

There are many IMRT planning and delivery systems. Fixed delivery 'step and shoot' techniques use five equally spaced coplanar fields with the MLC set in various positions as defined by the inverse treatment plan to create the beam modulation needed. Alternatively, dynamic therapy or tomotherapy may be used.

■ Conventional

Palliative treatment to the prostate may be given using opposing anterior and posterior beams and MLC shielding, planned by CT virtual simulation or with a conventional simulator.

Dose-fractionation

■ Curative radiotherapy

Prostate ± SV

Single phase
74 Gy in 37 daily fractions given in 7½ weeks.

Two phase
Phase 1: prostate + SV 56 Gy in 28 daily fractions given in 5½ weeks.
Phase 2: prostate 18 Gy in 9 daily fractions given in 11–13 days

With conformal planning and IMRT the dose to the prostate + SV can be increased to 64 Gy with a 10 Gy prostate boost, if OAR dose constraints are met.

Prostate + SV + pelvis

Phase 1: Pelvic nodes + prostate + SV 46 Gy in 23 daily fractions given in 4½ weeks.
Phase 2: Prostate + SV 10 Gy in 5 daily fractions given in 1 week.
Phase 3: Prostate 18 Gy in 9 daily fractions given in 11–13 days.

Alternative fractionation schedules (to the prostate alone)

50 Gy in 16 daily fractions of 3.1 Gy (Manchester regimen) given in 3½ weeks.
55 Gy in 20 daily fractions of 2.75 Gy given in 4 weeks.

Prostate bed

66 Gy in 33 daily fractions given in 6½ weeks.

■ Palliative radiotherapy

Extensive symptomatic prostatic disease

30 Gy in 10 daily fractions given in 2 weeks.
36 Gy in 6 weekly fractions of 6 Gy given in 6 weeks.

Bone pain

8 Gy single fraction.
20 Gy in 5 daily fractions in 1 week.

Lymph node or visceral disease

20 Gy in 5 daily fractions given in 1 week.
30 Gy in 10 daily fractions given in 2 weeks.

Breast bud radiotherapy

Prophylaxis 8 Gy single fraction.
Palliation 12 Gy in 2 daily fractions given in 2 days.

Treatment delivery and patient care

The patient is treated supine with a comfortably full bladder and after rectal voiding. Immobilisation systems are used with anterior and lateral laser lights to align midline and lateral skin tattoos to prevent lateral rotation. The isocentre is marked with reference to the anterior tattoo over the pubic symphysis.

Severe skin reactions are rare but may occur over the sacrum and natal cleft. If loose stools develop, a low residue diet is advised to prevent diarrhoea. Loperamide hydrochloride may be used for diarrhoea with care to avoid constipation. Mild proctitis and tenesmus are common and if severe, may be treated with steroid or local anaesthetic suppositories. Urinary symptoms of frequency, urgency and slow stream are common. Patients should remain well hydrated and a mid-stream urine should be examined to exclude infection. Patients with pre-existing obstructive problems may be helped by α-blockers such as tamsulosin. Cystitis may be helped by potassium citrate, cranberry juice or simple analgesia.

After radiotherapy, the incidence of grade 3 chronic intestinal sequelae requiring hospitalisation for diagnosis and/or minimal intervention is 3 per cent. Most cases occur within 3–4 years of treatment. A gastroenterologist should investigate rectal bleeding, diarrhoea, urgency and tenesmus. Argon plasma coagulation (APC), a non-contact thermal coagulation technique, applied endoscopically, can be used to treat chronic radiation proctitis. In very severe cases, formalin or a combination of APC and topical formalin can be useful.

The incidence of impotence is 30–50 per cent and may be reduced by excluding the penile bulb from treatment.

Verification

Electronic portal images are taken for the first 3–5 days of treatment and compared with DRRs from the planning CT scan, using bony landmarks, the beam edges and centre. The set-up error is calculated from any differences and may be corrected according to local protocol.

IGRT may improve accuracy of treatment delivery. The use of radio-opaque fiducial markers within the prostate allows variations arising from prostate movement to be identified and incorporated into the local protocol. Commercial systems such as Acculoc are available and have been shown to improve targeting of dose. Less invasive methods include the BATS ultrasound system and cone-beam CT scans taken before treatment to localise the prostate.

Diodes or TLD measurements on the first treatment day are used to measure dose delivered.

Prostate brachytherapy

Prostate brachytherapy is an excellent option for patients with localised low risk prostate cancer. Patients with intermediate risk prostate cancer can be treated with brachytherapy alone, but as the risk of disease outside the prostate capsule increases, EBRT alone or in combination with brachytherapy should be considered.

Indications for brachytherapy:

- life expectancy >10 years
- biopsy-confirmed adenocarcinoma prostate
- low risk disease: T1–T2a, PSA <10, GS 6
- intermediate risk disease: T1–T2a, PSA <15, GS 3 + 4 (low volume)
- prostate volume <50 mL (dynamic techniques can treat up to 90 mL).

It is important to select patients with no significant urinary outflow obstruction since they are at increased risk of urinary retention and morbidity following brachytherapy. Ideally patients should have an international prostate symptom score (IPSS) of <12 and urine flow rate Q_{max} of >15 mL/s.

■ LDR permanent seed brachytherapy

The most frequently used isotope is iodine-125. An alternative is palladium-103, which has a higher dose rate. The Seattle technique involves a planning study under general anaesthesia with the patient in the lithotomy position. A transrectal ultrasound (TRUS) probe is inserted into the rectum attached to a stepping unit that can advance or retract the probe (Fig. 28.9). Attached to the TRUS is a template, the coordinates of which are transposed onto the ultrasound images of the prostate. Serial ultrasound sections with 5 mm slices of the prostate from the base to the apex are captured onto the planning computer. The prostate, urethra (identified with the aid of aerosolised jelly) and rectum are outlined on the ultrasound images. A margin of 2–3 mm is added in all directions except posteriorly to form the PTV. A computer program is used to calculate the exact number and position of seeds required. It will also calculate where needles must be inserted in the template to achieve the desired distribution of seeds in the prostate. For treatment a second anaesthetic is needed, and with the patient and prostate in exactly the same position as in the planning study, needles are inserted through the template, and seeds implanted into the prostate using a stranded or loose seed technique.

It is difficult to replicate the planning position and the prostate moves when needles are inserted. To overcome this, the technique has now been modified into a single anaesthetic, single stage inverse planned procedure. Intraoperative dosimetry can now be planned from needle location. The Pötter technique involves inserting needles into the prostate at 1 cm intervals with a peripheral:central ratio of 3:1. The needle position is registered on the planning software with the ultrasound slices as above. Once the prostate volume has been outlined, the computer generates a plan within 45 s. Advanced dynamic dose calculation can capture seed position in real time continuously updating dosimetry as seeds are inserted. Any deviations from the plan can be corrected in real time before the end of the procedure.

Current standard reporting of dose is based on dosimetry from a CT scan performed 4 weeks after seed implantation when oedema has settled. Doses to the prostate, rectum and urethra are calculated. The V100 is the percentage of the

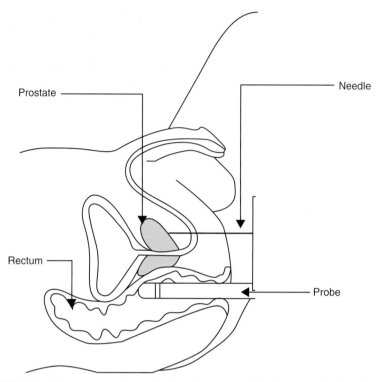

Figure 28.9 Technique for insertion of radioactive seeds into the prostate. Courtesy of Prostate Cancer Charity.

prostate volume that has received the 100 per cent prescription dose and should be >90 per cent. The D90 is the dose received by 90 per cent of the prostate volume and should be at least 90 per cent of the prescribed dose. The prostate V150 and V200 give a measure of the homogeneity of the dose distribution. The maximum rectal dose should be kept as low as possible. If it is less than 140 per cent of the treatment dose, the risk of proctitis is less than 1.2 per cent. The maximum urethral dose should be kept as low as possible, and should be less than 150 per cent of the treatment dose.

Using the same technique, LDR brachytherapy can be used for a boost treatment following EBRT to the prostate and pelvis.

■ HDR afterloading brachytherapy

HDR afterloading brachytherapy is performed under general anaesthesia using a stepping iridium-192 HDR machine. In contrast to LDR permanent seed implants, there is no calculated pre- or post-implant dosimetry, and dosimetry is defined by catheter position and dwell times. Large fraction sizes can be delivered which may have a biological advantage in prostate cancer. The technique reduces radiation exposure to the oncologist and other staff. The main use is as a boost treatment in conjunction with external beam radiotherapy. Afterloading catheters are inserted into the prostate through the perineum under TRUS guidance using a template that is sutured or fixed with adhesive to the patient. A CT scan is performed of the patient with the catheters in place and the dosimetry calculated on a 3D planning system. Several high dose fractions are then delivered in the HDR afterloading room and the patient remains an inpatient with an indwelling urinary catheter until the end of treatment. HDR monotherapy is performed in exactly the same way.

■ Dose-fractionation

Monotherapy

LDR 145 Gy (I-125), 125 Gy (Pa-103).
HDR 34–36 Gy in 4 fractions.

Combination therapy

LDR

EBRT: prostate ± pelvis 45 Gy in 25 daily fractions of 1.8 Gy given in 5 weeks.
Brachytherapy: 110 Gy (I-125), 90 Gy (Pa-103).

HDR

EBRT: prostate ± pelvis 45 Gy in 25 daily fractions of 1.8 Gy given in 5 weeks.
Brachytherapy: 17 Gy (Ir-192) in 2 fractions given in 24 hours.

key trials

Bolla M, Collette L, Blank L et al. (2002) Long-term results with immediate androgen suppression and external irradiation in patients with locally advanced prostate cancer (an EORTC study): a phase III randomised trial. *Lancet* **360**: 103–6.

Bolla M, van Poppel H, Collette L et al. (2005) Postoperative radiotherapy after radical prostatectomy: a randomised controlled trial (EORTC trial 22911). *Lancet* **366**: 572–8.

D'Amico AV, Manola J, Loffredo M et al. (2004) 6-month androgen suppression plus radiation therapy vs. radiation therapy alone for patients with clinically localised prostate cancer: a randomised controlled trial. *JAMA* **292**: 821–7.

Horwitz EM, Bae K, Hanks GE et al. (2008) Ten-year follow-up of Radiation Therapy Oncology Group protocol 92–02: a phase III trial of the duration of elective androgen deprivation in locally advanced prostate cancer. *J Clin Oncol* **26**: 2497–504.

Lawton CA, DeSilvio M, Roach M 3rd et al. (2007) An update of the phase III trial comparing whole pelvic to prostate only radiotherapy and neoadjuvant to adjuvant total androgen suppression: updated analysis of RTOG 94–13, with emphasis on unexpected hormone/radiation interactions. *Int J Radiat Oncol Biol Phys* **69**: 646–55.

Pollack A, Zagars GK, Starkschall G et al. (2002) Prostate cancer radiation dose response: results of the MD Anderson phase III randomised trial. *Int J Radiat Oncol Biol Phys* **53**: 1097–105.

Information sources

de Crevoisier R, Tucker SL, Dong L et al. (2005) Increased risk of biochemical and local failure in patients with distended rectum on the planning CT for prostate cancer radiotherapy. *Int J Radiat Oncol Biol Phys* **62**: 965–73.

Jackson ASN, Sohaiby SA, Staffurth JN et al. (2006) Distribution of lymph nodes in men with prostatic adenocarcinoma and lymphadenopathy at presentation: a retrospective radiological review and implications for prostate and pelvis radiotherapy. *Clin Oncol* **18**: 109–16.

Kupelian PA, Langen KM, Willoughby TR et al. (2008) Image-guided radiotherapy for localized prostate cancer: treating a moving target. *Semin Radiat Oncol* **18**: 58–66.

Memorial Sloane Kettering Prostate Cancer Nomogram. Available at www.mskcc.org

National Institute for Health and Clinical Excellence. (2008) *Prostate Cancer: Diagnosis and Treatment*. Clinical guidance 58. London, NICE. Available at www.nice.org.uk (accessed 9 December 2008).

Prostate Brachytherapy Video. Available at www.nyprostate.org

Prostate cancer risk management programme. Available at www.cancerscreening.nhs.uk/prostate/ (accessed 9 December 2008).

Roach M 3rd, Hanks G, Thames H Jr et al. (2006) Defining biochemical failure following radiotherapy with or without hormonal therapy in men with clinically localised prostate cancer: recommendations of the RTOG-ASTRO Phoenix Consensus Conference. *Int J Radiat Oncol Biol Phys* **65**: 965–74.

Taylor A, Rockall AG, Powell ME (2007) An atlas of the pelvic lymph node regions to aid radiotherapy target volume definition. *Clin Oncol* **19**: 542–50.

Bladder

29

Indications for radiotherapy

In the UK there are approximately 10 000 new cases of bladder cancer a year. The majority (85 per cent) are superficial bladder cancers confined to the mucosa with a 5-year survival rate of 80–90 per cent. However, 70 per cent recur and of these, 10–15 per cent develop muscle invasive bladder cancers within 5 years. Carcinoma *in situ* is usually more aggressive with up to 50 per cent progressing to muscle invasive cancers within 5 years. In the past 30 years, 5-year survival rates for muscle invasive bladder cancer have increased from 40 per cent to 60 per cent.

There has been a decrease in the use of radiotherapy as a single modality treatment and an increase in combined radical cystectomy and radiotherapy. There are no prospective randomised trials of radical cystectomy versus radiotherapy. When the effects of selection bias, stage migration due to clinical versus pathological staging and differences in prognostic factors are taken into account, there is little current evidence of a benefit of surgery over radiotherapy. Despite this, many still consider radical cystectomy to be the gold standard. Radical cystectomy involves *en bloc* removal of the pelvic lymph nodes and pelvic organs anterior to the rectum–bladder, urachus, and visceral peritoneum, with prostate and seminal vesicles in men and ovaries, fallopian tubes, uterus, cervix and vaginal cuff in women. Surgical techniques have improved including use of lower urinary tract orthotopic reconstructions. The best surgical series report 5-year recurrence free rates of 80 per cent for T2, N0, 55 per cent for T3, N0 and 30 per cent for Tx, N1 bladder cancer. Review of the world literature on outcomes following EBRT reports 5-year survival of 10–59 per cent for T2, 10–38 per cent for T3 and 0–16 per cent for T4 bladder cancers. A recent UK study has shown 5-year survival rates of 56.8 per cent after radical radiotherapy and 53.4 per cent after radical cystectomy in patients with invasive cancer, even though the patients undergoing radical cystectomy were significantly younger.

Ninety per cent of bladder cancers are urothelial (transitional cell) carcinomas (TCC), and 5 per cent are SCC. In areas where schistosomiasis is endemic, SCC constitutes up to 80 per cent of cases. Fewer than 5 per cent of cases are primary adenocarcinoma arising from the urachal remnant, small cell carcinoma, sarcoma, carcinosarcoma, lymphoma or melanoma. TCC is graded as G1 (well differentiated), G2 (moderately differentiated) and G3 (poorly differentiated). The tumour grade is an important predictor of tumour behaviour.

Bladder cancer is staged using the AJCC and TNM staging based on data from EUA and imaging. Tumours originate in the bladder epithelium and infiltrate deeply into the muscle layers, penetrating through the bladder wall into perivesical fat and adjacent pelvic organs. Lymphatic spread is first to the hypogastric, obturator, internal, external and common iliac lymph nodes and thence to the para-aortic and inguinal nodes. The risk of lymph node metastases relates to the depth of tumour invasion: 20 per cent for T1, 30 per cent for T2a and 60 per cent for T2b. More than a third of patients treated radically develop distant metastases within 18 months. Stage and grade of the tumour are the most important prognostic factors. The presence of extravesical spread (T3b) and lymph node involvement are poor prognostic factors. Nodal involvement is usually considered as an indication for palliative treatment in the UK.

■ Curative radiotherapy

Radical radiotherapy is an option for patients with T2a–T3b bladder cancer alone or in combination with chemotherapy. Good prognostic features are younger age, lower tumour stage, no pelvic lymph node involvement, normal renal function, no hydronephrosis, normal haemoglobin and complete transurethral resection of bladder tumour (TURBT). Patients must have good bladder function, no history of previous pelvic radiotherapy, surgery or infections and no inflammatory bowel disease. Cystectomy is preferable in patients with poor bladder function, a tumour within a bladder diverticulum, diffuse bladder involvement, multiple tumours, extensive carcinoma *in situ*, hydronephrosis, large tumours >5 cm with extravesical mass, and for SCC and adenocarcinoma. With good patient selection and accurate staging, radical radiotherapy is a good non-surgical curative option for invasive bladder cancer with bladder preservation.

Radical radiotherapy has been considered in the past for pT1 G3 high risk superficial bladder cancer as an alternative to cystectomy. A recent RCT has shown radiotherapy to be no better than conservative treatment in these patients.

There is no proven benefit to irradiating the pelvic lymph nodes, and chemotherapy, which is being increasingly used, may be adequate to treat metastatic disease when local radiotherapy is given.

■ Adjuvant radiotherapy

Studies of preoperative neoadjuvant radiotherapy have shown no benefit and there is no evidence for postoperative adjuvant radiotherapy, which is avoided because of the high risk of bowel toxicity.

■ Palliative radiotherapy

Palliative radiotherapy is useful for the relief of symptoms such as haematuria and pain for patients with T4 bladder tumours, pelvic nodal disease, bone and other distant metastases. Palliative short courses of pelvic radiotherapy may be appropriate for elderly patients with T2 and T3 bladder cancer who have significant comorbidities precluding radical treatment. They can be managed with repeated transurethral resection of a bladder tumour (TURBT), and palliative radiotherapy to the bladder and pelvis to control symptoms.

Sequencing of multimodality therapy

■ Neoadjuvant chemotherapy

Neoadjuvant chemotherapy before radical cystectomy or radiotherapy has been given with the aim of improving bladder preservation rates and survival. A meta-analysis has shown that neoadjuvant platinum-based chemotherapy increases 5-year overall survival significantly from 45 per cent to 50 per cent.

Fit patients with adequate renal function and no hydronephrosis should be considered for neoadjuvant chemotherapy.

■ Concurrent chemoradiotherapy

Concurrent chemoradiotherapy is currently being investigated and appropriate patients, such as those with solitary TCC tumours, no extensive carcinoma *in situ* and good PS, should be entered into clinical trials.

■ Adjuvant chemotherapy

Pathological staging is used to select patients for adjuvant chemotherapy after surgery. However this sequencing delays the systemic treatment of micrometastatic disease. There is no definite proof of benefit yet but studies are continuing.

Clinical and radiological anatomy

The bladder occupies the anterior portion of the pelvic cavity just superior and posterior to the pubic bone (Fig. 29.1).The base of the bladder is separated from the rectum by the vas deferens, seminal vesicles and ureters in men, and by the uterus and vagina in women. As the bladder distends, the neck remains fixed and the dome rises into the pelvic cavity. The bladder mucosa is lined with transitional epithelium. It appears smooth when full and has numerous folds when empty.

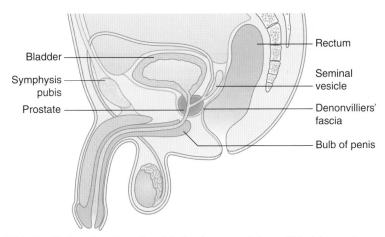

Figure 29.1 Sagittal section though pelvis to show prostate and bladder anatomy.

Assessment of primary disease

Patients are investigated with cystoscopy, TURBT, and bimanual pelvic examination under anaesthesia and urine cytology. Biopsies of the tumour should include muscle, and define the histological type, grade and depth of invasion. Random biopsies identify the presence of carcinoma *in situ*.

Diagrams of findings showing tumour location and extent at cystoscopy are very useful to aid planning. Ultrasound and intravenous urethrogram (IVU) are performed to detect other urothelial tumours and hydro-ureter secondary to obstruction of the ureteric orifices. MR scans show the local extent of disease in the pelvis and bladder better than CT. Alternatively, a CT scan of the abdomen and pelvis can be done. Chest X-ray will exclude large lung metastases. PET-CT is being investigated and may become the investigation of choice to stage for lymph node involvement and metastases.

Data acquisition

A CT scan is performed with the patient supine in the treatment position with arms folded across the chest with ankle supports to stabilise the legs and pelvis, and a knee support for comfort. The bladder should be emptied immediately before scanning and treatment, to reduce the volume irradiated and doses to normal tissues. The rectum should be empty to reduce organ motion and interfractional variations. A small volume of oral contrast is given 1 h before the planning CT scan to show the small bowel. The scan is performed with 3–5 mm slices from the lower border of L5 to the inferior border of the ischial tuberosities. An anterior tattoo is placed over the pubic symphysis and two lateral tattoos over the iliac crests to prevent lateral rotation with radio-opaque markers used for location on the scan. It is important to confirm on the planning scan that the patient has been able to empty the bladder. If there is a persistent large amount of residual urine on repeat CT scans, the patient requires intervention, which may include medication, a transurethral resection of the prostate (TURP) or as a last resort a urinary catheter. MRI is beneficial in planning partial but not whole bladder treatments and MRI/CT fusion may be useful.

Target volume definition

The current UK standard is treatment of the whole bladder and any extravesical component of the tumour.

The GTV is the primary bladder tumour, which is difficult to define on CT alone but MRI/CT fusion may help. Partial bladder approaches, which treat the whole bladder to a lower dose and boost the tumour alone, are currently being investigated. Detailed information from cystoscopy, bladder maps and diagnostic CT and MRI scans is needed for this technique.

The standard approach is to define the CTV as the GTV (primary tumour and any extravesical spread) and the whole bladder. In patients with tumours at the bladder base, the proximal urethra and in men the prostate and prostatic urethra are included on the CTV.

The PTV is the CTV with a 1.5–2 cm margin (Fig. 29.2). Studies have shown that the most significant bladder movement is in the cranial and AP directions and is random in time and direction. Bladder movement has been shown to occur in up to 60 per cent of patients as a displacement of over 1.5 cm between the bladder wall and the 95 per cent isodose. It is sensible therefore to grow the CTV by 1.5 cm to form the PTV around the normal outside bladder wall, but to grow the CTV by 2 cm to form the PTV around the primary bladder tumour and any extravesical spread. Tumours lying in the cranial part of the bladder are most at risk of moving out of the target volume and some authors recommend a margin of 3 cm from CTV to PTV around these bladder tumours. With improved image guidance these margins can be reduced. Care has to be taken with small bowel that may be stuck down to bladder tumours with extravesical spread. In these cases where small bowel is in close contact with tumour, a repeat planning CT scan can be performed to check whether the small bowel is mobile or the dose needs to be reduced.

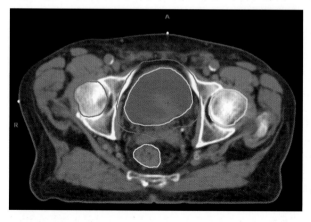

Figure 29.2 CT axial slice with CTV whole bladder, PTV and OAR. Rectum, yellow; femoral heads, green.

OAR should be outlined including rectum, femoral heads and small bowel. Recommended dose constraints are: rectum V50 <60 per cent, V60 <50 per cent; femoral heads V50 <50 per cent; small bowel V45 <250 cm^3.

For palliation of T4 tumours and pelvic nodal disease, the PTV must encompass the primary disease and its extension into the pelvis. If this volume is excessively large it can be reduced to cover only the area causing symptoms.

Dose solutions

■ Conformal

Forward planning is used to optimise a 3D conformal plan, usually with 10–15 MV photon beams, such as an anterior and two-wedged lateral or posterior oblique beams. The angle between the posterior oblique beams should be chosen to minimise dose to the rectum (Fig. 29.3).

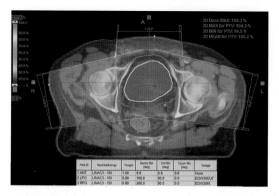

Figure 29.3 Axial CT slice showing conformal plan for whole bladder irradiation.

To minimise normal tissue irradiation, conformal MLC shielding is used. Doses to the rectum, femoral heads and small bowel should be kept as low as possible (see above). This is assessed by DVH constraints as shown in Figure 29.4, and the volume of small bowel receiving 45 Gy kept to a minimum.

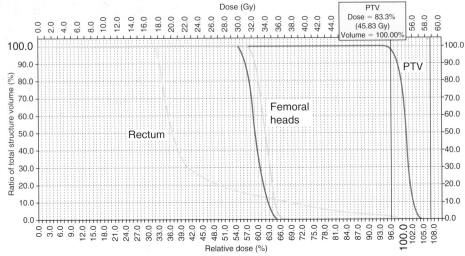

Figure 29.4 DVH for conformal plan for bladder cancer showing PTV, rectum and femoral heads.

With CT planning, a three-field technique as described above can be used for palliative treatments. In patients with extensive disease involving the rectum and pelvis, AP opposing beams can be designed using virtual simulation (Fig. 29.5).

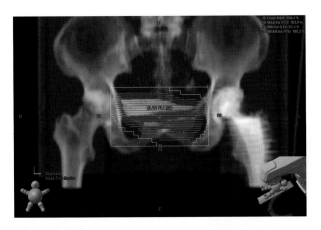

Figure 29.5 Virtual CT simulation showing DRR with volume for palliative treatment of bladder cancer.

■ Complex

IMRT with inverse planning has the potential to reduce the dose to normal tissues, allow the delivery of a synchronous boost needed for partial bladder irradiation and permit dose escalation to the tumour. However, IMRT for this tumour site requires excellent immobilisation, with IGRT to locate and minimise PTV at the time of treatment. It has been shown that without IGRT an isotropic margin of 3 cm is required, but with IGRT this can be reduced to 12 mm.

Conventional

Where CT planning is not available, the treatment can be simulated conventionally and the bladder visualised with contrast inserted into the bladder via an indwelling urinary catheter.

Dose-fractionation

■ Curative

Whole bladder

64 Gy in 32 daily fractions given in 6½ weeks.

■ Palliative

Whole bladder

21 Gy in 3 fractions given on alternate days in 1 week

or

36 Gy in 6 fractions of 6 Gy given once weekly for 6 weeks.

In most cases 21 Gy in 3 fractions on alternate days over 1 week is as effective as longer schedules for palliation as shown by the MRC BA09 trial. A weekly hypofractionated regimen of 6 Gy weekly for 6 fractions has been shown to effectively palliate symptoms in patients unfit for radical treatment and may be preferred by some patients.

Treatment delivery and patient care

Before radiation starts the patient should be made as fit as possible. Urinary infection should be treated, anaemia should be corrected to haemoglobin >12 g/dL and a low residue diet advised. Radiation cystitis is common; infection should always be excluded and a high fluid intake advised. Catheterisation should be avoided if possible to minimise the risk of infection. Mild proctitis and lethargy are common. Late side effects include fibrosis and shrinkage of the bladder, haematuria due to bladder telangiectasia, late bowel damage, vaginal dryness and stenosis in women and impotence in men.

Verification

The patient is immobilised as described above with an empty bladder and rectum and aligned using an anterior laser to check the midline and two lateral lasers to prevent rotation. The isocentre is marked with reference to the tattoo over the pubic symphysis for set-up. If an isocentre shift has to be performed, this is verified by comparison of EPI or simulator films with DRRs. TLD or diode measurement of dose delivered is performed on the first day of treatment.

The bladder is mobile and can change shape as well as position during treatment. Verification is therefore very important. The current standard is EPI comparing bony anatomy with the AP and lateral DRRs daily for the first 3–5 days, and then once weekly correcting for systematic errors. Verification that allows visualisation of soft tissues at the time of treatment delivery, such as kV cone beam imaging, MV imaging with tomotherapy and MV imaging of gold seed markers cystoscopically implanted into the bladder, will significantly improve the accuracy of radiotherapy to the bladder. ART, which modifies treatment plans to account for variations in individual patients, or gated radiotherapy based on delivery of treatment only when the bladder is in the correct position may be useful techniques.

key trials

Advanced Bladder Cancer Meta-analysis Collaboration (2003) Neoadjuvant chemotherapy in invasive bladder cancer: a systematic review and meta-analysis. *Lancet* **361**: 1927–34.

Advanced Bladder Cancer (ABC) Meta-analysis Collaboration (2005) Adjuvant chemotherapy in invasive bladder cancer: a systematic review and meta-analysis of individual patient data. Advanced Bladder Cancer (ABC) Meta-analysis Collaboration. *Eur Urol* **48**: 189–99.

Duchesne GM, Bolger JJ, Griffiths GO et al. (2000) A randomised trial of hypofractionated schedules of palliative radiotherapy in the management of bladder carcinoma: results of Medical Research Council trial BA09. *Int J Radiat Oncol Biol Phys* **47**: 379–88.

Harland SJ, Kynaston H, Grigor K et al. (2007) A randomised trial of radical radiotherapy for the management of pT1G3 NXM0 transitional cell carcinoma of the bladder. *J Urol* **178**: 807–13.

Tester W, Caplan R, Heaney J (1996) Neoadjuvant combined modality program with selective organ preservation for invasive bladder cancer: results of Radiation Therapy Oncology Group phase II trial 8802. *J Clin Oncol* **14**: 119–26.

Information sources

Alonzi R, Hoskin P (2005) Novel therapies in bladder cancer. *Clin Oncol* **17**: 524–38.

Bladder Cancer WebCafé. Available at: www.blcwebcafe.org

Harris SJ, Buchanan RB (1998) An audit and evaluation of bladder movements during radical radiotherapy. *Clin Oncol* **10**: 262–4.

Kotwal S, Choudhury A, Johnston C et al. (2008) Similar treatment outcomes for radical cystectomy and radical radiotherapy in invasive bladder cancer treated at a United Kingdom specialist treatment centre. *Int J Radiat Oncol Biol Phys* **70**: 456–63.

Logue J, McBain CA (2005) Radiation therapy for muscle-invasive bladder cancer: treatment planning and delivery. *Clin Oncol* **17**: 508–13.

McLaren DB, Morrey D, Mason MD (1997) Hypofractionated radiotherapy for muscle invasive bladder cancer in the elderly. *Radiother Oncol* **43**: 171–4.

NCRI Trials Portfolio. Available at: www.publincrn.org.uk

Redpath AT, Muren LP (2006) CT-guided intensity-modulated radiotherapy for bladder cancer: isocentre shifts, margins and their impact on target dose. *Radiother Oncol* **81**: 276–83.

Sengelov L, Von der Maase H (1999) Radiotherapy in bladder cancer. *Radiother Oncol* **52**: 1–14.

Shipley WU, Kaufman DS, Tester WJ et al. (2003) Overview of bladder cancer trials in the Radiation Therapy Oncology Group. *Cancer* **97**(8 suppl): 2115–19.

Testis

30

Indications for radiotherapy

Testicular cancer is the most common malignancy in young men, affecting about 2000 a year in the UK. Ninety per cent of patients present with low stage I–IIB disease. Eighty per cent have clinical stage I disease confined to the testis with normalised tumour markers after orchidectomy. The cure rate for clinical stage I testis cancer is expected to be 100 per cent. To achieve this, patients should be managed by experienced health professionals, using consensus guidelines such as those from the European Germ Cell Cancer Consensus Group (EGCCCG, see below), which outline the current standards of care.

Over 95 per cent of testicular cancers are germ cell tumours. Half of these are seminoma and half are non-seminomatous germ cell tumours (NSGCTs). NSGCTs are usually a mixture of teratoma, embryonal carcinoma, teratocarcinoma, choriocarcinoma and yolk sac tumour. Other rare testicular tumours include non-Hodgkin lymphoma, Sertoli and Leydig cell tumours. The treatment of non-Hodgkin lymphoma is discussed elsewhere and the management of Sertoli and Leydig cell tumours is surgical.

In seminoma the pathological risk factors for recurrence are tumour size >4 cm and rete testis invasion, whereas in NSGCT these are vascular and lymphatic invasion, the presence of embryonal carcinoma and the absence of yolk sac tumour.

Patients are staged according to the TNM classification of the UICC, and also according to the International Germ Cell Cancer Collaboration Group (IGCCCG) prognostic groups.

■ Seminoma

In stage I seminoma there are now three standard options for management following radical orchidectomy.

- surveillance
- para-aortic nodal radiotherapy (consider 'dog leg' radiotherapy to include the ipsilateral iliac and inguinal nodes in patients who have had previous inguinal/scrotal surgery or have distortion of lymphatic pathways)
- single course of carboplatin chemotherapy.

Surveillance studies have shown that only 15–20 per cent of patients relapse. Using the prognostic factors of rete testis involvement and tumour size >4 cm, the relapse rate is 32 per cent in patients with both risk factors, 15 per cent in patients with one risk factor and 12 per cent with no risk factors. Both adjuvant para-aortic nodal radiotherapy and a single course of carboplatin reduce the risk of relapse to

3–4 per cent. Surveillance involves intensive and prolonged restaging investigations over up to 10 years and is reliant on patient compliance, but may be useful where immediate treatment is contraindicated.

The following trials have influenced practice:

- MRC TE10: this trial randomised patients between treatment with para-aortic nodal radiotherapy or a dog leg field to a dose of 30 Gy in 15 fractions with no significant differences in outcome.
- MRC TE18: this trial randomised patients undergoing para-aortic nodal radiotherapy to receive 30 Gy in 15 fractions or 2 Gy in 10 fractions with no significant differences in outcome, but less toxicity with the lower dose.
- MRC TE19: this trial randomised patients to receive one cycle of carboplatin (AUC 7) or para-aortic nodal radiotherapy. At 7 years' follow-up, there was no difference in outcome.

In stage IIA seminoma, radiotherapy offers a high cure rate of 85–90 per cent. The current guidelines recommend radiotherapy to the para-aortic and ipsilateral iliac nodes to a dose of 30 Gy. In stage IIB seminoma, most patients receive chemotherapy, but current guidelines still consider an option of radiotherapy to the para-aortic and ipsilateral iliac nodes to a dose of 36 Gy.

Patients who relapse after initial treatment should be managed by experienced teams and entered into prospective randomised trials. The incidence of relapse after chemotherapy alone is low and radiotherapy may have a role for some patients with small and localised relapses. Radiotherapy may be used palliatively in patients with chemo-resistant disease.

Patients with testicular intraepithelial neoplasia (TIN) are treated with a surveillance strategy or orchidectomy in the UK. In Europe, radiotherapy to the testis of 20 Gy in 10 fractions over 2 weeks is also used.

■ NSGCT

Stage I patients are currently managed by orchidectomy and surveillance. Patients with more advanced or relapsed disease are treated with chemotherapy. Radiotherapy can have a palliative role in chemo-resistant disease for bulky inoperable disease, or cerebral, lymph node or bone metastases.

Clinical and radiological anatomy

Regional spread is predominantly lymphatic. From the testis it follows the testicular arteries to the para-aortic, renal hilar and retro-crural lymph nodes with involvement of the contralateral nodes occurring in 15–20 per cent. The typical 'landing zone' of left sided tumours is the left renal hilar and para-aortic region, and of right sided tumours is the inter-aortocaval and paracardiac area, as shown in Fig. 30.1.

The lymphatics from the scrotum drain to the inguinal lymph nodes but may be distorted by hernia repair, orchidopexy, scrotal surgery or pelvic infection.

Malignant teratomas also have a propensity for early vascular spread to the lungs and liver.

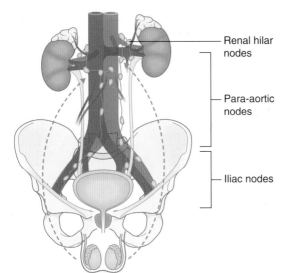

Renal hilar nodes

Para-aortic nodes

Iliac nodes

Figure 30.1 Lymphatic drainage of the testis.

Assessment of primary disease

The standard assessment should include a full clinical examination of the contralateral testis, lymph nodes areas (especially supraclavicular nodes and abdomen) and breasts to exclude gynaecomastia. Routine tests should include tumour markers AFP, β-hCG and lactate dehydrogenase, a baseline luteinising hormone (LH), follicle-stimulating hormone (FSH) and testosterone, chest X-ray, and CT scan of the chest, abdomen and pelvis with intravenous contrast. MRI is equally sensitive but less commonly used except for imaging brain metastases. FDG-PET is useful in assessing the significance of residual masses shown on CT after treatment. Patients should be advised on sperm storage.

Data acquisition

A CT scan of the abdomen is taken with the patient lying supine in the treatment position with arms by his sides. The head and legs are restrained with head rest, ankle and knee supports. Midline and lateral tattoos are used with laser lights to align the patient and prevent lateral rotation. Patients can be planned conventionally in a simulator, or using a CT scan for virtual simulation of the fields, which gives information on the soft tissue anatomy, and position of the renal pelvis.

Target volume definition

■ CT scanning

For stage I, the CTV includes lymph node areas at high risk of microscopic involvement i.e. para-aortic, renal hilar and retro-crural nodes bilaterally. Normal nodes are not visible on CT scans but intravenous contrast can be used to enhance renal blood vessels to help locate hilar nodes. If there has been previous scrotal surgery, the target volume also includes ipsilateral pelvic and inguinal lymph nodes (identified by contrast enhanced pelvic blood vessels) and the ipsilateral scrotal sac.

For stage II disease, GTV is defined by outlining enlarged (>1 cm) lymph nodes. CTV includes the nodal areas as for stage I, ensuring an adequate margin around the GTV. Both kidneys must be identified and outlined as critical normal organs, taking care to exclude a horseshoe kidney. Fig. 30.2 shows how virtual CT simulation can be used for accurate targeting of lymph nodes and design and shaping of fields to avoid normal kidneys.

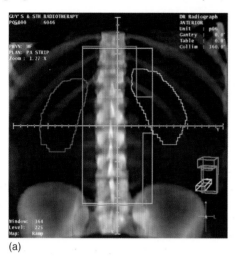 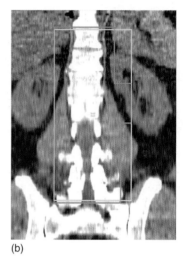

(a)   (b)

Figure 30.2 Virtual simulation for para-aortic nodal irradiation for seminoma of left testis. (a) Anterior DRR with kidneys outlined. (b) Coronal multiplanar reconstruction with MLC shielding to the kidneys.

■ Conventional simulation

Conventionally, the target volume for para-aortic nodal radiotherapy is defined by standard field sizes on a simulator:

- superior: lower border of T10
- inferior: lower border of L5
- lateral: to borders of transverse processes of vertebrae with inclusion of ipsilateral renal hilum.

The above field margins ensure inclusion of the para-aortic, renal hilar and retro-crural lymph nodes. The kidneys must be identified at planning by an IVU done in the simulator, and a horseshoe kidney excluded. As much normal kidney as possible should be excluded from the field using shielding.

In patients where the ipsilateral iliac nodes or ipsilateral iliac and inguinal nodes are to be treated, a larger rectangular field ('dog leg') is defined and shielding added to protect the kidneys, bladder and bowel as shown in Fig. 30.3. It is important to ensure adequate inclusion of lymph nodes lying at the mid level of the fifth lumbar vertebra between the para-aortic and pelvic nodes. Lead shields 1 cm thick are used to protect the remaining testis from scattered irradiation and preserve fertility. Measurements using TLDs have shown that the radiation dose to the testis can be reduced to 0.5–0.7 Gy. If scrotal irradiation is necessary because of previous scrotal surgery or tumour involvement of the tunica vaginalis, a scrotal field using electron therapy is used to treat the scrotal sac and lower inguinal nodes on the affected side.

This field is matched to a tattoo on the inferior border of the dog leg field. A lead cut-out is made to shield the penis and remaining testis.

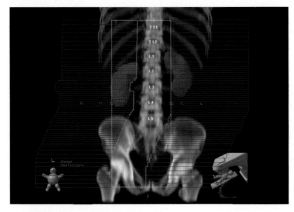

Figure 30.3 Virtual simulation for para-aortic, iliac and inguinal 'dog leg' irradiation for seminoma of right testis.

Dose solutions

Conformal CT planning is being developed. CT based fields tend to be wider than traditional fields and provide improved dosimetry to vessel-based target volumes. A high proportion of failures are marginal relapses which may be avoided by individualised CT-based planning. In practice, opposing anterior and posterior beams with individual shielding of renal parenchyma by MLC may give the best target volume coverage with lowest integral dose for this low dose treatment.

Conventionally, anterior and posterior fields are treated isocentrically on a linear accelerator. Perspex templates are used to define shielding to critical structures when extended dog leg fields are used. Calculations of the dose distributions for dog leg fields are made as for other irregular fields.

Low dose radiotherapy may give good palliation for metastases in sites such as brain and bone where chemotherapy is not appropriate.

Dose-fractionation

■ Seminoma stage I

20 Gy in 10 daily fractions given in 2 weeks.

■ Seminoma stage IIA

30 Gy in 15 daily fractions given in 3 weeks.

■ Seminoma stage IIB

36 Gy in 18 daily fractions given in 3½ weeks.

■ TIN

20 Gy in 10 daily fractions given in 2 weeks.

■ Palliative

20 Gy in 5 daily fractions given in 1 week.
30 Gy in 10 fractions given in 2 weeks.

Treatment delivery and patient care

The patient lies supine on the treatment couch with lasers used to align anterior and lateral tattoos. When dog leg irradiation is used, a template is needed to place lead shielding, or this is done more commonly now with MLC. Nausea and vomiting are common side effects and can be reduced with prophylactic antiemetics. If the patient has a history of peptic ulceration, a proton pump inhibitor should be prescribed with antiemetics. The skin reaction is mild. Patients should be offered sperm storage before treatment. They can be reassured that the para-aortic treatment does not result in any significant dose to the testis nor impair fertility in the long term. Dog leg fields and scrotal irradiation using testicular shielding do, however, give some dose (0.7 Gy and 1.5 Gy respectively) and patients should be counselled accordingly.

Verification

Treatment verification is carried out with EPI taken daily for the first 3 days and any systematic errors corrected. Diodes or TLD are used on the first treatment to check dose to isocentre and remaining testis.

key trials

Fosså SD, Horwich A, Russell JM *et al.* (1999) Optimal planning target volume for stage I testicular seminoma: a Medical Research Council randomised trial. Medical Research Council Testicular Tumour Working Group, TE10. *J Clin Oncol* **17**: 1146.

Jones WG, Fosså SD, Mead GM *et al.* (2005) Randomised trial of 30 versus 20 Gy in the adjuvant treatment of stage I testicular seminoma: a report on Medical Research Council Trial TE18, European Organisation for the Research and Treatment of Cancer Trial 30942 (ISRCTN18525328). *J Clin Oncol* **23**: 1200–8.

Oliver RT, Mason MD, Mead GM *et al.* (2005) MRC TE19 collaborators and the EORTC 30982 collaborators. Radiotherapy versus single-dose carboplatin in adjuvant treatment of stage I seminoma: a randomised trial. *Lancet* **366**: 293–300.

Information sources

Aparicio J, Germà JR, García del Muro X *et al.* (2005) Risk-adapted management for patients with clinical stage I seminoma: the second Spanish Germ Cell Cancer Cooperative Group study. *J Clin Oncol* **23**: 8717–23.

Huddart R, Kataja V (2008) ESMO Guidelines Working Group. Testicular seminoma: ESMO clinical recommendations for diagnosis, treatment and follow-up. *Ann Oncol* **19**(suppl 2): ii49–51.

Krege S, Beyer J, Souchon R *et al.* (2008) European consensus conference on diagnosis and treatment of germ cell cancer: a report of the second meeting of the European Germ Cell Cancer Consensus Group (EGCCCG): part II. *Eur Urol* **53**: 497–513.

Martin JM, Joon DL, Ng N *et al.* (2005) Towards individualised radiotherapy for Stage I seminoma. *Radiother Oncol* **76**: 251–6.

The Testicular Cancer Resource Centre. Available at: www.acor.org/TCRC/ (accessed 10 December 2008).

Warde P, Specht L, Horwich A *et al.* (2002) Prognostic factors for relapse in stage I seminoma managed by surveillance: a pooled analysis. *J Clin Oncol* **20**: 4448–52.

Penis

31

Indications for radiotherapy

Penis cancer is rare, with approximately 360 new cases per year in the UK, and should be treated in specialised centres. Over 95 per cent of tumours are SCCs. Penile cancer is staged by the AJCC TNM classification of 1997. In addition a commonly used staging system is that proposed by Jackson (Table 31.1).

Table 31.1 Staging system for carcinoma of the penis proposed by Jackson*

Stage	Characteristics
I	Tumour confined to glans and/or prepuce
II	Tumour extends onto shaft of penis
III	Tumour with malignant, but operable, inguinal lymph nodes
IV	Inoperable primary tumour extending off the shaft of the penis or inoperable groin nodes or distant metastases

*From: Jackson SM (1966) The treatment of carcinoma of the penis. *Br J Surg* **53**: 33–5. Reprinted with permission from Blackwell.

With advances in reconstructive surgical techniques, most patients (>85 per cent) are now treated with penile preserving surgery. The overall 5-year survival is 52 per cent, ranging from 66 per cent to 29 per cent in lymph node negative and positive disease, respectively. The local control rate with radical surgery is >90 per cent, and with brachytherapy or EBRT it is 65–85 per cent. Radiotherapy has a role in small early tumours as an alternative to penile preserving surgery in highly selected cases and is used palliatively in advanced inoperable cases.

Palpable mobile inguinal nodes are found in 30–50 per cent of patients at presentation, but half of these are due to infection rather than tumour. If tumour is confirmed by cytology or histology, an ipsilateral modified radical inguinal node dissection is performed with a dynamic sentinel node study on the contralateral side.

■ Curative radiotherapy

Electron beam radiotherapy can be used for very small stage I superficial tumours. Selected early stage I and II tumours <4 cm in size, and where there is invasion of the corpora cavernosa <1 cm, can be treated with interstitial brachytherapy.

EBRT can be used for selected stage II and III tumours in patients unfit for or refusing surgery.

■ Adjuvant radiotherapy

Adjuvant nodal radiotherapy can be used to reduce the risk of local recurrence after nodal dissection. Patients with a single positive node with extracapsular extension can be considered for adjuvant radiotherapy to the ipsilateral groin. Patients with involved multiple or bilateral inguinal nodes can be considered for adjuvant radiotherapy to the involved groin(s) and adjacent pelvic nodes.

■ Palliative radiotherapy

Palliative radiotherapy and chemotherapy can be used for advanced inoperable primary tumours or to treat fixed or fungating inguinal nodes or distant metastases.

Clinical and radiological anatomy

The penis is composed of two corpora cavernosa and the corpus spongiosum. Distally the corpus spongiosum expands into the glans penis, which is covered by a skin fold known as the prepuce. The prepuce and skin of the penis drain to the superficial inguinal lymph nodes. The glans penis and corpora have a very rich lymphatic supply, which drains to the deep inguinal and external iliac lymph nodes as shown in Fig. 31.1.

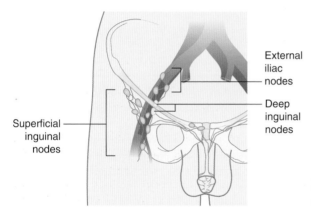

External iliac nodes

Deep inguinal nodes

Superficial inguinal nodes

Figure 31.1 Lymphatic drainage of the penis.

Assessment of primary disease

After histological confirmation of primary ± nodal disease, patients should have a full assessment including endoscopic examination of the urethra, cystoscopy, chest X-ray and CT scan of the abdomen and pelvis. In advanced cases, MRI of the pelvis and bone scans may be needed to complete staging.

Data acquisition

Patients are treated supine with arms folded comfortably across the chest. Treatment is planned with the box technique as described below, or using a planning CT scan with intravenous contrast of the inguinal and pelvic lymph node regions. Scans are taken from the lower border of L5 to 5 cm inferior to the ischial tuberosities using 3–5 mm slices.

Target volume definition and dose solutions

Very small superficial stage I tumours on the prepuce or glans, unsuitable for surgery or brachytherapy, can be treated with electron therapy as for SCC on the skin. A lead cut-out is made to treat the tumour with a 2 cm margin. An appropriate electron energy and thickness of bolus are chosen to give a skin dose of 100 per cent and ensure the tumour is covered at depth by the 90 per cent isodose.

For larger tumours, the CTV is the clinical and radiological GTV with a 2 cm margin proximally and distally, which in practice gives a PTV that covers the entire penis. To immobilise the penis, it is covered with a gauze Tubigrip and placed in a central cavity of a wax block within a hinged Perspex box. The box is closed, the gauze drawn up through a hole in the top and a wax plug is inserted to maintain the penis in position. The wax block allows even build up, and a homogeneous dose is obtained using opposing lateral fields treating isocentrically with 4 MV or 6 MV photons. The testes and groins are shielded from scattered irradiation by a lead sheet (Fig. 31.2).

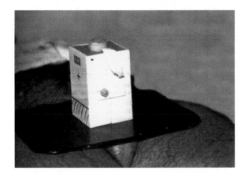

Figure 31.2 EBRT technique for carcinoma of the penile shaft.

Where the penis is short or retracted and cannot be treated with this technique, a CT planned volume is used to treat it with wax bolus and shielding to the testes. The typical arrangement is two anterolateral oblique 6 MV photon beams.

For inguinal and pelvic node adjuvant radiotherapy, pelvic blood vessels shown on a contrast-enhanced planning CT scan are used to define the nodal CTV and a 3D margin of 7–10 mm added to form a PTV (see Fig. 35.2, p. 405).

Conventionally, radiotherapy of the inguinal regions is defined by a field that extends laterally to the midpoint of the femoral neck, medially to the midline, inferiorly 2 cm below the inferior border of the ischial tuberosity and superiorly to a line joining the top of the anterior superior iliac spine to the pubic symphysis. Direct anterior or opposing anterior and posterior beams are used, with central shielding to cover the bladder and MLC shaping. If an anterior electron field is used, an additional margin will be needed to account for the wider penumbra of electrons.

In advanced cases, radiotherapy can be used to palliate pain and bleeding with a simple beam arrangement to the affected area.

■ Interstitial brachytherapy

Circumcision must be performed before implantation. The implant is performed under general anaesthesia following insertion of a urinary catheter. The planning target volume is defined as the GTV (palpable and visible tumour) with a margin of 1–2 cm. For small superficial tumours, a single plane implant may be considered, but for the majority, the entire circumference of the penis is enclosed in a two-plane implant. It is usual to use two or three sources in each plane and to maintain parallelism by the use of a small template (Fig. 31.3a). The separation between sources is usually 12–15 mm, but it may sometimes be up to 18 mm as determined by the thickness of the shaft of the penis.

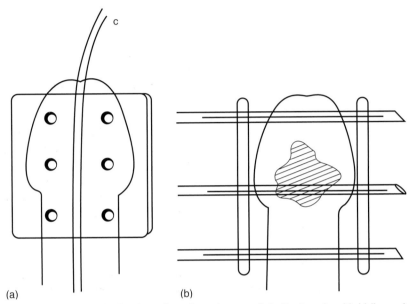

(a)　　　　　　　　　　　　　(b)

Figure 31.3 Technique for implantation of carcinoma of shaft of penis with iridium wires. (a) Rigid needles inserted through template. (b) Iridium wires held in position by template. c, catheter.

The implant is usually performed with the axis of implantation at right angles to the axis of the penis. Only a small part of the needle track is within the penis, and at the apex of the glans one or more needles may be entirely free in air but held in position by the template. The active length of iridium wire is usually 4–5 cm, which means that there is active wire extending through the skin on either side of the lesion (Fig. 31.3b).

Care must be taken not to pass the wires through the urethra, which can normally be avoided by making sure the catheter moves freely. In order to prevent radioactive material from coming into contact with the skin of the thigh or testes, the shaft of the penis is supported erect in a foam block. For those patients in whom it is important to preserve fertility, a 2 mm thick sheet of lead is placed over the thighs and testes.

Dose-fractionation

■ Primary tumour

Radical EBRT or electrons
64 Gy in 32 daily fractions given in 6½ weeks.

Brachytherapy
65 Gy to the 85 per cent reference isodose in 6–7 days.

■ Lymph nodes

EBRT or electrons

50 Gy in 25 daily fractions given in 5 weeks.

■ Palliative

30 Gy in 10 daily fractions given in 2 weeks.

Treatment delivery and patient care

For EBRT the patient is set up with the wax/Perspex block defining the area to be treated. Where no block is used, set-up uses lasers to align lateral pelvic tattoos.

Systemic antibiotics and circumcision may be needed prior to radiotherapy to control infection and prevent radiation-induced oedema and urethral obstruction. Treatment is poorly tolerated. Pain and difficulty passing urine are common. A high fluid intake is encouraged and midstream urine specimens sent regularly to exclude infection. Complications of both EBRT and brachytherapy include tissue swelling, moist desquamation, secondary infection, penile ulceration (8 per cent), penile necrosis (3–16 per cent) and urethral strictures (10–45 per cent).

Verification

With the block technique, treatment verification is done daily by ensuring adequate inclusion of the penis within the block and coverage by the treatment beams. EPI is used to verify other pelvic EBRT treatments with TLD or diode measurements. The anterior oblique field technique is checked using orthogonal EPI to verify the isocentre.

Information sources

Hadway P, Smith YC, Corbishley C *et al.* (2007) Evaluation of dynamic lymphoscintigraphy and sentinel lymph-node biopsy for detecting occult metastases in patients with penile squamous cell carcinoma. *BJU Int* **100**: 561–5.

Jackson SM (1966) The treatment of carcinoma of the penis. *Br J Surg* **53**: 33–5.

Mistry T, Jones RWA, Dannatt E *et al.* (2007) A 10-year retrospective audit of penile cancer management in the UK. *BJU Int* **100**: 1277–81.

Radiographics. Imaging of penile neoplasms. Available at: http://radiographics.rsnajnls.org/cgi/content/full/25/6/1629 (accessed 15 December 2008).

Sarin R, Norman AR, Steel GG *et al.* (1997) Treatment results and prognostic factors in 101 men treated for squamous carcinoma of the penis. *Int J Radiat Oncol Biol Phys* **38**: 713–22.

Smith Y, Hadway P, Biedrzycki O *et al.* (2007) Reconstructive surgery for invasive squamous carcinoma of the glans penis. *Eur Urol* **52**: 1179–85.

Solsona E, Algaba F, Horenblas S *et al.* (2004) European Association of Urology Guidelines. Available at: www.uroweb.org/fileadmin/tx_eauguidelines/penile (search via Google and click on [pdf] Erectile Dysfunction; accessed 15 December 2008).

St Georges Specialist Network Penis Cancer Guidelines (2007) Available at: www.sussexcancer.net/professionals/clinicalgroups/tumourgroups/urology/guidelines.asp (accessed 11 December 2008).

32 Cervix

Indications for radiotherapy

Cervical cancer is the second commonest female malignancy worldwide and is more common in developing countries. Its pathogenesis is associated with persistent papilloma virus infection, smoking, multiple sexual partners, parity and early coitus and childbirth, and 80–90 per cent are SCCs. Adenocarcinomas are commonly of endocervical type and are increasing in incidence. Anaplastic small cell tumours are aggressive with less than 50 per cent survival rate for stage I disease. Metastases from colon and breast and direct spread from uterine malignancies are also seen.

The choice of treatment for carcinoma of the cervix depends on the stage of the disease (FIGO), tumour volume and histology, probability of lymph node involvement and age and PS of the patient. Intraepithelial disease (cervical intraepithelial neoplasia [CIN]) is treated with superficial ablative techniques. Microinvasive stage Ia1 disease (no greater than 3 mm deep stromal invasion and no greater than 7 mm diameter) is treated with vaginal hysterectomy or excisional cone biopsy in young patients to preserve fertility.

■ Early stage disease

Stage Ia2 (3–5 mm deep stromal invasion and no greater than 7 mm diameter) and Ib1 (4 cm or less in size) are treated with radical hysterectomy and bilateral pelvic lymphadenectomy. In selected patients with tumours less than 2 cm who are keen to preserve fertility, radical vaginal trachelectomy (removal of cervix, the upper part of the vagina, and parametrial tissue) and laparoscopic pelvic lymphadenectomy may be carried out.

Stage Ib1 and IIa (tumour 4 cm or less) are treated equally effectively with radical surgery or combined radical EBRT and brachytherapy with both treatments giving 80–90 per cent 5-year survival rates.

Stage Ib2 or IIa tumours (>4 cm tumour size) have deep stromal invasion and an increased risk of parametrial and lymph node involvement. Surgery is performed in selected patients with large tumours, lymphovascular space invasion (LVSI) and adenosquamous or high grade histology, followed by postoperative radiotherapy. Ovarian transposition may minimise the chances of radiation-induced menopause.

Primary radical radiotherapy is preferable for other stage Ib2 and IIa patients. This avoids the increased morbidity seen when surgery is followed by postoperative radiotherapy. In patients who have residual macroscopic disease, positive surgical margins, parametrial involvement and positive lymph nodes, concomitant chemotherapy with radiotherapy improves local control and survival rates compared with postoperative radiotherapy alone, but late morbidity is also increased.

■ Locally advanced disease

Primary radiotherapy is the treatment of choice for locoregionally advanced disease with a careful balance of EBRT and brachytherapy to maximise dose to tumour and avoid normal tissues. Five-year survival rates with radiotherapy alone for stage IIb, IIIb and IVa disease are 65–75 per cent, 35–50 per cent and 15–20 per cent, respectively. Studies of combined chemoradiation with cisplatin ± 5FU have shown a 30–50 per cent decrease in risk of death from cervical cancer compared with extended field radiotherapy alone. However, patients with poor PS, impaired renal function and para-aortic node disease were excluded, making the results applicable to a selected population only. Similar good results have been shown with concurrent mitomycin and 5FU, but neoadjuvant chemotherapy shows no benefit when given before radiotherapy. Data from randomised trials show that cisplatin-based chemotherapy improves survival, especially in stage II disease. It is commonly delivered as a single agent, weekly during EBRT.

Where a vesico- or recto-vaginal fistula is present, a urinary diversion procedure or defunctioning colostomy should be performed prior to radiotherapy.

The role of para-aortic node irradiation is controversial with no survival advantage shown by the EORTC trial, but another study has reported 25–50 per cent long-term survival after treatment for microscopic disease but with increased morbidity.

■ Stage IVb metastatic disease

Short course pelvic radiotherapy is successful in relieving bleeding and pelvic pain in patients with metastatic disease. Palliative radiotherapy is used to relieve pain from bone secondaries and symptoms from brain and nodal metastases.

■ Occult disease

Patients who have cervical cancer detected as an incidental finding at simple hysterectomy for other reasons are usually treated postoperatively with chemo-radiation and vault brachytherapy as appropriate.

Clinical and radiological anatomy

Cervical cancer arises at the junction of the columnar epithelium of the endocervix and the squamous epithelium of the ectocervix. It spreads directly into cervical stroma presenting either as exophytic tumour protruding into the vagina or endocervical tumour expanding the cervix. Superiorly, spread is into the lower uterine segment, inferiorly to the vagina and laterally from paracervical spaces into the broad and utero-sacral ligaments and pelvic sidewalls. Rectal and bladder mucosal involvement is uncommon at presentation and occurs late (Fig. 32.1). The lymphatic plexus is rich, connecting with the lower uterine segment and laterally to the paracervical, parametrial, obturator, and internal and external iliac nodes (Fig. 32.2). Posterior tumours may spread to presacral, common iliac and para-aortic nodes along the ovarian vessels. Stage Ib tumours have 15–25 per cent risk of pelvic, and 5–15 per cent risk of para-aortic, nodal involvement, depending on tumour size, depth of stromal invasion and presence of LVSI. Blood spread is late with metastases seen in lungs, extrapelvic nodes, liver and bone as well as direct extension from para-aortic nodes to the lumbar vertebrae.

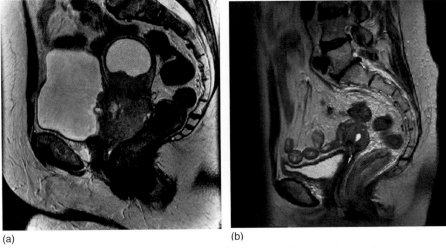

(a)   (b)

Figure 32.1 Sagittal MR scans of stage IVa SCC cervix with bladder invasion, biopsy-proven mucosal disease at cystoscopy, (a) before and (b) after radical EBRT and brachytherapy.

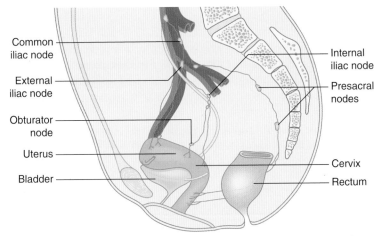

Figure 32.2 Lymphatic drainage of the cervix. Reproduced with permission from Johnston TB, Davies DV, Davies F (1958) *Grays Anatomy*, 32nd edn. Edinburgh: Churchill Livingstone.

Assessment of primary disease

Clinical assessment includes vaginal examination to inspect and palpate the extent of tumour in the cervix and vagina, and a bimanual examination to determine mobility and enlargement of the uterus. Vaginal spread is visualised using a speculum, and rectal examination defines involvement of parametrial tissues, utero-sacral ligaments and fixation to pelvic sidewalls. EUA is carried out in all patients, ideally jointly with surgical colleagues, with cervical biopsy, endocervical curettings and accurate assessment of the lesion according to the FIGO staging system. Insertion of radio-opaque markers such as gold grains into the lateral and AP extent of tumour can be used to aid target volume delineation and verify daily treatment delivery. Cystoscopy is performed to look for invasion of the bladder base mucosa, and proctoscopy where rectal invasion is suspected. CT scanning of the chest and abdomen is performed for staging and to assess the renal tract, and to detect ureteric obstruction or hydronephrosis, which may need stent placement prior to treatment. MRI is the modality of choice for detecting depth of cervical and uterine invasion and parametrial spread. CT and MRI detection of pelvic and para-aortic nodes has a low sensitivity, as nodes are designated involved when the short axis diameter is greater than 1 cm. When MRI is combined with ultra-small particles of iron oxide (USPIO) there is increased sensitivity of pelvic lymph node detection down to 3 mm. PET has a high sensitivity for detecting both nodal and distant metastases.

Data acquisition

■ CT scanning

With the change from 2D to 3D planning, CT scanning is now recommended for data acquisition. Patients are scanned supine with arms on the chest, knees and lower legs immobilised, and anterior and lateral tattoos marked with radio-opaque material aligned with lasers to prevent lateral rotation. For obese patients, a prone bellyboard immobilisation system may be used to allow small bowel to fall anteriorly away from the target volume. Clinical examination is made in the treatment position and inferior extent of tumour in the vagina marked with radio-opaque material. A protocol is used to maintain a constant bladder filling – 'comfortably full' – as variations in bladder volume have been shown to influence mobility and position of the uterus and cervix. For example, patients are asked to empty the bladder and drink 200 mL water 20 min before the scan and treatment each day.

CT scans are taken from the first lumbar vertebra to 5 cm beyond the vaginal introitus. Intravenous contrast is used to outline pelvic blood vessels to be used as surrogates for pelvic nodes in CTV delineation. It may also enhance the GTV-T. Oral contrast may be given to outline small bowel if IMRT is to be given.

EUA findings are used to optimise localisation of tumour margins along with diagnostic MRI and/or PET-CT scans co-registered with planning CT scans to define the AP part of the volume in particular (Fig. 32.3).

■ Conventional

Conventionally, the simulator is used to acquire patient data with the patient supine with arms on the chest, knee and lower leg immobilisation or alpha cradles to prevent pelvic rotation, and aligned using orthogonal laser beams with anterior and lateral tattoos marked with radio-opaque material. For obese patients, a prone bellyboard immobilisation system may be used to allow small bowel to fall anteriorly away from the target volume. Palpation of the primary tumour is carried out with the patient in the treatment position and the inferior border marked with radio-opaque material.

A protocol is used to maintain a constant bladder filling – 'comfortably full' – as variations in bladder volume have been shown to influence mobility and position of the uterus and cervix.

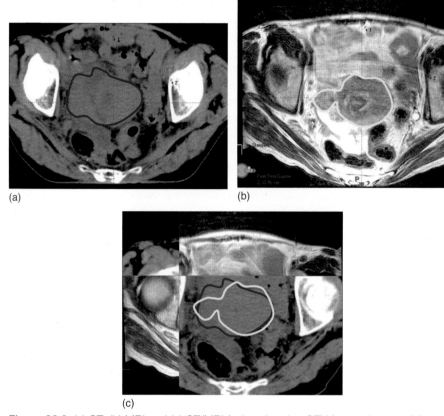

(a)
(b)
(c)

Figure 32.3 (a) CT, (b) MRI and (c) CT/MRI fusion showing GTV for carcinoma of the cervix. Courtesy of Professor R Reznek, Institute of Cancer, Barts and the London School of Medicine and Dentistry.

AP and lateral simulator films are taken. All clinical, surgical and histological data must be used as appropriate, along with any diagnostic CT or MRI information, showing tumour extent and the position of the kidneys, to define individualised treatment beams. Standard field borders using bony anatomical landmarks have been shown to include unnecessary normal tissue and may miss primary tumour or lymph nodes.

The upper border of the individualised treatment beam is at the lower margin of L4 to include distal common iliac nodes. The inferior border is 3 cm below the most inferior disease in the vagina as palpated or seen on MRI. Lateral borders are 2 cm outside the bony pelvic sidewalls. The anterior border must encompass the GTV-T as well as the common iliac nodes and is usually placed through the anterior third of the symphysis pubis. The posterior border is 2 cm from the GTV-T including posterior extension of tumour, utero-sacral ligaments and upper presacral nodes and is commonly situated 0.5 cm posterior to the anterior border of the S2/3 vertebral junction. Individualised shielding is employed in the anterior beam to the superior corners to exclude small bowel. Shielding to the inferior corners to protect femoral heads may mask the external iliac nodes and should be used sparingly. Lateral beams have shielding to sacral nerve roots posteriorly. For simulation of para-aortic nodal beams, intravenous contrast is required to localise kidneys for shielding.

Target volume definition

■ Primary radiotherapy

Primary radiotherapy is delivered to the primary cervical tumour (GTV with a margin for local microscopic spread [CTV-T]) as well as to potential sites of pelvic lymph node involvement (CTV-N), with or without concurrent chemotherapy. An initial course of EBRT is given to CTV-T and CTV-N to shrink the bulky primary tumour and make the geometry of subsequent intracavitary brachytherapy to CTV-T optimal. When intracavitary treatment is not feasible, e.g. due to obstruction of the cervical os, an EBRT boost is given to the residual GTV-T, with a 1–1.5 cm margin. If multiple uterine fibroids are present, primary surgery may be indicated, as brachytherapy may not be feasible.

CTV-T includes the primary GTV-T with potential microscopic spread to cervix, uterus, parametrial tissues, upper vagina, and broad and proximal utero-sacral ligaments. If posterior extension of cervical tumour is present, the entire utero-sacral ligaments and upper presacral nodes should be included. If following chemoradiation there is residual macroscopic disease on repeat imaging, an individualised EBRT boost to this disease in pelvic sidewall or nodes is performed, ensuring no overlap with brachytherapy doses.

CTV-N includes the pelvic lymph nodes, i.e. obturator, internal, external and common iliac, and upper presacral nodes. These are delineated by identifying contrast-enhanced pelvic blood vessels on each CT scan and using a 7 mm margin to create a 3D CTV (Fig. 32.4).

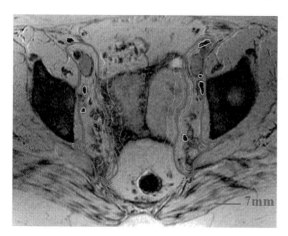

Figure 32.4 T2-weighted MRI after USPIO administration showing lymph nodes outlined in yellow. CTV delineation using 7 mm margin around contrast-enhanced pelvic blood vessels and nodal contours. (Blue lines show range of 3–15 mm margins.) Reproduced with permission from Taylor A *et al.* (2005) *Int J Radiat Oncol Biol Phys* **63**: 1604–12.

A typical CTV to PTV margin of 15–20 mm is used around the CTV-T to allow for organ motion of cervix and uterus and measured set-up uncertainties. For CTV-N organ motion occurs to a lesser extent and a 7–10 mm CTV to PTV margin is typically sufficient for set-up variations (Fig. 32.5).

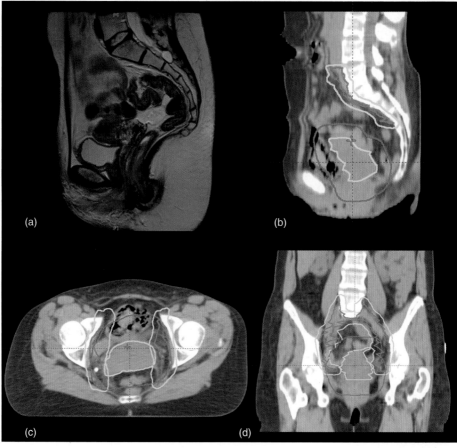

Figure 32.5 T2b carcinoma of the cervix: (a) sagittal T2-weighted MRI, (b) sagittal, (c) axial and (d) coronal CT scans with CTV and PTV for primary tumour and nodes (CTV-N in purple, PTV-N in green).

Virtual simulation can be used to define beams and shielding, using 3D tumour and normal organ information (Fig. 32.6). For 3D conformal radiotherapy and IMRT, tumour and normal organs are also outlined in 3D. Normal tissues to be contoured include bladder, rectum, small and large bowel, and the femoral heads.

■ Adjuvant radiotherapy

The GTV has been resected at surgery so the CTV-T comprises the surgical tumour bed including the vaginal vault and parametrial tissues. CTV-N contains obturator, internal, external and common iliac nodes. CTV-T is delineated using preoperative CT and MRI, operative diagrams and histological findings to include sites at high risk of recurrence. Pelvic lymph nodes (CTV-N) are delineated using CT contrast-enhanced blood vessels with a 7 mm margin. A CTV-PTV margin of 10–15 mm is used for CTV-T and a 7–10 mm margin for CTV-N to allow for organ motion and set-up errors.

Normal tissues to be contoured include bladder, rectum, small and large bowel, and the femoral heads.

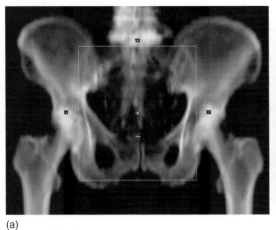
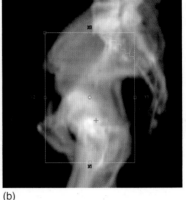

(a)   (b)

Figure 32.6 Virtual simulation of pelvic beams: (a) anterior BEV and (b) lateral BEV showing MLC shielding to sacral nerve roots.

■ Para-aortic radiotherapy

CT scanning is performed from the diaphragm to pelvis with intravenous contrast given to enhance blood vessels and kidneys and to locate the para-aortic nodes. Virtual simulation is used to design anterior and posterior beams, from the upper border of L1 to the L5/S1 junction, avoiding the kidneys laterally with MLC shielding and in continuity with pelvic beams when common iliac nodes are involved (Fig. 32.7). 3D volume outlining permits the use of IMRT.

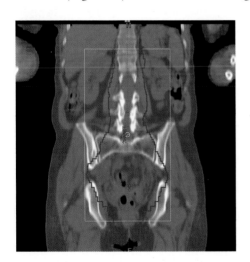

Figure 32.7 Virtual simulation of treatment beams for para-aortic and pelvic node irradiation with MLC shaping to shield kidneys.

■ Palliative radiotherapy

Symptoms of bleeding or pain from locally advanced cervical cancer can be alleviated with small volume, short-course radiotherapy. CT planning is used as described above, to localise the GTV alone with a 1.5–2 cm margin for the PTV. An arrangement of three to four beams is used to reduce toxicity as much as possible and can be produced after virtual simulation using 3D CT data.

Dose solutions

All patients selected for primary radiotherapy are treated by EBRT first to the primary tumour and pelvic lymph nodes. Shrinkage of the GTV leads to better geometry and closer application of the intracavitary sources, which deliver higher radiation doses to the tumour. The balance of dose from EBRT and intracavitary radiation is modified according to the stage and bulk of disease, and the risk or presence of pelvic lymph node involvement.

■ Conventional

High-energy photons (10–16 MV) are used for EBRT to spare superficial tissues and improve dose distributions. Conventionally, anterior, posterior and two lateral beams are usually used to spare the rectum with decreased weighting of the posterior beam (see Fig. 33.4, p. 389).

■ Conformal

Using 3D dose planning, MLC shaping is designed to spare normal tissues, where possible. Similarly, standard shielding can be used on simulated anterior, posterior and lateral beams to reduce dose to small bowel and sacral nerve roots.

■ Complex

IMRT techniques using five or seven photon beams may reduce dose to small bowel, rectum and bladder by shaping treatment to the pelvis. IMRT may also help to limit dose to pelvic bone marrow in patients undergoing chemoradiation. Organ motion studies have shown that the cervix and uterus position varies with both bladder and rectal filling by up to 20 mm. IGRT may be used to localise the target volume on a daily basis with a full IMRT implementation programme to ensure that it is delivered accurately and safely.

Brachytherapy

The principles of brachytherapy, differences between LDR, MDR and HDR, and ICRU Report No. 38 are described in detail in Chapter 5. Brachytherapy allows delivery of a very high dose to the central tumour volume to obtain maximal local control without exceeding the tolerance of surrounding normal tissues. It is feasible because the normal uterus and vaginal vault are relatively radio-resistant and there is rapid fall-off of dose at a distance from the cervix, protecting the adjacent rectum, bladder and small bowel. Gynaecological brachytherapy can be delivered at low, medium or high dose rate, or with pulsed brachytherapy, which uses many, closely spaced radiation fractions or pulses to mimic continuous LDR treatment.

■ GEC-ESTRO recommendations for image-based 3D brachytherapy

This method relies on CT and/or MR imaging rather than 2D orthogonal radiographs. Doses are prescribed to volumes rather than reference points. The

GEC-ESTRO group has recently published recommendations on target volume concepts and plan evaluation using DVHs. GTV, high risk (HR) CTV and intermediate risk (IR) CTV are defined with the bladder, rectum, sigmoid colon and small bowel as OAR (Fig. 32.8). The total dose, including EBRT dose, should be isoequivalent to 80–90 Gy in 2 Gy fractions for the HR CTV, and 60 Gy for the IR CTV. Doses of >87 Gy to the HR CTV have been associated with improved local control compared with doses below 87 Gy. Doses for 2 mL of tissue volume (D_{2cc}) for the OAR are calculated at 2 Gy per fraction. Isoequivalent doses of 80–90 Gy for the bladder and 70–75 Gy for the rectum and sigmoid colon are generally accepted.

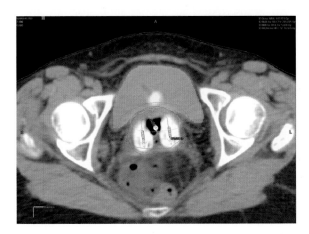

Figure 32.8 CT scan of patient with HDR brachytherapy applicators *in situ* and isodoses. HR (high risk) CTV cyan, IR (intermediate risk) CTV magenta.

■ The Manchester system for gynaecological brachytherapy

This system relies on prescribed doses to defined reference points. Manchester point A is defined as a point 2 cm lateral to the central uterine canal and 2 cm superior to the lateral fornix in the plane of the uterus. It lies within the paracervical tissues near the uterine artery and ureter, and was chosen to take into account the tolerance of adjacent dose-limiting normal structures. In practice, the prescribed dose of irradiation is specified at a point that is 2 cm above and 2 cm lateral to the flange of the intrauterine tube at the external os. This point is taken to be equivalent to Manchester point A. Point B is defined as being 3 cm lateral to point A, i.e. 5 cm from the midline on the lateral axis, and it is used to provide an indication of dose to the distal parametria. The ICRU Report No. 38 specifies reference points for the bladder and rectum. The bladder point is posterior to the catheter balloon filled with 7 mL of contrast solution. The rectal point is 0.5 cm posterior to the most posterior packing or posterior sarface of the ovoids.

■ Applicators used in gynaecological brachytherapy

A number of different applicators are available for use with an intact uterus. A central intrauterine tube is used with a vaginal applicator, which can consist of a cylinder, ovoids or a ring. Applicators have been developed that contain holes for interstitial needles, which may be used to produce better coverage of inner parametrial disease.

Vaginal vault brachytherapy can be delivered using a vaginal cylindrical applicator or vaginal ovoids. Both are available in varying diameters/sizes. Ovoids produce a better dose distribution if coverage of the parametrial soft tissues is required, whereas cylindrical applicators mainly treat the vaginal mucosa. Doses are prescribed to 0.5 cm from the surface of the applicator.

■ Example of LDR/MDR applicator insertion technique

After examination under general or spinal anaesthesia and urinary catheter insertion, the uterine cavity is measured with a sound. The cervical canal is dilated and a central uterine tube of appropriate length is inserted. The vaginal applicators are then positioned and fixed to the tube. Vaginal packing is used to distance OAR from the applicator and to prevent rotation of the applicators. The applicators can be further secured using labial sutures or bandaging. 2D or 3D imaging can then be performed.

■ Fractionated HDR delivery technique

The principles of applicator insertion are the same as those for LDR/MDR. A Schmidt's sleeve can be placed or sutured into the cervical canal, which may facilitate reinsertion of the applicators without anaesthesia for subsequent fractions. A rectal retractor can be used instead of or as well as vaginal packing to create distance between the applicators and rectum. A perineal bar is another method used to secure the applicator position.

Dose-fractionation

■ Primary radiotherapy

Stage IB2 and IIA

EBRT
45 Gy in 25 daily fractions of 1.8 Gy given in 5 weeks followed by intracavitary brachytherapy.

Intracavitary brachytherapy
LDR

27 Gy to point A single insertion.

or

HDR

14 Gy in 2 fractions given in 5–8 days to point A.

Stage IIB or above

EBRT
50.4 Gy in 28 daily fractions of 1.8 Gy given in 5½ weeks followed by intracavitary brachytherapy.

Intracavitary brachytherapy
LDR

22.5–25 Gy to point A single insertion.

HDR

21 Gy in 3 fractions over 5–8 days to point A.

Concurrent chemotherapy (weekly cisplatin $40\,mg/m^2$) is given for both high risk early stage disease and locally advanced tumours unless patients are medically unfit for chemotherapy or have a GFR $<50\,mL/min$. Overall treatment time should not exceed 56 days including brachytherapy and should ideally be 49 days or less.

■ EBRT boost to central tumour when brachytherapy not feasible

15 Gy in 8 daily fractions

or

20 Gy in 11 daily fractions.

Total dose 65 Gy (in 2 Gy equivalent).

■ EBRT boost to residual macroscopic disease

5.4 Gy in 3 daily fractions of 1.8 Gy
or
10.8 Gy in 6 daily fractions of 1.8 Gy.

■ Adjuvant radiotherapy

EBRT

45 Gy in 25 daily fractions of 1.8 Gy given in 5 weeks.
50.4 Gy in 28 daily fractions of 1.8 Gy in 5½ weeks if macroscopic residual disease.

Concurrent chemotherapy is administered if there are positive surgical margins, positive pelvic nodes or parametrial involvement and treatment time should not exceed 56 days.

Intracavitary brachytherapy to vaginal vault

LDR
15 Gy at 0.5 cm from surface of applicator.
20 Gy at 0.5 cm from surface of applicator given in a single application if macroscopic residual vault disease.

HDR
8 Gy at 0.5 cm from surface of applicator in 2 fractions
or
12 Gy in 3 fractions if positive vaginal surgical margin.

■ Para-aortic node radiotherapy

Adjuvant radiotherapy

45 Gy in 25 daily fractions of 1.8 Gy given in 5 weeks.

■ Palliative treatment

Whole pelvis or para-aortic nodes

20–30 Gy in 5–10 daily fractions given in 1–2 weeks.
8–10 Gy in 1 fraction for haemostasis.

Treatment delivery and patient care

Patients are aligned with tattoos and laser lights using an identical set-up to that for localisation in the CT scanner or simulator. When given concurrently, chemotherapy is given every 7 days with radiotherapy delivered 1–2 h later with strict scheduling compliance. Overall treatment time should be as short as possible and delays avoided so that for SCC it does not exceed 56 days and ideally is 49 days or less. These are category 1 patients and any unscheduled gaps in treatment are rectified by treating at the weekend or by using 2 fractions in 1 day with a minimal interval of 6 h. Intracavitary brachytherapy should follow EBRT as planned without delay.

Patients are reminded to follow the bladder filling protocol to ensure reproducibility of treatment and reduce side effects. Acute side effects may be increased when radiotherapy is combined with concurrent chemotherapy. Diarrhoea may occur during EBRT of the pelvis, and is treated with loperamide hydrochloride and a low residue diet. If diarrhoea worsens and/or abdominal pain occurs, treatment may need to be suspended. Urinary frequency and dysuria may occur, and a urine specimen should be taken to exclude infection. Rectal bleeding and painful defecation may occur. Patients undergoing para-aortic nodal irradiation should receive prophylactic antiemetics to prevent nausea and vomiting. A good fluid intake should be encouraged and patients should avoid smoking. Severe perineal or natal cleft skin reactions are treated with 1 per cent hydrocortisone cream. Studies have shown that haemoglobin should be maintained at 12 g/dL or above, as locoregional recurrence rates are higher in anaemic patients. Premenopausal patients will lose ovarian function, and hormone replacement therapy may be given to improve menopausal symptoms and prevent osteoporosis. Vaginal hydration gels and dilators are used to help reduce vaginal shortening and stenosis. Psychosexual counselling may be helpful. Chronic fatigue, urinary or faecal urgency or incontinence and pelvic pain are uncommon late effects of pelvic radiotherapy and require special care.

Verification

Portal films or EPIs are taken on the first 3–5 treatment days and compared with DRRs or simulator images within a verification strategy protocol. Any systematic errors of >5 mm are identified and corrected and weekly EPIs then taken. Exit dosimetry using diodes is performed on the first day in all patients.

Key trials

Keys HM, Bundy BN, Stehman FB *et al.* (1999) Cisplatin, radiation and adjuvant hysterectomy compared with radiation and adjuvant hysterectomy for bulky stage IB cervical carcinoma. *N Engl J Med* **340**: 1154–61.

Morris M, Eifel PJ, Lu J *et al.* (1999) Pelvic radiation with concurrent chemotherapy compared with pelvic and para-aortic radiation for high-risk cervical cancer. *N Engl J Med* **340**: 1137–43.

Peters WA, Liu PY, Barrett RGW *et al.* (1999) Cisplatin, 5-fluorouracil plus radiation therapy are superior to radiation therapy as adjunctive therapy in high risk, early stage carcinoma of the cervix after radical hysterectomy and pelvic lymphadenectomy: report of a phase III inter group study. *Gynecol Oncol* **72**: 443.

Rose PG, Bundy BN, Watkins EB *et al.* (1999) Concurrent cisplatin-based radiotherapy and chemotherapy for locally advanced cervical cancer. *N Engl J Med* **340**: 1144–53.

Whitney CW, Sause W, Bundy BN *et al.* (1999) Randomised comparison of fluorouracil plus cisplatin versus hydroxyurea as an adjunct to radiation therapy in stage IIB-IVA carcinoma of the cervix with negative para-aortic lymph nodes: a Gynecologic Oncology Group and Southwest Oncology Group study. *J Clin Oncol* **17**: 1339–48.

Information sources

Cancer Backup (2007) Pelvic radiotherapy in women: possible late effects. Available at: www.cancerbackup.org.uk

Green J, Kirwan J, Tierney J *et al.* (2005) Concomitant chemotherapy and radiation therapy for cancer of the uterine cervix. *Cochrane Database Syst Rev* CD002225.

Haie-Meder C, Pötter R, Van Limbergen E *et al.* (2005) Recommendations from Gynaecological (GYN) GEC-ESTRO Working Group (I): concepts and terms in 3D image based 3D treatment planning in cervix cancer brachytherapy with emphasis on MRI assessment of GTV and CTV. *Radiother Oncol* **74**: 235–45.

Pötter R, Haie-Meder C, Van Limbergen E *et al.* (2006) Recommendations from Gynaecological (GYN) GEC ESTRO Working Group (II): concepts and terms in 3D image based treatment planning in cervix cancer brachytherapy: aspects of 3D imaging, radiation physics, radiobiology, and 3D dose volume parameters. *Radiother Oncol* **78**: 67–77.

Sedlis A, Bundy BN, Rotman MZ *et al.* (1999) A randomised trial of pelvic radiation therapy versus no further therapy in selected patients with stage IB carcinoma of the cervix after radical hysterectomy and pelvic lymphadenectomy: a Gynecologic Oncology Group Study. *Gynecol Oncol* **73**: 177–83.

Taylor A, Rockall AG, Reznek RH *et al.* (2005) Mapping pelvic lymph nodes: guidelines for delineation in intensity-modulated radiotherapy. *Int J Radiat Oncol Biol Phys* **63**: 1604–12.

Taylor A, Rockall AG, Powell ME (2007) An atlas of the pelvic lymph node regions to aid radiotherapy target volume definition. *Clin Oncol* **19**: 542–50.

33 Uterus

Indications for radiotherapy

A total abdominal hysterectomy with bilateral salpingo-oophorectomy is the mainstay of treatment for all tumours of the corpus uteri, of which adenocarcinoma of the endometrium of endometrioid type is the most common. Histological staging and prognostic factors are determined from the surgical specimen and are used to guide adjuvant treatment.

For low risk patients (stage IA and IB, grade I–2) relapse-free survival is 95 per cent with surgery alone, and neither lymphadenectomy nor adjuvant EBRT is indicated. Vaginal vault brachytherapy may be considered in some patients with stage IB grade 2 disease where there is lymphovascular space invasion (LVSI).

For intermediate risk patients (with stage IA–IB grade 3 without LVSI, IC grade I and 2, stage IIA grade I–2, age 60 or over) there is a 15–25 per cent risk of locoregional relapse after surgery, which can be reduced to around 5 per cent with postoperative pelvic radiotherapy. The PORTEC-2 trial randomised these patients between postoperative pelvic radiotherapy and vaginal brachytherapy to see if local control can be maintained, with a reduction in toxicity of treatment and improvement in quality of life. Vaginal vault brachytherapy may be the treatment of choice if no difference in overall pelvic failure and survival is shown.

High risk patients include those with two or more of the following risk factors: stage T1C (invasion of more than 50 per cent of myometrium), grade 3 disease, and LVSI. For these patients lymph node involvement is around 35 per cent and overall 5-year survival 55–60 per cent. Other poor prognostic features are serous papillary or clear cell histology, which often present with advanced disease, and involvement of the cervix (stage II). Bilateral pelvic lymph node dissection (BPLND) is performed for accurate staging but has not been shown to confer any survival advantage for high risk early stage patients. Pelvic radiotherapy after surgery improves locoregional control. However, high risk patients and those with locally advanced disease die of metastatic spread, so the addition of concurrent and adjuvant chemotherapy is being investigated in a randomised trial (PORTEC-3). A vaginal brachytherapy boost is given in addition to EBRT to improve local control in patients with histological involvement of the cervical stroma.

The behaviour of serous tumours is more like that of primary ovarian cancer, so omentectomy is performed in addition to BPLND. Chemotherapy may play a role in adjuvant treatment in addition to EBRT.

Radiotherapy may be used as a primary treatment for more advanced or inoperable disease or in the rare instance when the patient is unfit for surgery. Five-year survival rates of 70–75 per cent are obtained for stage II, 50 per cent for stage III and 25 per cent for stage IV disease.

Rarer tumours include carcinosarcomas, leiomyosarcomas, endometrial stromal sarcomas (which are mainly low grade), and squamous cell carcinomas. Surgery is the mainstay of treatment for these tumours, with adjuvant pelvic EBRT given with proven benefit for carcinosarcomas and SCCs and for local control only in selected cases of leiomyosarcomas and endometrial stromal sarcomas.

Sequencing of multimodality treatment

Multicentre trials are currently assessing the value of concurrent chemotherapy with radiotherapy, followed by adjuvant chemotherapy with platinum drugs and taxanes, for high risk and advanced stage endometrial carcinoma. These regimens are being compared with pelvic radiotherapy alone to establish outcomes in terms of locoregional relapse and survival, as well as the toxicity profile and effect on quality of life. Chemotherapy can also be given before pelvic radiotherapy.

Clinical and radiological anatomy

The uterus is supported by the levator ani muscles and is commonly anteverted and inclined forwards at an angle of 90° to the axis of the vagina (Fig. 33.1). The myometrial wall of the body of the uterus is lined by endometrium and covered externally by a reflection of the peritoneum. The base of the bladder is closely applied to the anteroinferior part of the uterus, and posteriorly the pouch of Douglas lies between the posterior fornix and the rectum. Loops of small bowel may lie in the pouch of Douglas, limiting the dose of irradiation which can be given.

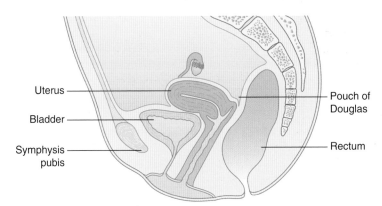

Figure 33.1 Regional anatomy of the uterus.

Tumour may infiltrate locally through the myometrium and parametrium to involve other pelvic organs including into the peritoneal cavity, or it may extend inferiorly to the endocervix and vagina. Lymphatic drainage from the corpus passes through the broad ligament to the obturator, external iliac and presacral lymph nodes, and via the round ligament to the superficial inguinal lymph nodes (Fig. 33.2). Spread may also occur in the ovarian vessels to the para-aortic nodes, and by retrograde lymphatic spread to the lower third of the vagina, particularly posterior to the urethra. If the endocervix is involved, lymphatic spread occurs through paracervical and parametrial pathways to pelvic lymph nodes. Serous tumours spread like ovarian tumours trans-coelomically. The most common sites for distant metastases are the lungs, liver, bone and brain.

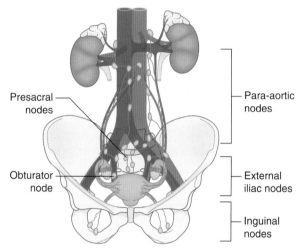

Presacral nodes

Para-aortic nodes

Obturator node

External iliac nodes

Inguinal nodes

Figure 33.2 Lymphatic drainage of the uterus.

Assessment of nodal involvement by CT and MRI are both dependent on size criteria (usually a short axis lymph node diameter greater than 1 cm), but the sensitivity is only 40–70 per cent. MRI with intravenous contrast agent USPIO (ultra-small particles of iron oxide) improves the sensitivity of detecting pelvic nodal metastases down to 3 mm with maintained specificity. PET has a high sensitivity for detecting both nodal and distant metastases.

Assessment of primary disease

Patients commonly present with postmenopausal bleeding. They first undergo a transvaginal ultrasound examination. Assessment then involves hysteroscopy and biopsy to make a histological diagnosis. MRI is more sensitive than CT at identifying the presence of myometrial invasion (Fig. 33.3) and determining its depth (e.g. whether greater than 50 per cent), and cervical involvement, as well as at detecting pelvic and para-aortic lymph nodes for accurate preoperative staging. All patients with moderate or high grade tumours on biopsy should therefore undergo MRI at diagnosis to select patients for referral to specialist centres for BPLND. Assessment of patients for adjuvant radiotherapy should take into account all surgical and histological information including stage, grade, histological subtype, presence of LVSI, and positive lymph nodes or positive washings collected at surgery. Inguinal lymph nodes are assessed by palpation, although involvement of enlarged nodes can only be proved by histological or cytological examination. It is uncommon and related to invasion of the lower third of the vagina.

CT scan of the chest and abdomen is performed for high grade uterine sarcomas to exclude distant metastases because of the risk of early haematogenous spread.

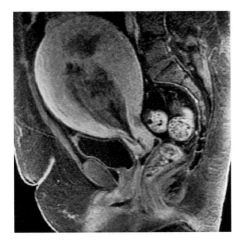

Figure 33.3 Sagittal T1-weighted MR scans showing a T1c endometrial carcinoma infiltrating into the outer half of the myometrium.

Data acquisition

■ CT scanning

Most patients referred for radiotherapy require adjuvant pelvic EBRT following surgery. With the change from 2D to 3D planning, CT scanning is now recommended for data acquisition. Patients are scanned in the treatment position supine with arms on the chest, knees and lower legs immobilised. Anterior and lateral tattoos are aligned with lasers to prevent lateral rotation and marked with radio-opaque material. For obese patients, the prone bellyboard may be used to allow small bowel to fall anteriorly away from the target volume. A protocol is used to maintain a constant bladder filling 'comfortably full' to push the small bowel superiorly. For example, patients are asked to empty the bladder and drink 200 mL water 20 minutes before the scan and treatment each day. The introitus is marked with radio-opaque material.

CT scans are taken from the superior border of L3 to 5 cm beyond the vaginal introitus. Intravenous contrast can be used to visualise primary tumour and uterus if still *in situ* and pelvic blood vessels, and thereby design target volumes for pelvic nodes most accurately. In this situation image registration with diagnostic MRI is especially useful to localise gross tumour in the uterus and/or nodes. Oral contrast is given to outline small bowel if IMRT is to be given.

■ Conventional

Conventionally the simulator is used to acquire data with the patient supine with arms on the chest, knee and lower leg immobilisation or alpha cradles to prevent pelvic rotation. The patient is aligned using orthogonal laser beams with anterior and lateral tattoos marked with radio-opaque material. For obese patients, a prone bellyboard immobilisation system may be used to allow small bowel to fall anteriorly away from the target volume. A protocol is used to maintain constant bladder filling 'comfortably full' as described above.

The vaginal vault is marked with a radio-opaque tampon for adjuvant treatment. In the rare cases where surgery has not been feasible, palpation of the primary tumour is carried out with the patient in the treatment position and the inferior border marked with radio-opaque material.

AP and lateral simulator films are taken. All clinical, surgical and histological data must be used, with any diagnostic CT or MRI information showing tumour extent, to design individually placed beam borders. The use of standard borders using bony anatomical landmarks has been shown to include unnecessary normal tissue and may miss primary tumour or lymph nodes.

Target volume definition

■ Adjuvant radiotherapy

CT planning

There is no GTV postoperatively and CTV-T includes the vaginal vault and parametrial tissues. CTV-N includes the obturator, external and internal iliac nodes and additional common iliac lymph nodes when indicated. CTV-T and -N are delineated using preoperative CT and MRI, operative diagrams and histological findings to include sites at high risk of recurrence. Guidelines have been proposed for standardised nodal CTV definition using CT scans with contrast-enhanced pelvic blood vessels (surrogate for lymph nodes) with a 7 mm margin.

A typical CTV-PTV margin of 10–15 mm is added for CTV-T and 7 mm for CTV-N to allow for organ motion and set-up errors, and is individualised depending on known results of departmental set-up variations.

Normal tissues to be contoured include bladder, rectum, small bowel and the femoral heads.

Conventional

The superior border is usually at the L5/S1 junction to include external and internal iliac nodes. If these nodes are positive, the border is at the lower margin of L4, individualised to include distal common iliac nodes. The inferior border is placed to include the upper half of the vagina for adjuvant treatment, or 3 cm below the most inferior disease in the vagina as palpated or seen on MRI. Lateral borders are 2 cm outside the bony pelvic sidewalls. The anterior border must encompass the CTV-N as well as GTV-T (if present) and is placed through the anterior third of the symphysis pubis. The posterior border is commonly situated 0.5 cm posterior to the anterior border of the S2/3 vertebral junction, but this is varied according to surgical and histological findings. Individualised shielding is employed in the anterior beam to the superior corners to exclude small bowel. Shielding to the inferior corners to protect femoral heads may mask the external iliac nodes and should be used sparingly. Lateral beams have shielding to sacral nerve roots posteriorly (Fig. 32.6b, p. 377).

A tattoo is placed at the centre of the volume with two lateral pelvic tattoos to aid alignment and reproducibility of the patient position.

■ Primary radiotherapy

Non-surgical patients with stage I and II disease may have multiple comorbidities which limit the volume that can be treated radically. The GTV for uterine tumours is defined on clinical examination and with MRI. The CTV-T includes the whole uterus, cervix, ovaries, parametrium and upper half of vagina. Involved nodes are detected by CT, MRI or MRI with USPIO. If the whole vagina is involved, the inguinal nodes may need to be included in the CTV-N. A CTV-PTV margin of 10–15 mm is commonly used to allow for set-up uncertainty and physiological movement of the corpus and bladder.

■ Palliative radiotherapy

For patients with locally advanced inoperable stage III/IV disease, the treatment intent is often palliative. Neoadjuvant chemotherapy may be considered followed by EBRT individualised to the gross extent of tumour in uterus, cervix, parametrial tissues, any vaginal extension and involved lymph nodes with a 2 cm margin.

OAR

The bladder, rectum, femoral heads and small bowel are delineated, and the sigmoid colon if utero-vaginal brachytherapy is used.

Intracavitary brachytherapy

Vault brachytherapy can be delivered using either a vaginal cylindrical applicator (Fig. 33.4) or vaginal ovoids. Both are available in varying diameters/sizes. Ovoids will treat the upper third of the vagina in most patients whereas cylindrical applicators can be loaded to treat any length of vagina required.

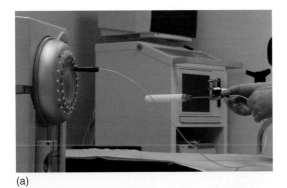

(a)

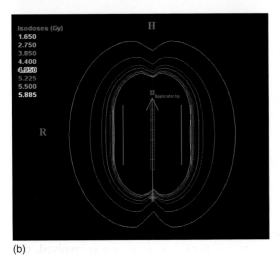

Isodoses (Gy)
1.650
2.750
3.850
4.400
4.950
5.225
5.500
5.885

H

R

Applicator tip

(b)

Figure 33.4 (a) Vaginal cylinder applicator for HDR brachytherapy with (b) dose distribution from an applicator 3 cm (W) × 3 cm (dwell length) prescribed at 0.5 cm from surface.

A central uterine tube ± vaginal applicator is commonly used to treat the primary tumour in the unoperated patient.

■ Para-aortic radiotherapy

See Chapter 32.

Dose solutions

■ Conventional

A 'brick' arrangement with four beams is commonly chosen (anterior, posterior and lateral opposing wedged beams), or where possible the posterior beam is omitted to reduce rectal dose. Higher energy photons (8–16 MV) are commonly employed and individual shielding used in superior corners of the anterior beam to exclude small bowel and reduce normal tissue dose. Care should be taken that any shielding of inferior corners to exclude femoral heads does not also shield external iliac nodes. Shielding to the sacral nerve roots may be used posteriorly in the lateral beams.

■ Conformal

With 3D target volume localisation, 3D dose planning can be used with individual shaping of each beam using MLC or shielding blocks to spare normal tissues. One anterior, two lateral opposing and one partially weighted posterior beam are commonly used (Fig. 33.5). Conformal radiotherapy and systematic target volume definition significantly reduces dose to the rectum and bladder compared with conventional solutions, as well as avoiding geographical miss.

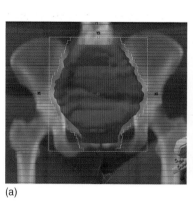
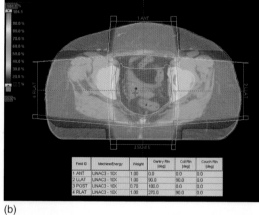

(a)   (b)

Figure 33.5 Postoperative radiotherapy for endometrial carcinoma. (a) DRR with anterior BEV. (b) Axial slice colourwash of the dose distribution using four-beam arrangement.

■ Complex

Pelvic IMRT (Fig. 33.6) has been shown to reduce the dose to bladder, rectum and small bowel by 20–50 per cent. This is especially important in the

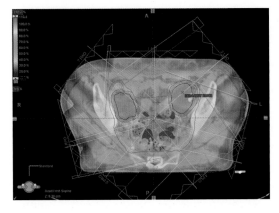

Figure 33.6 Stage IIIc carcinoma of endometrium with inoperable pelvic nodes – IMRT plan for postoperative EBRT.

postoperative situation, with reduction in acute and late morbidity. It may help to limit dose to pelvic bone marrow in patients undergoing chemoradiation.

Dose-fractionation

■ Adjuvant radiotherapy

External beam irradiation

45–50.4 Gy in 25–28 daily fractions of 1.8 Gy given in 5–5½ weeks.

Vaginal vault brachytherapy as boost after EBRT for patients with cervical involvement

LDR

10–15 Gy at 0.5 cm from the surface of the applicator.

HDR

8 Gy in 2 fractions at 0.5 cm from the surface of the applicator given at least 2 days apart.

Vaginal vault brachytherapy as sole adjuvant treatment for selected intermediate risk patients

LDR

30 Gy at 0.5 cm from the surface of the applicator.

HDR

22 Gy in 4 fractions at 0.5 cm from the surface of the applicator given at least 2 days apart.

■ Primary radiotherapy

Unoperated stage I and II disease

EBRT

45 Gy in 25 daily fractions of 1.8 Gy given in 5 weeks followed by intracavitary irradiation.

Intracavitary irradiation

LDR 20 Gy to point A single insertion

or

HDR 12 Gy in 3 fractions.

Inoperable stage III disease

EBRT

50.4 Gy in 28 daily fractions of 1.8 Gy given in 5½ weeks followed by intracavitary irradiation.

Intracavitary irradiation

LDR 22.5 Gy to point A single insertion

or

HDR 14 Gy in 2 fractions.

EBRT boost

Rarely, if intracavitary treatment is not feasible EBRT may be followed by an additional dose to the GTV using a conformal plan.

15–20 Gy in 8–11 daily fractions of 1.8 Gy given in 1½–2 weeks.

Intracavitary radiotherapy alone for primary disease, if unfit for EBRT

LDR

50 Gy given in 2 fractions in 15 days.

HDR

33 Gy in 5 fractions given in 15 days.

■ Para-aortic radiotherapy

45 Gy in 25 daily fractions of 1.8 Gy given in 5 weeks.

■ Palliative radiotherapy

20 Gy in 5 fractions given in 1 week.
30 Gy in 10 fractions given in 2 weeks.
8–10 Gy as a single fraction for haemostasis.

Treatment delivery and patient care

The patient is treated using the same position, immobilisation system and bladder filling protocol as for localisation, aligned using three skin tattoos and orthogonal laser lights.

Acute side effects may be increased when radiotherapy is combined with concurrent chemotherapy. Diarrhoea or abdominal discomfort may occur during EBRT, and is usually controlled by a low residue diet and loperamide hydrochloride. If these symptoms are severe, treatment may be interrupted to allow recovery. Care of the perineal skin is advised, but erythema and desquamation are now uncommon with 10–16 MV beams, unless the lower vagina is affected. Severe perineal or natal cleft skin reactions are treated with 1 per cent hydrocortisone cream and Intrasite gel.

Less commonly rectal discomfort or bleeding, urinary frequency or dysuria may occur and a urinary specimen should be taken to exclude infection.

A good fluid intake should be encouraged.

The risk of lymphoedema is increased when EBRT is given to patients who have undergone BPLND. Premenopausal patients will lose ovarian function, and hormone replacement therapy may be given to improve menopausal symptoms and prevent osteoporosis. Psychosexual counselling may be helpful, as well as vaginal hydration gels and dilators to improve vaginal function. Chronic fatigue, urinary or faecal urgency or incontinence and pelvic pain are uncommon late effects of pelvic radiotherapy and require special care.

Verification

Portal images are taken on the first 3 days of treatment using EPIs or portal films and compared with simulator or DRR images with a verification strategy protocol. Any systematic errors of >5 mm are identified and corrected, and weekly EPIs then taken. Exit dosimetry using diodes is performed on the first day in all patients.

Treatments in large patients may show a high random error and then daily portal imaging may be necessary.

---

key trials

Creutzberg CL, van Putten WL, Warlam-Rodenhuis CC *et al*. (2004) Postoperative Radiation Therapy in Endometrial Carcinoma (PORTEC) Trial. Outcome of high-risk stage IC, grade 3, compared with Stage I endometrial carcinoma patients. *J Clin Oncol* **22**: 1235–41.

Kitchener H, Redman CW, Swart AM *et al*. (2006) ASTEC – A Study in the Treatment of Endometrial Cancer: a randomised trial of lymphadenectomy in the treatment of endometrial cancer. *Gynecol Oncol* **101**: S21 (abstract).

Nout RA, Putter H, Jürgenliemk-Schulz IM *et al*. (2008) Vaginal brachytherapy versus external beam pelvic radiotherapy for high-intermediate risk endometrial cancer: results of the randomised PORTEC-2 trial. *J Clin Oncol* **26**(suppl): abstract LBA5503.

Information sources

Churn M, Jones B (1999) Primary radiotherapy for carcinoma of the endometrium using external beam radiotherapy and single line source brachytherapy. *Clin Oncol* **11**: 255–62.

Kong A, Johnson N, Cornes P *et al*. (2007) Adjuvant radiotherapy for stage I endometrial cancer. *Cochrane Database Syst Rev* (**2**): CD003916.

Small W Jr, Mell LK, Anderson P *et al*. (2008) Consensus guidelines for delineation of clinical target volume for intensity-modulated pelvic radiotherapy in postoperative treatment of endometrial and cervical cancer. *Int J Radiat Oncol Biol Phys* **71**: 428–34.

34 Vagina

Indications for radiotherapy

Primary carcinomas of the vagina are rare, with 80 per cent occurring in women over 60 years as SCCs. Clear cell adenocarcinomas of the vagina are seen in young women who are exposed to oestrogen therapy *in utero*. More commonly, tumours found in the vagina are an extension from primary cervical, vulval or urethral tumours, local spread from the rectum or bladder or metastatic lymphatic or vascular deposits from endometrial, breast or lung carcinomas. Surgery is the mainstay of treatment for malignant melanomas of the vagina, which have a high incidence of distant metastases and poor overall survival rates.

Vaginal intraepithelial neoplasia (VAIN) is treated with local laser ablation, excision or radiotherapy. Surgery is preferred in younger patients with intraepithelial 'field change' as this can be associated with cervical or anal cancers. It also avoids a radiation-induced menopause. Older patients with multifocal or multiply recurrent disease, or those who are unsuitable for organ-preserving surgery, can be equally effectively treated with vaginal brachytherapy.

Radiotherapy is the treatment of choice for most patients with vaginal tumours, because radical surgery may cause loss of function of bladder and/or rectum. Small, superficial, stage I lesions less than 3 cm in size are treated with brachytherapy alone. All other stages of the disease require either combined EBRT and brachytherapy or EBRT alone to treat the primary tumour and lymph nodes. Concurrent chemotherapy with cisplatin is used for locally advanced disease.

Radiotherapy gives overall survival rates of 44–77 per cent, 34–48 per cent, 14–42 per cent, and 0–18 per cent for stage I, II, III and IV disease, respectively. Most relapses after radiotherapy occur locally and cure rates are dose dependent. Maximal conformality of treatment is therefore an advantage. Palliative EBRT is given to control bleeding or pain from advanced primary tumours or vaginal metastases. Intracavitary or interstitial brachytherapy can also be used for palliation of vaginal mucosal disease and is particularly useful in patients with malignant melanoma.

Surgery has a role in selected patients with stage I disease, and usually involves a radical upper vaginectomy and bilateral pelvic lymphadenectomy with radical hysterectomy if the uterus has not previously been removed. Adjuvant radiotherapy should be considered if surgical margins are close or positive. Pelvic exenteration with vaginal reconstruction is sometimes chosen for more advanced stages, residual or recurrent disease. Surgery is the treatment of choice if a vesico-vaginal or recto-vaginal fistula is present at diagnosis. Ovarian transposition before radiotherapy can help to preserve ovarian function in the premenopausal patient.

Clinical and radiological anatomy

More than 50 per cent of vaginal tumours arise in the upper third of the vagina and from the posterior vaginal wall and spread laterally into paravaginal tissues (Fig. 34.1). They invade directly into the adjacent bladder and rectum. Lymphatic spread from the upper part of the vagina is to the lower cervix, obturator and hypogastric nodes, from the posterior wall to presacral and para-rectal deep pelvic nodes and from the anterior wall to the lateral pelvic wall nodes. The lymphatics of the lower third of the vagina drain by vulval lymphatics to the inguino-femoral and iliac nodes. Lower third tumours can also directly invade the urethra or anus. Of patients with stage II disease, 25–30 per cent have positive pelvic nodes, necessitating EBRT as well as brachytherapy.

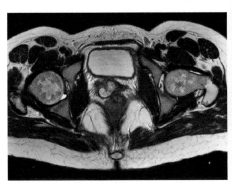

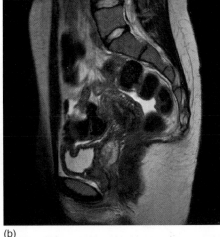

(a)   (b)

Figure 34.1 T2-weighted MR images of a patient with stage II clear cell adenocarcinoma of the vagina arising in the right posterior wall of the upper third. (a) Axial and (b) sagittal views.

Assessment of primary disease

Clinical examination of the entire vaginal mucosa and cervix is made by colposcopy and multiple biopsies taken from any suspicious areas as well as the primary tumour. For patients with invasive carcinoma, staging and assessment must include cystoscopy, hysteroscopy, endometrial curettage, cervical biopsy, bimanual examination and sigmoidoscopy where indicated. The inguino-femoral region is examined for lymphadenopathy and needle aspiration of palpable nodes performed to obtain cytology. CT or MRI can be used to detect ureteric obstruction and lymph node involvement, which do not influence the FIGO staging system but are used to plan treatment. Tumour stage (FIGO) is the most important prognostic factor, with tumour grade, volume extent within the vagina and presence of lymphovascular invasion all influencing survival. Adenocarcinomas and tumours of the lower third of the vagina have a worse prognosis.

Data acquisition

■ CT scanning

Patients are scanned supine with legs abducted where appropriate to reduce perineal skin reactions. Movement is limited by leg immobilisation with anterior and lateral tattoos used to prevent lateral rotation. Radio-opaque markers are placed by clinical examination in the treatment position at the inferior extent of vaginal tumour to define the inferior GTV margin and at the introitus (Fig. 34.2). Variations in bladder volume have been shown to influence mobility and position of the uterus, cervix and vagina and a protocol should therefore be used to maintain a constant bladder filling – 'comfortably full'. Patients are asked to empty the bladder and drink 200 mL water 20 min before the scan and before treatment each day. Patients should be encouraged to empty their bowels regularly before CT scanning and daily treatment. Intravenous contrast is used to enhance pelvic blood vessels, which are used as surrogates for pelvic lymph nodes when designing the CTV-N. CT scans are acquired from L3 to 5 cm below the introitus.

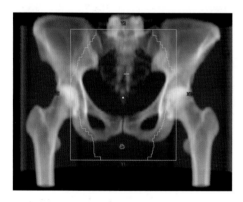

Figure 34.2 DRR with radio-opaque marker at the introitus to show anterior BEV.

Target volume definition

■ CT planning

GTV-T is the primary vaginal tumour as defined by clinical examination, EUA, and co-registered MRI or CT scans. CTV-T includes the entire vagina, cervix and surrounding paravaginal tissues. For tumours of the lower third, the introitus is also included.

CTV-N includes different pelvic lymph nodes below the common iliac nodes depending on the site of the primary tumour:

- for tumours of the upper two-thirds of the vagina – obturator, external and internal iliac, presacral and para-rectal lymph nodes
- for tumours of the lower third of vagina – inguino-femoral and distal external iliac nodes
- for tumours involving the posterior vaginal wall – presacral and para-rectal deep pelvic nodes.

These are delineated by identifying contrast-enhanced pelvic blood vessels on each CT scan and using a 7 mm margin to create a 3D CTV-N.

A typical CTV to PTV margin of 10–15 mm is used around the CTV-T to allow for organ motion of cervix and vagina and measured set-up uncertainties. For CTV-N, organ motion occurs to a lesser extent and a 7 mm CTV to PTV margin is usually sufficient for set-up variations (Fig. 34.3). Bladder, rectum, small bowel and femoral heads are all outlined as OAR. For brachytherapy:

$$CTV\text{-}T = GTV\text{-}T + 2 \text{ cm margin.} \tag{34.1}$$

After EBRT, brachytherapy is used to deliver a further localised high-dose boost to residual GTV for stage I and II disease. When volume of residual tumour precludes brachytherapy (e.g. stage III disease), repeat imaging is used to define a new GTV-T. Further EBRT is given using a conformal plan with a 15–20 mm margin for the CTV-T and a further 10 mm margin for the PTV.

■ Conventional

Patient positioning, immobilisation and bladder protocol are used as described above. Where CT is not available for planning, all clinical, surgical, histological and radiological data must be used to define tumour extent before locating the beam borders using a simulator. Palpation of the primary tumour is carried out with the patient in the treatment position and the inferior tumour extent and introitus marked with radio-opaque material. AP and lateral simulator films are taken.

For tumours of the upper two-thirds of the vagina, the CTV includes the whole vagina, cervix and obturator, external and internal iliac, presacral and para-rectal lymph nodes. The superior border of the beam is at the L5/S1 junction, lateral borders are 20 mm lateral to the bony pelvic sidewall and the inferior border is at the introitus. The anterior border should encompass the GTV-T and iliac nodes superiorly and is usually at the anterior one-third of the symphysis pubis. The posterior border is 20 mm from the GTV-T including posterior extension of tumour and internal iliac nodes and is commonly situated 5 mm posterior to the anterior border of the S2/3 vertebral junction. When tumours involve the posterior wall of the vagina, presacral and para-rectal deep pelvic nodes are included, and the border should be placed posterior to these nodes and the GTV.

For tumours of the lower third of the vagina the volume includes the whole vagina, introitus, para-vaginal tissues, inguino-femoral and distal external iliac nodes. The superior border is at the upper acetabulum to include inguinal nodes, inferior border 30 mm below the introitus and lateral borders cover the femoral heads to include femoral nodes.

Dose solutions

■ EBRT

For all tumours of the vagina, a conformal plan is used (Fig. 34.3) with MLC or standard shielding to avoid normal organs, especially small bowel and posterior rectum. IMRT may provide the best solution for pelvic nodal treatments.

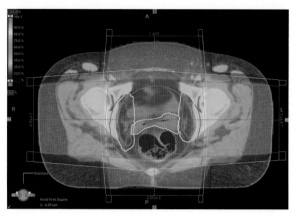

Figure 34.3 Axial CT scan of a patient with a vaginal tumour showing CTV and PTV of primary and nodes (CTV purple, PTV green) with dose distribution.

For conventional treatment of upper vaginal tumours, four MV beams are commonly used, e.g. anterior, posterior and two lateral; for lower third tumours, where CTV-N includes inguinal nodes, anterior and posterior opposing beams can be used, unequally weighted to spare the rectum and increase dose anteriorly to the inguino-femoral regions.

■ Brachytherapy

Cylindrical vaginal applicators can be used to deliver intracavitary brachytherapy for VAIN or superficial tumours that are less than 5 mm deep, either at diagnosis or after EBRT. Where tumours are more than 5 mm deep, either at diagnosis or after EBRT, interstitial brachytherapy is required. Interstitial implants using the Paris system are described in Chapter 5. Brachytherapy for tumours of the upper third of the vagina is delivered with the same technique as for cervical carcinomas, with a central intrauterine tube and vaginal applicators, as discussed in Chapter 32. A brachytherapy boost to tumours of the middle and lower third of the vagina, limited to the posterior wall, can be delivered using cylindrical applicators in both the vagina and rectum.

■ Palliation

For palliation of locally advanced fixed and fungating vaginal tumours, either EBRT or, when technically feasible, brachytherapy can be given. Radiotherapy is limited to the GTV with a 15 mm CTV margin to reduce toxicity using a conformal plan where possible or CT-simulated opposing beams.

Dose-fractionation

■ EBRT

Primary tumour and lymph nodes

45–50.4 Gy in 25–28 daily fractions of 1.8 Gy given in 5–5½ weeks.

External beam boost if brachytherapy not feasible

15–20 Gy in 8–11 daily fractions of 1.8 Gy given in 1½–2 weeks.

■ Brachytherapy

Brachytherapy alone

LDR

For VAIN, 60 Gy using intracavitary technique at 5 mm from surface of applicator. For superficial invasive disease, 65–70 Gy using intracavitary technique at 5 mm from surface of applicator in two insertions approximately 2 weeks apart.

For invasive disease, 65–70 Gy to 85 per cent isodose using an interstitial technique according to the Paris system.

HDR

33 Gy in 6 fractions given in 10–19 days.

Using intracavitary technique, prescribed at 5 mm from the surface of applicator. Using interstitial technique, prescribed to 85 per cent isodose using Paris system.

Brachytherapy after EBRT

LDR

15–20 Gy at 5 mm from the surface of applicator or to point A if using intracavitary technique.

If there are applicators in the vagina and rectum, 15–20 Gy are prescribed at the MPD between the surfaces of the two applicators.

20–25 Gy to 85 per cent isodose using Paris system using interstitial technique.

HDR

11 Gy in 2 fractions or 16.5 Gy in 3 fractions using either intracavitary or interstitial techniques.

■ Palliative treatment

EBRT

20 Gy in 5 daily fractions given in 1 week
  or
30 Gy in 10 daily fractions given in 2 weeks.
8–10 Gy as a single fraction for haemostasis.

> LDR brachytherapy 20–30 Gy.
> HDR brachytherapy 18–24 Gy in 3–4 fractions.

Treatment delivery and patient care

Patients are treated with the same bladder and bowel protocol and immobilisation devices as at CT scanning or simulation and aligned using three tattoos and laser lights to avoid lateral pelvic rotation. Care must be taken to check that the inferior border of the treatment encompasses the distal extent of tumour.

Acute perineal and natal cleft skin reactions are common and can be severe, and are treated with 1 per cent hydrocortisone cream. If moist desquamation occurs, treatment may need to be suspended and Intrasite gel used to promote healing, with diamorphine for pain control. Diarrhoea, abdominal pain, cystitis, proctitis and rectal bleeding may occur. Infections are excluded, loperamide hydrochloride prescribed and a low residue diet advised, as appropriate. Patients should be warned in advance of the 4–10 per cent risk of vesico-vaginal or recto-vaginal fistulae, which may occur particularly with more advanced tumours invading bladder or rectal wall. Patients should be encouraged to use vaginal rehydration gels and dilators to maintain vaginal function once treatment is completed as vaginal fibrosis can lead to narrowing and shortening of the vagina. There is an 11 per cent risk of necrosis of the femoral heads at 5 years when opposing anterior and posterior beams are used in an elderly population to treat inguinal nodes.

Verification

Portal films or EPIs are taken daily for the first 3–5 days to calculate any systematic errors. Corrections are made to reduce the systematic error to <1 mm and a weekly imaging protocol is then followed. Exit dosimetry is carried out using silicon diodes on the first treatment day to verify dose delivered.

Information sources

Chyle V, Zagars GK, Wheeler JA *et al.* (1996) Definitive radiotherapy for carcinoma of the vagina: outcome and prognostic factors. *Int J Radiat Oncol Biol Phys* **35**: 891–905.

Mock U, Kucera H, Fellner C *et al.* (2003) High-dose-rate (HDR) brachytherapy with or without external beam radiotherapy in the treatment of primary vaginal carcinoma: long term results and side-effects. *Int J Radiat Oncol Biol Phys* **56**: 950–7.

Perez CA, Grigsby PW, Garipagaoglu M *et al.* (1999) Factors affecting long term outcome of irradiation in carcinoma of the vagina. *Int J Radiat Oncol Biol Phys* **44**: 37–45.

Pingley S, Shrivastava SK, Sarin R *et al.* (2000) Primary carcinoma of the vagina: Tata Memorial Hospital experience. *Int J Radiat Oncol Biol Phys* **46**: 101–8.

Vulva

Indications for radiotherapy

Patients with carcinoma of the vulva commonly present with early stage T1, T2, N0 squamous cell carcinoma at a mean age of 70 years. Surgery is the mainstay of treatment, ranging from wide local excision (WLE) for early stage disease to radical vulvectomy for large or multicentric lesions, those within 1 cm of the midline or involving the labia minora. Overall 5-year survival rates of 95 per cent for stage I and 85 per cent for stage II disease are obtained. Unilateral or bilateral inguino-femoral lymph node dissection (LND) is recommended where the primary tumour invades more than 1 mm into the stroma and is chosen according to the size and laterality of the primary tumour. For small, lateralised tumours, defined as lying with a medial margin >1 cm from the midline, contralateral lymph node metastases are rarely seen in the absence of an ipsilateral metastasis, so unilateral LND may be performed. Where groin nodes are involved at surgery, radiotherapy is given to the inguino-femoral and pelvic lymph nodes, as randomised trial evidence has shown that pelvic radiotherapy is superior to elective pelvic node dissection. Lymph node metastasis is the single most important prognostic factor and results in a 50 per cent reduction in long-term survival.

■ Node negative

Adjuvant radiotherapy to the vulva alone is given to improve local control in patients undergoing WLE where the tumour shows a histological margin of less than 5 mm, re-excision is not possible and nodes are negative. If macroscopic residual disease is shown in the vulva in node negative patients after WLE, a radical local excision or vulvectomy is performed to obtain complete clearance. If this is not possible, radiotherapy is given with or without chemotherapy.

■ Node positive

Postoperatively, adjuvant EBRT is given to inguino-femoral and pelvic lymph nodes when there are one or more macroscopically involved nodes, two or more microscopically involved nodes, or evidence of extracapsular spread.

Primary radiotherapy ± chemotherapy may be used for patients who are unfit for surgery or with locally advanced disease, with or without subsequent surgery. Studies are examining the role of more conservative surgery combined with irradiation in selected patients with good prognosis in order to preserve bladder and/or rectal function and improve quality of life.

Palliative radiotherapy is given for fungating disease, pain or bleeding at the primary site or to the inguino-femoral regions. There is no role for radiotherapy in patients with vulval intraepithelial neoplasia (VIN), which represents a field change and is treated with surgery.

Sequencing of multimodality therapy

For stage III and IVA disease, primary concurrent chemoradiation with cisplatin ± 5FU in patients with adequate renal function (GFR >50 mL/min) is currently being investigated, followed 4–6 weeks later by surgery. No randomised trial data are available yet comparing this with primary radiotherapy alone. Toxicity is undoubtedly greater for the combined treatment but the response rates are promising.

Clinical and radiological anatomy

The vulva consists of the mons pubis, labia majora, labia minora, clitoris and Bartholin's glands. Most tumours of the vulva involve the labia majora. SCC spreads to the superficial inguinal and then deep femoral nodes in about 20–30 per cent of patients presenting with early stage disease. Of these, 20 per cent are shown to have pelvic lymph node metastases in addition. Tumour involvement of the midline structures of the vulva, e.g. clitoris, may lead to bilateral groin node spread, which is also present in 25–30 per cent of the patients with a positive ipsilateral groin node. Occasionally there is direct spread to the pelvic nodes via internal pudendal vessels. Direct local spread to the vagina, urethra, anus, bladder, rectum and pelvic bones is less common than lymph node spread. Blood-borne metastases to lung and bone are uncommon.

Assessment of primary disease

Careful clinical examination of the vulva and whole perineum is essential, with multiple biopsies of any suspicious areas performed as well as a deep biopsy of the primary tumour to assess depth of invasion. Excision of the entire lesion is not advised as planning of subsequent treatment may then be difficult. Inspection of the cervix and cervical cytology should also be carried out because of the multi-centric pattern of disease.

SCCs account for 90 per cent of vulval tumours and, rarely, melanomas, adenocarcinomas and basal cell carcinomas are seen. Extent of the primary tumour is assessed by clinical examination and MRI (Fig. 35.1). The inguino-femoral region is examined for lymphadenopathy. Fine needle aspiration of palpable nodes is performed (with or without ultrasound guidance) to distinguish between malignancy and infection. CT scanning can be used to stage pelvic lymph nodes, but MRI with ultra small particles of iron oxide (USPIO) shows increased sensitivity for detecting disease in normal sized nodes. Sentinel node biopsy is being investigated and results correlated with full inguino-femoral lymphadenectomy.

Data acquisition

Patients are immobilised supine with legs abducted as much as possible, on a CT scanner or simulator using lateral tattoos to prevent pelvic rotation. Where CT is

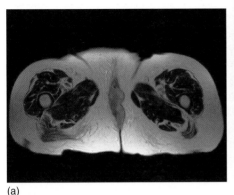
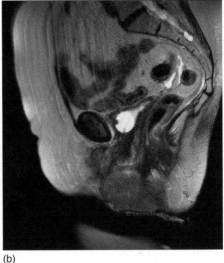

(a)   (b)

Figure 35.1 Stage III carcinoma of the vulva showing disease around the urethral catheter suggestive of urethral involvement. (a) Axial and (b) sagittal T2-weighted MR scans.

available, it can be used to identify the primary tumour and inguino-femoral and pelvic lymph nodes, using intravenous contrast to outline blood vessels. CT is especially useful for measuring depth of lymph nodes when selecting electron beam energies.

Using a simulator for locally advanced disease, clinical examination in the treatment position is essential with radio-opaque material used to mark limits of the macroscopic tumour and lymph nodes. The introitus should be marked with radio-opaque material in all patients to aid localisation of the inferior border of the CTV or field margin.

Target volume definition

When the margin of WLE is less than 5 mm, if re-excision is not possible and bilateral inguino-femoral LND is negative, radiotherapy is given to the vulva alone. This is usually done with the patient in the lithotomy position, immobilised using stirrups and poles, using detailed EUA findings and histopathology results to define the target volume including the depth. The GTV has been excised and the CTV includes the excision scar and remaining vulval tissues.

Following surgical excision and when nodal irradiation is indicated, the CTV includes the remaining vulva, inguino-femoral nodes, and distal external and internal iliac lymph nodes. Inguinal, femoral and iliac blood vessels can be used as surrogates for nodes and a 7 mm margin created around vessels to define CTV-N. The CTV-PTV margin used is dependent on measured set-up errors within each department.

If the simulator is used, the superior border is placed above the acetabulum to include distal external and internal iliac nodes, the inferior border 2 cm inferior to the vulval marker, and lateral borders defined by palpation to the outer inguinal ligament at the anterior superior iliac spine or to cover the femoral heads.

For locally advanced disease, the GTV of the primary tumour and lymph nodes are outlined with a 2 cm margin for the CTV-TN. The CTV for elective nodal irradiation is delineated as described above.

Dose solutions

Radiotherapy to the vulva alone is delivered with the patient in the lithotomy position, using electron therapy with good apposition of the applicator and bolus to ensure adequate skin dose to macroscopic disease.

For photon therapy to the vulva and lymph nodes, the patient lies supine. The target volume is irregular, lying anteriorly at the vulva and inguinal nodes, with deep extension to the femoral and pelvic lymph nodes. Treatment is usually given with conformal radiotherapy using four beams (Fig. 35.2) as this reduces toxicity compared with anterior and posterior opposing photon beams since bowel and rectum can be shielded. If opposing fields are used, unequal weighting, such as 2:1 anterior to posterior, may be used to increase dose to the anterior structures but this arrangement may give unacceptable hot-spots. Bolus may be needed to ensure adequate dose to gross primary tumour or positive surgical margins, particularly with the skin sparing effect of higher energy beams.

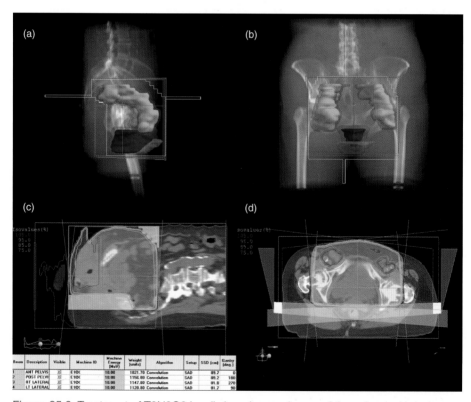

Figure 35.2 Treatment of T3N2G2 locally invasive carcinoma of the vulva and inguino-femoral and pelvic nodes showing GTV, CTV and PTV with bolus (pink), on (a) lateral and (b) anterior DDRs and (c) sagittal and (d) axial CT scans with 4 beam configuration. Courtesy of Dr Frances Calman and Marium Naeem.

For locally advanced disease, additional treatment is given to the primary tumour and palpable lymph nodes with a 2 cm margin. This can be done with reduced anterior and posterior opposing photon beams or a perineal electron beam localised to the primary vulval site and delivered in the lithotomy position. Inguino-femoral nodes lie at a depth of 5–8 cm and a direct electron beam can be used for this boost treatment with energy chosen using CT planning. Electron therapy may be optimally combined with photons to ensure adequate treatment at depth. Care should be taken to avoid overlap between electron beams used to treat the vulva and boost treatment to the groin nodes.

Interstitial radiotherapy may be useful as a boost treatment in selected patients, particularly if the lower vagina is involved by tumour.

Dose-fractionation

■ Adjuvant radiotherapy to vulva alone, node negative, surgical margin <5 mm

Electron therapy
45 Gy in 25 daily fractions of 1.8 Gy given in 5 weeks.

■ Adjuvant radiotherapy to vulva alone, node negative, residual macroscopic disease

Electron therapy
45 Gy in 25 daily fractions of 1.8 Gy given in 5 weeks.

Boost to residual disease
15 Gy in 8 daily fractions of 1.875 Gy given in 1½ weeks.

Total dose
60 Gy in 33 daily fractions given in 6½ weeks.

■ Adjuvant radiotherapy to vulva, inguinal and pelvic nodes, node positive

EBRT
45–50.4 Gy in 25–28 daily fractions of 1.8 Gy given in 5–5½ weeks.

Electron therapy
Boost to inguinal nodes if multiple positive nodes or extracapsular spread:

15 Gy in 8 fractions of 1.875 Gy in 1½ weeks.

Total dose
60–65.4 Gy in 33–36 daily fractions given in 6½ weeks.

VULVA

■ Primary radiotherapy to primary tumour and nodes (may be given as concurrent chemoradiation for inoperable, locally advanced disease)

EBRT

45–50.4 Gy in 25–28 daily fractions of 1.8 Gy given in 5–5½ weeks.

Subsequently surgery is performed if possible or further radiotherapy to the primary tumour and involved nodes given.

Electron therapy

Boost to primary tumour and palpable nodes:

15–20 Gy in 8–11 daily fractions of 1.8 Gy given in 2½ weeks

or

interstitial therapy to give a boost dose of 20 Gy to primary tumour.

Total dose

60–65.4 Gy in 33–36 daily fractions.

■ Recurrent disease

EBRT

45 Gy in 25 daily fractions of 1.8 Gy given in 5 weeks.

Electron therapy

Individualised boost:

15–20 Gy in 8–11 daily fractions of 1.8 Gy

or

interstitial therapy to give a boost dose of 20 Gy to primary tumour.

Total dose

60–65 Gy in 33–36 daily fractions.

Recurrent disease in the inguinal region only, if patient not fit for pelvic radiotherapy.

50 Gy in 20 fractions using an individualised combination of photons and electrons.

■ Palliative treatment

Photon or electron therapy

20 Gy in 5 daily fractions given in 1 week.
30 Gy in 10 daily fractions given in 2 weeks.
8–10 Gy in a single fraction for haemostasis.

Treatment delivery and patient care

Care must be taken in aligning the patient, using immobilisation of the lower limbs and lateral tattoos to prevent pelvic rotation.

Acute reactions of the vulval skin are common and can be severe. They should be treated with 1 per cent hydrocortisone cream. If moist desquamation occurs, treatment may need to be suspended and Intrasite gel used to promote healing with diamorphine given for pain relief. Urinary frequency and dysuria, and proctitis and diarrhoea are other possible side effects, which should be treated symptomatically. Late vulval fibrosis and atrophy may occur and vaginal rehydrating gel can be helpful. Lymphoedema can occur in up to 30 per cent of patients when inguino-femoral surgery and radiotherapy are combined. Urethral stenosis can also occur as a late effect. Limiting the total vulval dose to 65 Gy or less reduces the risk of skin necrosis. There is an 11 per cent risk of necrosis of the femoral heads at 5 years, if opposing anterior and posterior beams are used in an elderly population. This is reduced by conformal planning.

Verification

A series of daily portal or EPI films is taken to assess the systematic and random error rates and a correction strategy agreed. Checks must be made that all visible and palpable disease is encompassed as planned by the dose solution chosen. Exit dosimetry is carried out using silicon diodes or TLD on the first day of treatment to verify dose delivered.

Information sources

Barnes EA, Thomas G (2006) Integrating radiation into management of vulva cancer. *Semin Radiat Oncol* **16**: 168–76.

Busch M, Wagener B, Schaffer M *et al.* (2000) Long term impact of post operative radiotherapy in carcinoma of the vulva FIGO I/II. *Int J Radiat Oncol Biol Phys* **48**: 213–18.

de Hullu JA, van der Avoort IAM, Oonk MHM *et al.* (2006) Management of vulvar cancers. *Eur J Surg Oncol* **32**: 825–31.

Homesley HD, Bundy BN, Sedlis A *et al.* (1986) Radiation therapy versus pelvic node resection for carcinoma of the vulva with positive groin nodes. *Obstet Gynecol* **68**: 733–40.

IGCS. *Guidelines for Vulva Cancer.* Available at: www.kenes.com/igcs/posters/P01d.htm (accessed 12 December 2008).

Montana GS, Thomas, GM, Moore DH *et al.* (2000) Preoperative chemo-radiation for carcinoma of the vulva with N2/N3 nodes: a Gynaecologic Oncology Group study. *Int J Radiat Oncol Biol Phys* **48**: 1007–13.

Pecorelli S, Ngan HYS, Hacker NF (2006) Staging classifications and clinical practice guidelines of gynaecologic cancers. *Suppl Int J Gynecol Obstet* **70**: 207–312.

Tyring SK (2003) Vulvar squamous cell carcinoma: guidelines for early diagnosis and treatment. *Am J Obstet Gynecol* **189**: S17–23.

36 Sarcoma

Indications for radiotherapy

Bone and soft tissue sarcomas are uncommon tumours (<1 per cent of all cancers). More than 50 per cent arise in the extremities, 35 per cent in trunk, abdomen and retroperitoneum, and 10–15 per cent in other miscellaneous sites. Staging systems are shown in Table 36.1.

Table 36.1 Staging systems for soft tissue sarcomas

Tumours may be staged using the TNM system and grading		
I	Grade 1–2	T1a–T2b
II	Grade 3–4	T1a–1b, T2a
III	Grade 3–4	T2b–T3
IV	Any grade, any T, with metastases to nodes	
or elsewhere or more commonly as		
I	Low grade of any size or depth	
II	High grade of <5 cm of any depth	
III	High grade >5 cm deep	
IV	Any grade with metastases	

Grading takes into account mitotic count (<3, 3–20 or >20 mitoses /10 high power fields), necrosis and size.

A large number of tumour types (>50) are recognised by histological examination, immunocytochemistry, cytogenetics and molecular pathology techniques but the histological subtype is of relatively little significance in planning radiotherapy. Tumour size and anatomical site, which affect resectability, and tumour grade, are the most significant prognostic factors. Deep rather than superficial tumour situation, and recurrence after previous complete excision confer a worse prognosis.

Osteosarcoma and chondrosarcoma are treated with surgery with or without chemotherapy. They are radio-resistant tumours and if surgery is impossible, consideration should be given to referring the patient to an appropriate centre for proton therapy. If radiotherapy has to be given, local control requires high doses even after surgery or adjuvant chemotherapy.

Ewing's sarcoma and rhabdomyosarcoma are discussed in Chapter 37.

Surgery is the most effective treatment to ensure cure of soft tissue sarcomas, and the first intervention should remove all tumour with a wide margin. If tumours cannot be completely excised (without amputation of the limbs) radiotherapy will improve local control rates.

After complete excision of low grade stage I tumours with a >1 cm clear margin, no further treatment is needed. It is not yet clear whether radiotherapy is advantageous after complete excision of small (<5 cm) high grade tumours.

Postoperative radiotherapy is given after complete excision of high grade tumours which are more than 5 cm in diameter, and for all grades and sizes of tumours after incomplete excision.

Inoperable tumours are treated with initial radiotherapy, with surgery subsequently if marked tumour shrinkage makes this possible. In some sites, surgery will never become feasible and radical radiotherapy is then the treatment of choice. Chemotherapy may also be given initially in this situation to try to reduce tumour bulk.

All patients who present with locally recurrent disease or whose initial excision has been performed without proper staging and assessment will require postoperative radiotherapy with or without re-excision.

Desmoid tumours which arise in young people should be treated by wide local excision. However, sometimes relentless local progression of symptomatic disease or repeated recurrence after inadequate excision may need to be treated with radiotherapy. Giant cell tumours of bone should be treated surgically unless this is impossible. Lymphoma of bone is usually treated with chemotherapy alone. Bone lesions of Langerhans' cell histiocytosis are sensitive to low doses of radiotherapy but since their malignant nature is uncertain, curettage or intralesional steroids are preferred.

Radiation induced soft tissue sarcomas may be treated with radiotherapy as part of the planned management if appropriate. Such decisions must always be taken by the multidisciplinary team who are able to balance risks and benefits for individual patients.

Palliation may be achieved with shorter regimens and higher dose/fraction, although doses of less than 40 Gy in 3 weeks are unlikely to be adequate to relieve symptoms or prevent local progression.

Sequencing of multimodality therapy

Chemotherapy may be used adjuvantly after surgery to try to prevent metastases in high risk disease and has been shown to produce marginal benefit for local control and survival. It may be given as first treatment to shrink inoperable primary tumours.

The timing of radiotherapy in relation to surgery is important. Preoperative therapy has the advantage of a well-defined tumour volume with no risk of spillage of tumour cells which would require wider treatment margins. Blood supply is uninterrupted. For retroperitoneal tumours, preoperative radiotherapy may reduce toxicity to the bowel which is displaced by tumour but postoperatively falls into the surgical bed that has to be treated.

Clinical trials have shown that this approach produces comparable or better tumour control rates than postoperative EBRT. It may increase the probability of delay in wound healing. If preoperative EBRT is given, an interval of 4–6 weeks should elapse between EBRT and surgery.

A boost to the tumour bed by brachytherapy at the time of surgery or subsequently may improve local control rates. Intraoperative electron beam therapy has been used for retroperitoneal sarcoma and produces better local control rates and less bowel toxicity but with high rates of neuropathy.

Clinical and radiological anatomy

As soft tissue sarcomas may occur in any part of the body, detailed protocols must consider site-specific factors as well as sarcoma-related ones. Relevant anatomical details can be found in the various other chapters of this book. Spread is commonly haematogenous to lungs or through lymphatics to regional lymph nodes.

Assessment of primary disease

Careful clinical examination of the whole body is followed by plain X-ray for bone tumours to localise the tumour and assess the stability of the bone. For all patients, the tumour is scanned with ultrasound and/or CT scanning, and a biopsy is done at the same time under imaging control to plan treatment preoperatively. Both CT and MR scans are used diagnostically to assess relation of tumour to bone (CT) and to other soft tissues, most importantly nerves and blood vessels (MRI) (Fig. 36.1). CT scans are used to rule out metastases in the lungs, which are the commonest site of metastatic spread except in epithelioid sarcoma (regional nodes), and angiosarcoma where subdermal spread makes treatment volume definition difficult.

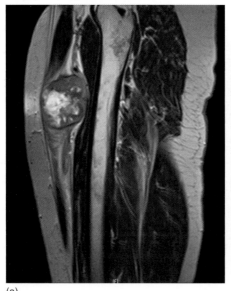
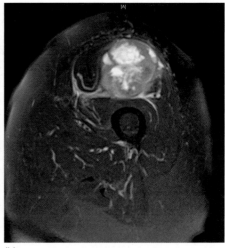

(a)   (b)

Figure 36.1 Preoperative MR scan of pleomorphic sarcoma in left vastus lateralis in (a) coronal and (b) axial views.

Data acquisition

■ Immobilisation

Immobilisation techniques will vary with different tumour sites, but for the common tumours in upper or lower limbs, individually prepared vacuum bags or Perspex shells are used. Laser lights are used to minimise rotational movement, and cranio-caudal movement should be prevented by appropriate foot or hand restraints.

■ CT planning

If possible, preoperative and pre-radiotherapy CT scans should be taken with the limb in the same position, and pre- and postoperative CT and/or MRI co-registered for planning. However, changes in muscle configuration following surgery and the position of the scar will alter appearances significantly and it is essential for surgeon and radiation oncologist to plan jointly all treatments for optimal local control and functional outcome.

Target volume definition

Postoperatively, a CTV must be designed which includes the initial GTV, any likely sites of tumour dissemination from surgery (such as scar) and a margin to encompass potential microscopic spread, which will vary for different tumour types from 20 mm to 50 mm (Fig. 36.2). Clips placed at surgery may be helpful. With improved imaging, a GTV-CTV margin of 20 mm may be adequate. Optimum treatment volume sizes are being studied (in the VORTEX trial). Incomplete excision of very large tumours (which may be 15–20 cm long in the limbs) may make the CTV planned this way prohibitively large, and it may not be possible to encompass scars and excision margins in full. EBRT may then be restricted to areas of bulky residual disease, for example around vessels or nerves.

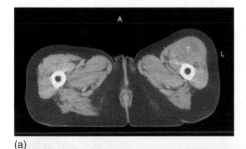

(a)

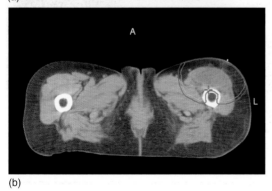

(b)

Figure 36.2 Axial CT scans: (a) preoperative showing same tumour (T); and (b) postoperative with CTV and PTV.

A CTV-PTV margin of 5–10 mm is added for set-up variability. In sites (such as ribs) where respiration is important, techniques appropriate to these sites should be used. OAR will also vary depending on the primary tumour site, and tolerance doses should be noted from relevant chapters. PRVs depend on balancing relative risks of recurrence or normal tissue toxicity in individual cases.

Dose solutions

■ Conformal

As long as 3D imaging and planning are available, all treatments should be planned conformally, even though in some cases, beam arrangements may still be simple (Fig. 36.3).

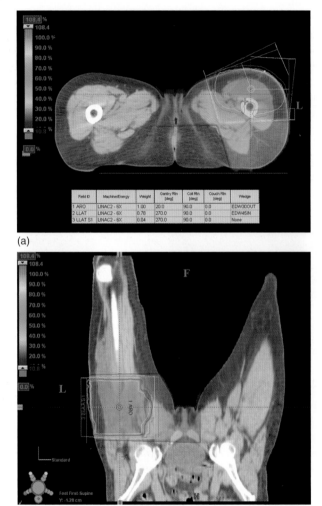

(a)

(b)

Figure 36.3 (a) Axial and (b) sagittal dose distribution for treatment of tumour.

■ Complex

IMRT is particularly useful for soft tissue sarcomas arising in sites such as the retroperitoneum where a steep dose gradient (for example between tumour and kidney) is needed or where a concave or convex dose distribution will spare vital tissues such as spinal cord. If respiratory movement is significant, a method of gating should be considered (see Chapter 2).

Conventional

Treatment plans will need to be individualised although simple arrangements of opposing or wedged pairs of beams may be used for limb lesions. Care should be taken in this case to leave a strip of normal tissue unirradiated on one or both sides of the limb to prevent late lymphoedema from fibrosis of lymphatic channels.

Radiation to a joint should be avoided if possible.

Brachytherapy

Catheters are inserted into the tumour bed at the time of surgery, thus ensuring that they are correctly placed using the Paris rules (Chapter 5). They are not loaded until the sixth postoperative day to permit wound healing. With low dose rate iridium wire, 45 Gy are given over 4–6 days as the only radiotherapy, or as a boost of 15–20 Gy before 45–50 Gy EBRT. This approach may be particularly useful for re-irradiation treatments.

Dose-fractionation

Postoperatively

66 Gy in 33 daily fractions given in 6½ weeks.

This dose is recommended for maximal tumour control although it will be associated with a risk of functional impairment from fibrosis. Delivery of some of this dose by brachytherapy may be beneficial (15–20 Gy).

Preoperatively

50 Gy in 25 daily fractions given in 5 weeks.
10–16 Gy in 5–8 daily fractions given in 5–10 days as a postoperative boost if the surgical margins are positive.

Inoperable tumours using conformal, IMRT with concomitant boost, or shrinking field techniques

GTV

66 Gy in 33 daily fractions given in 6 ½ weeks.

CTV

50 Gy in 25 daily fractions given in 5 weeks.

Doses may have to be adjusted to give as high a dose as is compatible with surrounding normal tissue tolerance.

Palliative treatments

40–45 Gy in 15–17 daily fractions of 2.67 Gy given in 3–3½ weeks if normal tissue tolerance permits.

Langerhans' cell histiocytosis

8–10 Gy in 4–5 daily fractions given in 1 week.

■ Giant cell tumour of bone

45 Gy in 25 daily fractions of 1.8 Gy given in 4–5 weeks.

Verification

Simulator films or DRRs are compared with port films or EPIs and doses are verified with lithium fluoride dosimeters or diodes.

Treatment delivery and patient care

For lesions in the upper part of the adductor compartment in the thigh or the sacral region, testis and natal cleft should be excluded or shielded.

Skin reactions should be prevented by good skin care and reactions treated with aqueous or 1 per cent hydrocortisone cream. For retroperitoneal sarcomas, antiemetics will be needed and loperamide for diarrhoea in pelvic/abdominal tumours. Neuropathy may occur if high doses are used. Late effects of muscle fibrosis can be reduced by physiotherapy to encourage movement during and for 6–8 weeks after treatment. Pathological fracture is commoner after postoperative than preoperative radiotherapy (9 per cent compared with 2 per cent).

key trials

O'Sullivan B, Davis AM, Turcotte R *et al.* (2005) Preoperative versus postoperative radiotherapy in soft-tissue sarcoma of the limbs: a randomised trial. *Lancet* **359**: 2235–41.

Pisters PW, Harrison LB, Leung DH *et al.* (1996) Long-term results of a prospective randomised trial of adjuvant brachytherapy in soft tissue sarcoma. *J Clin Oncol* **14**: 859–68.

Rosenberg SA, Tepper J, Glatstein E *et al.* (1982) The treatment of soft-tissue sarcomas of the extremities: prospective randomised evaluations of (1) limb-sparing surgery plus radiation therapy compared with amputation and (2) the role of adjuvant chemotherapy. *Ann Surg* **196**: 305–15.

VORTEX, UK-opened 01/02/06. A Randomised Phase 3 Trial Comparing a Two-Phase Conventional Radiotherapy Treatment with that of a Single Phase Treatment to Selectively Spare Normal Tissue and Increase Limb Function without Compromising Local Control in Soft Tissue Sarcomas.

Yang JC, Chang AE, Baker AR *et al.* (1998) Randomised prospective study of the benefit of adjuvant radiation therapy in the treatment of soft tissue sarcomas of the extremity. *J Clin Oncol* **16**: 197–203.

Information sources

Pervais N, Colterjohn N, Farrokhyar F *et al.* (2008) A systematic meta-analysis of randomised controlled trials of adjuvant chemotherapy for localised soft tissue sarcoma. *Cancer* **113**: 573–81.

Sarcoma Meta-analysis Collaboration (1997) Adjuvant chemotherapy for localised resectable soft-tissue sarcoma of adults: meta-analysis of individual data. *Lancet* **350**: 1647–54.

Weiss SW, Goldblum JR (2007) *Enzinger and Weiss's Soft Tissue Tumors*. Edinburgh: Elsevier.

Paediatric tumours

General considerations

■ Indications for radiotherapy

Children who are cured of cancer have a long life expectancy and treatment-related complications may be more severe than in adults. Although many paediatric tumours are very radio-sensitive, current protocols of treatment are designed to try to reduce toxicity of treatment for those who can be cured and to increase intensity of chemotherapy for those with poor outcome. Radiotherapy is therefore only used where it cannot effectively be replaced by surgery and chemotherapy. In very young children, even when radiotherapy will improve cure rates, it is often now deferred until the child is older and toxicity will be reduced because of greater maturity of organs and tissues.

Normal tissues in the period of development are more radio-sensitive than adult normal tissues, and the relative sparing effect of low dose per fraction for late morbidity is therefore exploited using doses per fraction of 1.2–1.8 Gy. Sequential studies in various tumour types have led to reductions in total dose and target volumes. Nevertheless, radiotherapy is still an important component of curative therapy for many tumour types and remains a valuable tool for easy and effective palliation.

■ Sequencing of multimodality treatment

Radiotherapy is usually given after chemotherapy and/or surgery and therefore the effects expected from radiotherapy alone may be modified.

■ Assessment of primary disease

All patients must be treated in specialist centres, using agreed national or international protocols. Management must be discussed at an appropriate multidisciplinary team meeting. As new drugs with potential synergistic or additive effects with radiotherapy are used, radiation doses may need to be reduced further for safety. Baseline assessment of any normal organ function that may be affected by treatment must be undertaken to be used in monitoring long-term effects.

■ Data acquisition

Immobilisation

Play therapists and specially trained nurses and radiographers are essential for preparation of all children for radiotherapy. Close collaboration is needed between paediatric and radiation oncologists. For very young children, adequate immobilisation may be difficult to achieve without anaesthesia, which increases the complexity of organising treatment. Dedicated and experienced anaesthetists and designated theatre sessions are needed to assure that treatments can be given safely and at the appropriate times. With adequate preparation, most children older than 3 years will learn to cope with the treatment satisfactorily without anaesthesia. Immobilisation is achieved with thermoplastic or Perspex shells or vacuum moulded bags as appropriate. Play specialists may help experienced mould room staff in making adjustments to normal practice to allow children who were initially apprehensive to become more at ease with the process.

CT scanning

With the patient immobilised in the treatment position, CT scans are acquired through the region of interest with 3–5 mm slice thickness. Diagnostic images may be co-registered with planning scans, which should include not only the whole tumour but the whole of any relevant OAR.

■ Dose solutions

Treatment should always be as conformal as possible using CT and MRI as appropriate if available. However, other considerations such as maintaining symmetry and minimising dose outside the treatment volume may lead to simple beam arrangements. IMRT solutions may produce better dose distributions for some tumours, and better sparing of OAR (for example in the head and neck where parameningeal sarcomas may be very close to the visual apparatus). However, they may result in increased low doses to larger volumes. There is concern about the potential risk of further increasing incidence of second malignancies.

It is important to maintain symmetry of growth of the musculoskeletal system by treating vertebrae across their whole width including the transverse processes and avoiding unfused epiphyses wherever possible. Treatment to one side of the neck only may result in asymmetry of muscle growth. Sometimes, taking all these factors into account, treatment with simple opposing MLC shaped beams may remain the best choice. Full DVHs of OAR must be obtained (see Chapter 4).

■ Dose-fractionation

Children should be treated by specialist teams working in collaboration with larger international and national groups. Details of treatment prescriptions are given in constantly revised protocols of the UK, European and American collaborative groups, which should always be consulted.

■ Treatment delivery and patient care

If anaesthesia is needed, treatment should be given early in the morning to ensure that the necessary period of fasting before general anaesthesia happens during the night to avoid mealtimes. Attention must be paid to maintaining good nutritional status especially if treatment causes anorexia, nausea or vomiting. Central line access is needed. Medication for specific side effects for each tumour site is detailed in relevant chapters. Appropriate adjustments in dosage are made according to the weight of the child. The radiation oncologist should be involved in the follow-up of any child treated with radiotherapy to document late toxicity, the expression of which may be modified by continuing changes in chemotherapy practice.

■ Verification

EPIs are taken on the first day of treatment and for 3 days and sometimes weekly throughout treatment to ensure reproducibility, especially if the child is awake during treatment. Diodes or TLDs are used to verify doses delivered.

Wilms' tumour

■ Indications for radiotherapy

Wilms' tumour occurs in about 8 per million children (80–90 cases per year in the UK), 70 per cent before the age of 4 and 90 per cent before age 7. The majority of Wilms' cases are sporadic but there is a strong association between Wilms', aniridia, genitourinary malformation and mental retardation in the WAGR (Wilms' tumour, aniridia, genitourinary abnormalities and mental retardation) syndrome, and in overgrowth syndromes such as Beckwith–Weidemann and hemihypertrophy. Results of a series of randomised studies in Europe and the USA confirmed that:

- preoperative radiotherapy reduces the risk of tumour rupture with increase in disease-free survival, but not overall survival
- preoperative chemotherapy is as effective as preoperative radiotherapy
- 8 weeks' chemotherapy is adequate for stage I disease and short treatments are as good as long ones
- two drugs (vincristine and actinomycin) are better than one
- addition of a third drug (doxorubicin) improves outcome for poor prognosis disease.

Both actinomycin and doxorubicin are radio-sensitisers, so should not be given at the same time as radiotherapy.

Treatment of this tumour is multimodal with surgery and chemotherapy, and in some cases radiotherapy. Actual sequencing of treatment varies between American and European studies, which have also used slightly different staging systems. The risk of biopsy tract seeding led the European groups to advocate chemotherapy without biopsy but American groups have been concerned about the 10 per cent incidence of misdiagnosis based on imaging alone.

Treatments are stratified by stage, histological subtype and by treatment response into low, intermediate and high risk groups. Preoperative radiotherapy has been replaced by chemotherapy. Postoperative radiotherapy at a low dose is given to patients with stage III favourable histology disease.

Those with unfavourable histology are treated with a higher dose. Those with intermediate group disease are currently treated with radiotherapy and chemotherapy with or without doxorubicin. If there is residual lung tumour after preoperative chemotherapy in a child with metastases, whole lung radiotherapy should be given. Radiotherapy is used for high risk primary tumour whatever the chemotherapy response. This is given to the whole abdomen and pelvis if there is diffuse tumour or gross rupture. Radiotherapy may also be used to treat liver metastases which are unresectable or show incomplete response to chemotherapy, and to treat bone and brain metastases regardless of chemotherapy response.

Survival rates are high – 90 per cent for stages I and II and 70 per cent for stage IV, so there has been a major emphasis on reducing treatment and its toxicity and on identifying disease with a poor prognosis for intensification of treatment. Current studies are concerned with developing case adapted treatment based on prognostic factors.

■ Assessment of primary disease

The commonest presentation is with an asymptomatic abdominal mass (75 per cent), with pain (44 per cent), fever and haematuria occurring less commonly. The diagnosis must be differentiated from neuroblastoma by measurement of catecholamines and ultrasound and MRI. Staging includes chest X-ray and/or CT scan of the chest and measurement of renal function by DMSA scan.

■ Target volume definition

GTV is defined as the tumour volume after chemotherapy but before surgery using co-registered MR-CT scans where available (Fig. 37.1). The CTV is the GTV + 10 mm. Care is taken to irradiate the vertebrae symmetrically taking the volume across the midline. PTV is individualised taking into account departmental measurements of systematic errors.

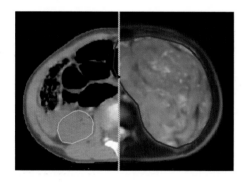

Figure 37.1 Fused CT/MR images of Wilms' tumour of left kidney.

■ Dose solutions

Conformal

With virtual simulation or 3D definition of the GTV, AP/PA beam arrangements with MLC shaping are often still appropriate to produce symmetrical irradiation of the vertebrae, avoid the contralateral kidney and minimise whole body doses (Fig. 37.2).

Complex

IMRT is rarely needed and conformal treatment is often adequate.

■ Dose-fractionation

Stage III favourable

10.8 Gy in 6 fractions of 1.8 Gy given in 1½ weeks.

Stage III intermediate

14.4 Gy in 8 daily fractions of 1.8 Gy given in 1½ weeks.

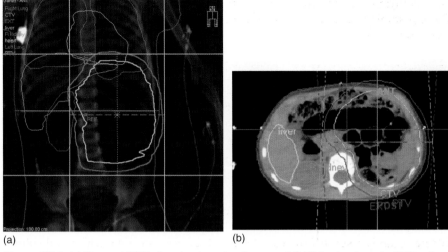

Figure 37.2 (a) Coronal DRR showing target volume and OAR for treatment of Wilms' tumour of left kidney. (b) Axial CT scan showing AP/PA beam arrangement.

Boost
10.8 Gy in 6 daily fractions of 1.8 Gy if node positive or macroscopic residual disease.

Stage II, III high risk
25.2 Gy in 14 fractions of 1.8 Gy daily given in 2½ weeks.

Boost
10.8 Gy in 6 fractions of 1.8 Gy to macroscopic residual disease.

Whole abdomen and pelvis
21 Gy in 14 daily fractions of 1.5 Gy given in 2½ weeks with kidney shielding at 12 Gy.

Whole lung (Fig. 37.3)
15 Gy in 10 daily fractions of 1.5 Gy given in 2 weeks with lung correction.

Possible boost
10.8–14.4 Gy in 6–8 daily fractions of 1.8 Gy to residual disease after surgery.

Partial liver
21 Gy in 14 daily fractions of 1.5 Gy given in 2½ weeks.

Dose constraints to OAR
- Whole lung – 15 Gy
- Heart – 15 Gy
- Ovary/testis – as low as possible (<5 Gy)
- Liver – 20 Gy to <50 per cent of total liver volume

If multiple areas need to be treated (i.e. flank plus lungs and/or liver) the treatments should be simultaneous to avoid the overlap of fields which would occur if the different areas were to be treated sequentially.

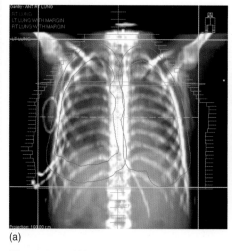
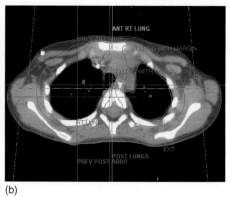

(a) (b)

Figure 37.3 Whole lung irradiation. (a) Coronal DRR. (b) Axial CT scan showing AP/PA beam arrangement. All images courtesy of Dr M Gaze.

Neuroblastoma

Neuroblastoma is the most common extracranial solid tumour in children, with 80 per cent presenting before the age of 4 and 90 per cent before age 10 with a median of 22 months.

■ Indications for radiotherapy

Tumours are now grouped by image-defined risk factors and histology, and survival is influenced by age and stage with overall 5-year survival rates of 44 per cent. Histology ranges from ganglioneuroma, which resembles normal organ architecture and requires little if any treatment, to undifferentiated neuroblastoma with MYCN amplification, which carries a poor prognosis. Neuroblasts are known to be radio-sensitive *in vitro* but show variable sensitivity *in vivo*. There are few well-controlled trial data to define the role of radiotherapy but review of studies undertaken showed reduction of risk of local relapse of between 22 per cent and 81 per cent. A study of chemotherapy alone versus chemotherapy and radiotherapy has shown improved overall survival rates when both modalities are used (41 per cent vs. 73 per cent). Indications for radiotherapy are shown in Table 37.1.

As these tumours may arise from a number of different sites, individualised planning must take into account all relevant normal tissue tolerances and possible late side effects.

Table 37.1 Role of radiotherapy in treatment of neuroblastoma

	Radiotherapy	No radiotherapy
Age <18 months	? Stage IV + MYCN >10	Localised disease + MYCN >10; stage IV + MYCN <10
Age >18 months	Localised disease + MYCN >10; stage IV	? Localised disease + MYCN <10

Sequencing of multimodality treatment

Multimodality treatment includes initial chemotherapy followed by surgery, often high dose chemotherapy and consideration of radiotherapy by EBRT, finishing with immunotherapy with retinoic acid.

Studies are now looking at combinations of chemotherapy (topotecan), MIBG (meta-iodobenzylguanidine) and EBRT and patients are referred to specialised centres for these combinations. High dose chemotherapy is now preferred to TBI for stage 4 (International Neuroblastoma Staging System, INSS) or stage M (International Neuroblastoma Risk Group Staging System, INRGSS) disease.

Assessment of disease

Thirty-five per cent of neuroblastomas arise in the adrenal gland, 30 per cent from paraspinal ganglia, 19 per cent from the posterior mediastinal sympathetic chain and the rest in the neck or other sites. They originate from the primitive adrenergic neuroblast of neural crest tissues. Prognosis depends on histological type and differentiation and measurement of MYCN amplification and loss of heterozygosity (LOH) on chromosome 1p and 11q. Diagnosis is made on the basis of tumour imaging and measurement of urinary catecholamines, with biopsy to confirm histological subtype and for estimation of molecular markers of prognosis. MYCN is not just a marker of prognosis but also determines risk stratification and therefore influences the selection of treatment.

Target volume definition

The GTV is defined as the post-chemotherapy but presurgical volume shown by CT scanning.

> CTV = GTV + 10 mm
> PTV = CTV + 5 mm or according to departmental protocols.

Consideration of potential growth impairment may require CTV volumes to extend across the midline to preserve symmetry and care must be taken since some organs may be displaced following surgery. Beam sizes will be at least 6 cm.

Dose solutions

Simple opposing beam arrangements may give adequate tumour coverage and minimal normal tissue dose, but shaping should be achieved with MLC if available. Because of multiple constraints and the proximity of vital organs, inverse planning and use of IMRT may be necessary to achieve an optimal plan.

Dose-fractionation

21 Gy in 14 daily fractions of 1.5 Gy given in 2½ weeks.

Radioactive labelled MIBG can be a useful treatment if scanning shows good uptake in tumour; 4 Gy to the whole body is given in two doses, the first determined by body weight (444 MBq/kg). The actual whole body dose (WBD) achieved is then measured and the second dose adjusted to achieve the final desired WBD of 4 Gy.

Rhabdomyosarcoma

■ Indications for radiotherapy

Seventy per cent of rhabdomyosarcomas occur before the age of 10 with the peak incidence at 2–5 years of age. Radiotherapy improves local control rates compared with chemotherapy alone and is still necessary for cure in many patients.

Concern about the late effects of radiotherapy has led to much reduced use, although it is still important for local control for tumours of unfavourable histology or site or those larger than 5 cm. Primary chemotherapy after initial biopsy is tailored to known prognostic factors and many combinations of drugs and alternating regimens are used. Surgery may be used for residual easily resectable macroscopic disease. Where complete remission of disease is obtained with chemotherapy, radiotherapy is deferred until relapse. If complete remission cannot be achieved by cosmetically and functionally satisfactory surgical excision after chemotherapy, radiotherapy may be given as part of the initial treatment. Treatment decisions are always influenced by the need to minimise effects on normal tissues and studies are still underway to refine the indications for each component of the multimodality treatment.

■ Assessment of primary disease

These tumours may arise in many different sites in the body. Site of origin is a significant prognostic factor. Favourable sites include the orbit, head and neck (non-parameningeal) and paratesticular tumours. Unfavourable sites are parameningeal, extremities, bladder/prostate, abdomen, pelvis, retroperitoneum and trunk.

Histological subtype is also of prognostic significance with alveolar and pleomorphic histology being associated with poorer outcomes than embryonal types.

Staging is according to the American Intergroup Rhabdomyosarcoma Study definition:

1 – completely resected localised disease
2 – gross resection, microscopic residual
3 – incomplete resection, gross residual disease
4 – metastatic disease.

Risk groups are defined based on staging, site, size, age and histological type.

■ Data acquisition, target volume definition and dose solutions

CT scanning and MRI are used to plan treatment with the patient in an appropriate immobilisation device for the tumour site. General principles of planning are applied depending on the site involved (see relevant chapters).

For treatment of residual disease after chemotherapy with or without surgery, the GTV is taken as the pre-chemotherapy volume in most cases. Exceptions include where a mass protruded into a body cavity without invasion (e.g. chest wall lesion extending into pleural cavity displacing lung) and has now shrunk back.

Some tumour sites such as orbit and limb are electively irradiated because of a high risk of local relapse. GTV for treatment of relapse is defined by the volume before re-induction chemotherapy. A CTV margin of 5 mm is allowed. PTV margin is chosen according to site and departmental protocols.

The most conformal plan should be designed with careful MLC shielding of normal tissues. Brachytherapy may be considered for vaginal tumours.

■ Dose-fractionation

Treatment of primary disease residual after chemotherapy

45 Gy in 25 daily fractions of 1.8 Gy given in 5 weeks.
Boost if indicated for bulky residual disease after chemotherapy/surgery.
9 Gy in 5 daily fractions of 1.8 Gy given in 1 week to macroscopic residuum.

Ewing's sarcoma

■ Indications for radiotherapy

Chemotherapy is essential for control of systemic disease which is the commonest cause of failure. All patients are treated within national or international protocols which use primary multi-agent chemotherapy, followed wherever possible by surgical excision. Radiotherapy is an effective agent, which has produced similar local control rates to surgery in randomised trials. Surgery is preferred for selected sites where complete excision is feasible. Radiotherapy may be added after incomplete excision and is a useful treatment for palliation of local disease when a child presents with metastases or after failure of chemotherapy. Longer-term trials are needed to determine optimal combinations of local treatment. Local radiotherapy to the tumour site gives results equivalent to irradiation of the whole bone.

■ Assessment of disease

Ewing's sarcoma in bone and its soft tissue variant, peripheral primitive neuroectodermal tumour, are characterised by a diagnostic (t11; 22) (q24; q12) chromosomal translocation. They occur commonly in the limbs or chest wall (formerly known as Askin tumours) and pelvis, and present with pain, swelling and sometimes systemic symptoms of fever and weight loss. They are diagnosed, as other sarcomas, by MRI (which clearly demonstrates the extent of soft tissue involvement which is a common finding), CT scanning and biopsy. Staging investigations must rule out metastases in bone, lungs, bone marrow, lymph nodes and other soft tissues. Lesions at a distance from the primary tumour may be found (skip lesions). Volume of tumour and site are important prognostic factors, with bulky pelvic lesions carrying the worst prognosis.

■ Data acquisition, target volume definition and dose solutions

Planning is carried out using the relevant principles outlined in site-specific chapters. MRI co-registered with CT scans gives the best definition of tumour extent. GTV is defined as the pre-chemotherapy extent of disease. CTV is created by adding a margin of 2–3 cm around the tumour for a first phase of treatment and a boost given to the GTV with a smaller CTV margin of 2 cm. Since extension is primarily along the marrow cavity, it may be appropriate to create anisotropic margins with the greatest expansion in the long axis of the bone. Conformal planning is used to give optimal dose distribution with sparing of normal tissues including a strip of tissue along a limb to prevent oedema. Small bowel and bladder must be outlined when treating large pelvic lesions.

■ Dose-fractionation

Radiotherapy alone for local control

45 Gy in 25 daily fractions of 1.8 Gy given in 5 weeks.

Boost
10.8 Gy in 6 daily fractions of 1.8 Gy.

Radiotherapy after surgery

45 Gy in 25 daily fractions of 1.8 Gy given in 5 weeks.

■ Treatment delivery and patient care

Principles are discussed in relevant site specific chapters. Careful multidisciplinary surveillance is important during treatment. Diarrhoea and frequency of micturition may occur with pelvic irradiation. Gentle exercise should be encouraged during treatment of limb lesions to minimise fibrosis.

Lymphomas

■ Indications for radiotherapy

There has been a gradual reduction in use of radiotherapy for lymphomas in childhood with the development of new effective chemotherapy combinations and increasing sophistication in diagnosis on the basis of molecular markers. In Hodgkin lymphoma, benefit has been shown in the DHL-HD studies for IFRT of 20–25 Gy in some groups. The UK HD3 study compared chemotherapy and radiotherapy in stage 1 disease and showed equivalence in terms of tumour control. In view of the high risk of second tumours after radiotherapy, chemotherapy is now preferred. Radiotherapy is used to treat PET positive residual disease after chemotherapy; it may be given for palliation or as salvage therapy after chemotherapy failure.

■ Target volume definition

- GTV 1 = pre-chemotherapy disease extension
- GTV 2 = boost to post-chemotherapy disease extent (PET +)
- CTV = GTV + 5 mm margin
- PTV = according to tumour site based departmental protocols and adjacent critical tissues

■ Dose solutions

- Conventional – AP/PA opposing beams.
- Conformal – outline all nodes on CT planning scans, use MLC shaped beams.
- Complex – this is not usually appropriate or necessary but may be considered for bulky abdominal disease or that in proximity to vital organs.

■ Dose-fractionation

PTV 1

19.8 Gy in 11 daily fractions of 1.8 Gy given in 2½ weeks.
(1.5 Gy fractions may be used for very young children or very large volumes).

PTV2

10 Gy in 5 daily fractions given in 2 weeks.
The testes should always be shielded during treatment of infra-diaphragmatic disease.

Langerhans' cell histiocytosis

This is a disease in which it is believed that a common, as yet unidentified, pathogen triggers an aberrant immune response leading to lesions in single sites, or in multiple sites in the same system (for example bone), or several systems (skin, bone, lung, brain, etc.). These lesions are known to be radio-sensitive but immune modulating systemic treatment is now preferred to radiotherapy, which has a minor role for palliation of severe pain. For localised disease requiring treatment where surgery is impossible, or to abort severe functional deficits, as in the treatment of spinal cord compression, doses of 6–10 Gy in 1.5 Gy per fraction have been recommended.

Information sources

Websites of various international and national collaborative groups are recommended for up-to-date details of treatment protocols:

Children's Cancer and Leukaemia Group (CCLG) (UK) – www.cclg.org.uk

Children's Oncology Group (COG) – www.childrensoncologygroup.org

International Society of Paediatric Oncology (SIOP) – www.siop.nl

National Cancer Institute (NCI) – www.cancer.gov/clinical trials; clinical trials home page of the National Cancer Institute (accessed 15 December 2008).

Pinkerton R, Matthay K, Shankar AG (eds) (2007) *Evidence-based Pediatric Oncology*, 2nd edn. Blackwell Publishing, Oxford.

38 Systemic irradiation

Indications for systemic irradiation

■ Total body irradiation

The indications for allogeneic bone marrow or stem cell transplantation with total body irradiation (TBI) as part of the conditioning are diminishing as more effective high dose chemotherapy regimens have been developed and the late effects of radiation are more widely recognised, especially in children.

Current indications for TBI as part of the conditioning regimen include the treatment of young adults (<40–45 years) with:

- high risk acute myelocytic leukaemia (AML) in first remission
- second remission AML (standard risk)
- second remission acute lymphocytic leukaemia (ALL) if there is a human leucocyte antigen (HLA) compatible sibling donor
- first remission ALL with CNS involvement or Philadelphia chromosome positivity
- low grade lymphoma after chemotherapy failure
- childhood AML/ALL in second or subsequent remissions.

The aim of treatment is to reduce the number of any residual malignant cells and to permit engraftment of the re-infused donor marrow or stem cells. For tumour control, the total dose of radiation should be as high as possible within the limits of normal tissue tolerance. Ease of engraftment is related to the type of marrow or stem cells infused. Less immune suppression is needed when the patient's own cells are re-infused than when fully compatible donor cells are used. High doses of TBI appear to facilitate engraftment of cells that are not fully compatible, although this type of procedure is less commonly used now.

■ Half body irradiation

High dose single fraction half body irradiation (HBI) is sometimes given as palliative treatment for widespread painful bony metastases from carcinomas, usually of the breast, bronchus or prostate, and can afford good symptomatic relief, although survival is not prolonged.

Fractionated systemic irradiation is now rarely used for non-Hodgkin lymphoma because new drugs are more effective. If used, sequential HBI is better tolerated than TBI and is therefore preferred.

Assessment of disease

Patients are treated according to national or international protocols and the radiation oncologist must have access to these and to discussions of the relevant multidisciplinary team to ensure the radiation is given appropriately, at the correct time. Remission of the disease should be obtained where possible before TBI and stem cell transplant is used. For patients with ALL, 'boosts' may be given in conjunction with TBI to sanctuary 'sites', either prophylactically or when there has been a previous relapse in these areas.

Patients with lymphoma who achieve a good response after chemotherapy but who have residual tumour at sites of initial bulky disease have also been treated with local boosts to these areas. However, TBI is less commonly used for these patients now. TBI given after previous mediastinal or cranial irradiation will be associated with a higher rate of complications.

In other situations, boosts may be given safely and most conveniently in a few treatments before TBI. Total doses are determined according to the age of the patient, the time interval since previous irradiation and the type and amount of previous chemotherapy. Young age, short time interval (less than 6 months) and high doses of chemotherapy are generally associated with increasing toxicity.

Because the chemotherapy component of conditioning will vary from one drug (cyclophosphamide, melphalan) to various drugs in combination, the oncologist must remain familiar with local haematological protocols and take into account any potential interactions with radiotherapy. The doses specified here as within normal tissue tolerance are when TBI is used in combination with cyclophosphamide.

Data acquisition

■ Conventional

TBI

A vacuum bag is prepared in which the patient can lie comfortably on their side during treatment. The patient's height and the required beam dimensions are determined and measurements of body thickness (separation) are taken at multiple sites (head, neck, upper and lower lung, mediastinum, abdomen, pelvis, thigh, ankle) to calculate dose distribution and define dose prescription point at the maximum lung dose.

HBI

The patient lies in the supine position with head supported on a comfortable head rest. Beams extend from the head or the feet to cover the upper or lower half of the body. The other border of the field is determined by the site of any disease, but is usually at the level of the iliac crests. Lateral tattoos are placed over the iliac crests and used to match beams if necessary.

■ Complex

If treatment is to be given with IMRT or tomotherapy techniques, CT scans of the whole or half body should be obtained.

Target volume definition

There is no GTV if the patient is treated in complete clinical remission and the CTV is the whole body. Since with a conventional technique, beams of radiation are used which extend beyond the patient at all points, a PTV is not defined. If additional radiation is to be given to sites at high risk of microscopic residual disease such as the testes, brain or mediastinum, which results in a cumulative dose higher than that which can be given to the whole body, these may be designated as additional CTVs with a dose specified. OAR such as the lungs, kidneys and eyes may be shielded in some techniques and for complex treatment solutions should be outlined to obtain DVHs and design MLC shielding.

Dose solutions

■ TBI – conventional

For treatment, the patient lies on one side facing a linear accelerator placed at an extended distance to allow an adequate single beam to cover the whole body. The collimator is rotated so that the maximum size of the diagonal of the beam (usually about 140 cm) can be obtained. A Perspex shield placed at the edge of the treatment couch between the patient and the machine provides skin build up (Fig. 38.1). As leukaemic cells may infiltrate the skin, skin sparing is undesirable. The arms may be positioned across the chest to act as bolus and help reduce lung doses. AP–PA opposing beams are used to achieve an adequate MPD.

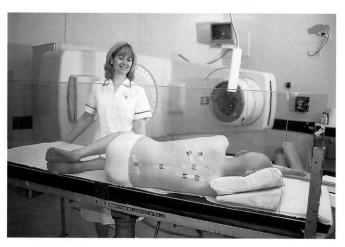

Figure 38.1 Patient positioned at extended focus–skin distance for total treatment with dosemeters positioned on back for measurement of upper and lower lung, mediastinal, abdominal and pelvic doses.

A number of different TBI regimens have been shown to be safe and effective, using the endpoints of engraftment, tumour control and incidence of pneumonitis, the most common dose-limiting toxicity. From radiobiological first principles, a TBI regimen should use the highest tolerable dose to control tumour, and an LDR or fraction size to minimise normal tissue damage. Variability in parameters of the tumour, growth characteristics, radio-sensitivity and differences in the number of occult residual cells at the time of TBI make it difficult to determine the best schedule for any individual patient. However, study data from

Seattle, and the UK Medical Research Council protocols, suggest that doses of 12–14.4 Gy are safe and effective. Beam arrangements are not critical although it is desirable to treat the whole body as a single volume.

Opinion is divided about the need to achieve a homogeneous dose distribution. Some centres attempt to obtain homogeneity using tissue compensators for areas such as the feet, between the legs, and neck where doses will otherwise be high. There are, however, usually no consequences of these higher doses, which are within tolerance of the relevant areas of the body. Some groups attempt to shield lungs and kidneys as pneumonitis is a common and severe complication, and renal function needs to be preserved as much as possible since many nephrotoxic drugs are used in these patients. However, shielding at extended FSD in a patient who is not well immobilised may lead to undesired shielding of potential sites of leukaemic cell infiltration and has not been shown to reduce rates of lung complications.

■ TBI – complex

With more modern linear accelerators, field in field compensation, using open fields with segmentation of the beam to give higher or lower doses where required, and full IMRT (as for example may be delivered with tomotherapy) may permit an optimised whole body dose distribution with relative shielding of some organs. CT planning is then needed for adequate dosimetry and to determine how much dose attenuation is needed for specific areas. However, leukaemic cells may involve any organs of the body and doses need to be as high as tolerable to afford maximal leukaemic cell kill. There is so far no clear evidence that these more sophisticated techniques have led to improvements in outcome.

■ Half body – conventional

Treatment is given with a linear accelerator working at an extended FSD to give an adequate beam size. The patient lies supine on the couch with legs bent if necessary, and treatment is given with opposing lateral beams. If the patient is short, an adequate field size may be obtained with them lying prone and then supine on a mattress on the floor using anterior and posterior beams. With this technique, the upper part of the body is treated with a gantry angle of 0° while the lower half is treated with the gantry rotated 24° away from the junction, to minimise overlap of beams and give a slightly larger beam size. If both halves of the body are to be treated, the two beams should be matched as discussed in Chapter 2.

Dose-fractionation

■ TBI

Using a 6–10 MV linear accelerator beam at extended FSD, or rotational therapy:

■ Children
14.4 Gy in 8 fractions of 1.8 Gy specified as the maximum lung dose, treating twice daily over 4 days with as long an interval as possible between fractions (minimum 6 h).

- Adults

12 Gy in 6 fractions of 2 Gy specified as the maximum lung dose, treating twice daily for 3 days with as long an interval as possible between fractions (minimum 6 h).

Where there has been no previous cranial or testicular irradiation and a full prophylactic dose is indicated, a boost may be given in the 3 days preceding total body irradiation:

- Cranial boost

Opposing lateral beams are used without immobilisation or shielding, using Reid's baseline (external outer canthus of eye to external auditory meatus) since subsequent cataract is likely anyway from TBI.
5.4–6 Gy in 3 daily fractions.

- Testicular boost

A single direct beam of orthovoltage radiation or electrons is used with the penis taped as far out of the field as possible and the legs apart to avoid the skin of the thighs.
5.4–6 Gy in 3 daily fractions.

- Mediastinal boost (bulk disease with residuum after chemotherapy – no previous radiation)

10–10.8 Gy in 5–6 daily fractions.

■ HBI (single fraction)

Upper half body

6 Gy MPD at the centre of the beam in the mediastinum (with lung correction) given in a single fraction.

Lower half body

8 Gy MPD in a single fraction specified at the midpoint of the pelvis.

■ Fractionated HBI

3 Gy in 10 daily fractions given in 2 weeks (0.3 Gy/fraction).

If treatment to the other half of the body is to be given subsequently, an interval of 6–8 weeks should elapse to allow time for bone marrow recovery.

Treatment delivery and patient care

During the first fraction of TBI, diodes or lithium fluoride dosemeters are placed on the front and back of the patient in the positions shown in Figures 38.1 and 38.2. These remain in place throughout the first fraction. Before the next fraction is given, measured doses are analysed to ensure that they are within tolerance. The prescription treatment dose is specified as the maximum lung dose as this is the dose-limiting normal tissue. For each fraction, treatment is delivered with opposing anterior and posterior beams by rotating the couch.

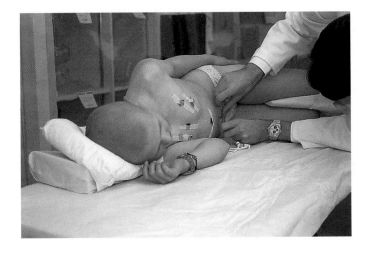

Figure 38.2
Dosemeters placed
on front of patient in
positions
corresponding to
those in Figure 38.1.

Although these patients are immunosuppressed and at risk of infection, special sterile precautions have been shown to be unnecessary. Premedication with steroid and antiemetics (5-HT antagonist) given 30 min before each fraction will reduce nausea and vomiting. Parotid swelling is common within the first 24 h of irradiation but subsides spontaneously. Subsequent dry mouth and disturbance of taste may persist for up to a year. Mild diarrhoea occurs from 4–5 days after the start of treatment. Reversible hair loss, if not already present, starts after 10–14 days. Recovery of engrafted cells begins from day 7–21. A somnolence syndrome of anorexia, lassitude, nausea or headache may occur from 6 to 8 weeks after treatment and is self-limiting. Sterility may be expected but has not proved absolutely inevitable and hormone replacement therapy will be needed for many patients. Cataract is usual after several years.

Pneumonitis with cough and breathlessness from radiation alone occurs in <5 per cent of patients treated with this schedule. However, chest symptoms are common. Their aetiology is multifactorial and effective treatment depends on accurate diagnosis. The incidence of second malignancies after TBI and stem cell transplantation increases with each year of survival and lifetime surveillance is essential.

Verification

Doses to this irregular volume are measured by placing lithium fluoride dosemeters or diodes in anterior and posterior pairs in various parts of the body and checking dose distributions in the first fraction of the treatment. Cover of the body is assured by checking the light beam on the wall behind the patient.

key trials

Thomas ED, Clift RA, Hersman J *et al.* (1982) Marrow transplantation for acute nonlymphoblastic leukemia in first remission using fractionated or single-dose irradiation. *Int J Radiat Oncol Biol Phys* **8**: 817–21.

Information sources

Aristeia C, Tabiliob A (1999) Total-body irradiation in the conditioning regimens for autologous stem cell transplantation in lymphoproliferative diseases. *Oncologist* **4**: 386–97.

Kim TH, Khan FM, Galvin JM (1980) A report of the work party: comparison of total body irradiation techniques for bone marrow transplantation. *Int J Radiat Oncol Biol Phys* **6**: 779–84.

Leiper AD (1995) Late effects of total body irradiation. *Arch Dis Child* **72**: 382–5.

Soule BP, Simone NL, Savani BN (2007) Post-transplant events – pulmonary function following total body irradiation (with or without lung shielding) and allogeneic peripheral blood stem cell transplant. *Bone Marrow Transplant* **40**: 573–8.

Wheldon TE, Barrett A (2001) Radiobiological modelling of the treatment of leukaemia by total body irradiation. *Radiother Oncol* **58**: 227–33.

Appendix

List of abbreviations

5FU	5-fluorouracil
5-HT	5-hydroxytryptamine
ABC	active breathing control
AFP	α-fetoprotein
AP/PA	anteroposterior/posteroanterior
APER	abdomino-perineal resection of rectum
ART	adaptive radiotherapy
BED	biological effective dose
β-hCG	β subunit of human chorionic gonadotrophin
CEA	carcinoembryonic antigen
CFRT	conformal radiotherapy
CLD	central lung distance
CLND	completion lymph node dissection
CNS	central nervous system
CSF	cerebrospinal fluid
CSRT	craniospinal radiotherapy
CT	computed tomography
CTV	clinical target volume
DAHANCA	Danish head and neck cancer group
DCIS	ductal carcinoma *in situ*
D_{max}	dose at the depth of maximum build up
DMSA	dimercaptosuccinic acid–kidney scan
DRE	digital rectal examination
DRR	digitally reconstructed radiograph
DVH	dose–volume histogram
EBRT	external beam radiotherapy
EBV	Epstein–Barr virus
EGFR	epithelial growth factor receptor
ENT	ear, nose and throat
EORTC	European Organisation for Research and Treatment of Cancer
EPID/EPI	electronic portal imaging device/image
EUA	examination under anaesthesia
EUS	examination under ultrasound control
FDG	[^{18}F]2-fluoro-2-deoxy-D-glucose
FIGO	Federation Internationale de Gynecologie et d'Obstetrique
FNA	fine needle aspiration/aspirate
FSD	focus skin distance
GEC-ESTRO	Groupe Européenne de Curiétherapie – European Society of Therapeutic Radiation Oncology
GFR	glomerular filtration rate
GTV	gross tumour volume
Gy	gray
HBI	half body irradiation
HDR	high dose rate
HER2	antigen expressed in some breast cancers, of prognostic significance in determining response to Herceptin
HNPCC	hereditary non-polyposis colorectal carcinoma
HVL	half value layer
ICRU	International Commission on Radiation Units
IFRT	involved field radiotherapy
IGRT	image-guided radiotherapy
IMRT	intensity-modulated radiotherapy
INRT	involved node radiotherapy

IORT	intraoperative radiotherapy	% DD	percentage depth dose
IVU	intravenous urogram	PET	positron emission tomography
kV	kilovolts	PRV	planning organ at risk volume
LDR	low dose rate	PS	performance status
LENT-SOMA	Late Effects on Normal tissues – Subjective, Objective, Management and Analytic scales	PTV	planning target volume
		RCT	randomised controlled trial
		RPA	recursive partition analysis
		RTOG	Radiation Therapy Oncology Group
LOH	loss of heterozygosity		
LVSI	lymphovascular space invasion	SCC	squamous cell carcinoma or spinal cord compression
MALT	mucosa-associated lymphoid tissue		
		SF	surviving fraction
MeV	mega electron volts	SPECT	single photon emission computed tomography
MIBG	meta-iodobenzylguanidine		
MLC	multi-leaf collimation/collimator	SSD	source skin distance
MPD	midplane dose	TBI	total body irradiation
MRI	magnetic resonance imaging	TLD	thermo-luminescent dosemeters/dosimetry
MRS	magnetic resonance spectroscopy		
		TNM	Tumour, Nodes, Metastases
MV	mega volts	TPS	treatment planning system
MYCN	antigen expressed in neuroblastoma	TSEBT	total skin electron beam therapy
NCI-CTC	National Cancer Institute – Common Toxicity Criteria	UICC	Union Internationale Contre le Cancer
NTCP	normal tissue complication probability	USPIO	ultra-small particles of iron oxide
OAR	organs at risk	WBD	whole body dose
OPG	orthopantogram	WHO	World Health Organization
PCI	prophylactic cranial irradiation	WLE	wide local excision
PEG	percutaneous endoscopic gastroscopy		

Index